EPIDEMIOLOGY IN OLD AGE

EPIDEMIOLOGY IN OLD AGE

Edited by

SHAH EBRAHIM

Royal Free Hospital School of Medicine, University of London

and

ALEX KALACHE

Aging and Health Programme, World Health Organization, Geneva

Published by the BMJ Publishing Group
in collaboration with the
World Health Organization

© BMJ Publishing Group 1996

First published in 1996
by the BMJ Publishing Group, BMA House, Tavistock Square,
London WC1H 9JR

British Library Cataloguing in Publication Data

A catalogue record for this book is available
from the British Library

ISBN 0-7279-0948-7

Printed and bound in Great Britain by
Latimer Trend & Company Ltd., Plymouth

Contents

Contributors

Professor Elizabeth M Badley
Arthritis Community Research and Evaluation Unit, Wellesley Hospital Research Institute, 160 Wellesley Street East, Toronto, Ontario M4Y 1J3, Canada

Professor Margret M Baltes
Free University of Berlin, Universitatsklinikum Benjamin Franklin, Department of Gerontopsychiatry, Ulmenallee 32, 14050 Berlin, Germany

Dr Martin Blanchard
University Department of Psychiatry, Royal Free Hospital School of Medicine, London NW3 2PF, UK

Dr Ruth Bonita
University Geriatric Unit, Faculty of Medicine and Health Sciences, North Shore Hospital, Takapuna, Auckland 9, New Zealand

Dr Ann Bowling
Centre for Health Informatics and Multiprofessional Education, University College London Medical School, Whittington Hospital Campus, London N19 5NF

Dr Carol Brayne
Department of Community Medicine, Institute of Public Health, University of Cambridge, University Forvie Site, Cambridge CB2 2SR, UK

Professor Chris J Bulpitt
Department of Geriatric Medicine, Hammersmith Hospital, Du Cane Road, London W12 0HS, UK

Professor John Campbell
Department of Medicine, University of Otago, PO Box 913, Dunedin, New Zealand

Dr Iain Carpenter
Centre for Health Services Studies, George Allen Wing, University of Kent, Canterbury, Kent CT2 7NF, UK

Professor Ann Cartwright
University Department of Public Health, Royal Free Hospital School of Medicine, London NW3 2PF, UK

Professor David Challis
Personal Social Services Research Unit, Cornwallis Building, University of Kent, Canterbury, Kent CT2 7NF, UK and Department of Psychiatry, Mathematics Tower, University of Manchester, Oxford Rd, Manchester, M13 9PL, UK

Dr Lin-Yang Chi
Department of Community Medicine, Institute of Public Health, University of Cambridge, University Forvie Site, Cambridge CB2 2SR, UK

Professor Mike Clarke
Department of Public Health and Epidemiology, Faculty of Medicine, University of Leicester, 22–28 Princess Road West, Leicester LE1 6TP, UK

Dr Alain Colvez
INSERM CJF 93-06, Hôpital Saint-Charles, 300 rue Auguste Broussonet, 34295, Montpellier cedex 5, France

Mr Cam Donaldson
Health Economics Research Unit, University Medical Buildings, Foresterhill, Aberdeen AB9 2ZD, UK

Professor Shah Ebrahim
University Department of Public Health, Royal Free Hospital School of Medicine, London NW3 2PF, UK

Ms Shelley Farrar
Health Economics Research Unit, University Medical Buildings, Foresterhill, Aberdeen AB9 2ZD, UK

Professor Gerda G Fillenbaum
Center for the Study of Ageing and Human Development, Duke University Medical Center, PO Box 3003, Durham, NC 22710, USA

Dr Astrid Fletcher
Department of Epidemiology and Population Sciences, London School of Hygiene and Tropical Medicine, Keppel Street, London WC1E 7HT, UK

Dr Katia Gilhome Herbst
45 Balfour Road, Highbury, London N5 2ND, UK

Dr J A Muir Gray
Anglia and Oxford Regional Health Authority, Old Road, Headington, Oxford OX3 7LF, UK

Professor J Grimley Evans
Division of Clinical Geratology, Nuffield Department of Medicine, Radcliffe
Infirmary, Oxford OX2 6HE, UK

Dr Emily Grundy
Age Concern Institute of Gerontology, King's College, Cornwall House,
Waterloo Road, London SE1 8WA, UK

Dr Rowan H Harwood
Department of Health Care of the Elderly, Queen's Medical Centre,
University Hospital, Nottingham NG7 2UH, UK

Dr Irene Higginson
Department of Public Health and Policy, London School of Hygiene and
Tropical Medicine, Keppel Street, London WC1E 7HT, UK

Professor David J Hunter
Nuffield Institute for Health, University of Leeds, 71–75 Clarendon Road,
Leeds LS2 9PL, UK

Dr Alex Kalache
Aging and Health Programme, World Health Organization, CH-1211
Geneva 27, Switzerland

Professor Robert L Kane
Institute for Health Services Research, University of Minnesota School of
Public Health, D-351 Mayo (Box 197), 420 Delaware Street SE,
Minneapolis, MN 55455, USA

Professor Kay-Tee Khaw
Clinical Gerontology Unit, University of Cambridge, Addenbrooke's
Hospital, Cambridge CB2 2QQ, UK

Dr Kevin Kinsella
Aging Studies Branch, International Programs Center, US Bureau of the
Census, Washington, DC, 20233-0001, USA

Professor Tom Kirkwood
School of Biological Sciences, 239 Stopford Building, Oxford Road,
Manchester M13 9PT, UK

Professor James Lindesay
Department of Psychiatry, University of Leicester, Leicester General
Hospital, Gwendolen Road, Leicester LE5 4PW, UK

Dr Cath McGrother
Department of Public Health and Epidemiology, Faculty of Medicine, University of Leicester, 22–28 Princess Road West, Leicester LE1 6TP, UK

Professor Klim McPherson
Health Promotion Sciences Unit, Department of Public Health and Policy, London School of Hygiene and Tropical Medicine, Keppel Street, London WC1E 7HT, UK

Dr Stefania Maggi
National Research Council for Italy, Program for Research on Aging, via Pancaldo 21, 50100 Firenze, Italy

Professor Michael Marmot
Department of Epidemiology and Public Health, University College London School of Medicine, 1–19 Torrington Place, London WC1E 6BT, UK

Dr Darwin C Minassian
Centre for Preventive Eye Health, Institute of Ophthalmology, Bath Street, London EC1V 9EL, UK

Dr Samer Z Nasr
UCLA School of Medicine, Multicampus Program of Geriatric Medicine and Gerontology, VA Medical Center, Sepulveda, CA 91343, California, USA

Dr Nawab Qizilbash
Memory Trials Research Group, Department of Clinical Geratology, University of Oxford, Radcliffe Infirmary, Oxford OX2 6HE, UK

Ms Linda Rothman
Arthritis Community Research and Evaluation Unit, The Wellesley Hospital Research Institute, 160 Wellesley Road, Toronto, Ontario M4Y 1J3, Canada

Professor Laurence Z Rubenstein
UCLA School of Medicine, and Director, Geriatric Research Education and Clinical Center, VA Medical Center, Sepulveda, CA 91343, California, USA

Dr Kasturi Sen
The Oxford Centre for Environment Ethics and Society, Mansfield College, Oxford, OX1 3TF, UK

Dr Alberto Spagnoli
Laboratory of Geriatric Neuropsychiatry, Institute di Ricerche "Mario Negri", via Eritrea 62, 20157 Milan, Italy

Dr John M Starr
Department of Geriatric Medicine, Western General Hospitals NHS Trust, Edinburgh EH4 2XU, UK

Professor Alvar Svanborg
Section of Geriatric Medicine, University of Illinois at Chicago, 840 South Wood Street, Chicago, Illinois 60612, USA

Professor Cameron G Swift
Department of Health Care of the Elderly, King's College School of Medicine and Dentistry, London SE22 8PT, UK

Dr Renato P Veras
Instituto de Medicina Social, Universidade Aberta da Terceira Idade, Rua Sao Fransisco Xavier 524, 10th Floor, Rio de Janeiro, Brazil, 20559–900

Professor Archie Young
University Department of Geriatric Medicine, Royal Free Hospital School of Medicine, London NW3 2PF, UK

Foreword

Population ageing represents a triumph of social development and public health. From a demographic perspective, the view of ageing as a crisis[1] must be rejected: ageing has a lead time of decades and provides societies with the opportunity to prepare themselves with appropriate policies and programmes. The real crisis is in the present day to day lives of many elderly people and their carers. Health policies are needed to tackle the problems faced both by those already in old age and by future cohorts of elderly people.

The importance of a population perspective and the central role of epidemiology in understanding the causes, concomitants, and development of policy for an ageing population has been realised by the World Health Organization for many years. This has prompted an active interest in health care for elderly people and the promotion of research on ageing,[2] and has highlighted the uses of epidemiology in scientific research.[3] Reports on ageing[4][5] produced over the past decade and more have emphasised the need to plan specific services for elderly people, and to ensure that comprehensive health and social services are developed and that health promotion, disease prevention, and disability postponement are given due emphasis. The plan of action produced by the Vienna international assembly on ageing,[6] convened by the United Nations, provided the framework for many activities—community based health care, a focus on health promotion and self care, and advocacy for elderly people in scientific and professional organisations. This framework is now being received in the light of celebrations of 1999 as the international year of older persons.

An innovative programme—Aging and Health—was initiated by the WHO's division of health promotion, education, and communication in 1995. This programme seeks to face up to the new challenges in both developing and developed countries and includes the following elements: emphasis of the human life course; health promotion; health information; and cultural, gender, intergenerational, and ethical perspectives. Specific activities proposed will involve the creation of an updated, accessible information centre on ageing; the promotion of regular national surveys of elderly people; advocacy; evaluation and development of community rehabilitation programmes; strengthening of family care and self care; and training and research. The emphasis of the activities of this programme is on healthy ageing and policy development.

The pace and patterns of ageing in developing countries are without precedent and are occurring within a different context from that of the developed countries of the world. We are now entering a new era where it is becoming essential that ageing *worldwide* is taken seriously and that the necessary research findings are collated, gaps in our knowledge are identified and filled, and health and social policies, which will ultimately be of benefit to all of us, are developed. This book provides a solid background of information about ageing, disease, and health care, and health policy implications. It is intended that the book should be widely disseminated, form a resource for educational programmes, and ensure that knowledge—which is power—is available to all.

Ilona Kickbush
Director,
Division of Health Promotion, Education and Communication,
World Health Organization,
Geneva

1 World Bank. *Averting the old age crisis. Policies to protect the old and promote growth.* Oxford: Oxford University Press, 1994. (World Bank policy research report.)
2 Heikkinen E, Waters WE, Brezinski ZJ, editors. *The elderly in eleven countries. A sociomedical survey.* Copenhagen: WHO, 1983. (Public health in Europe 21.)
3 World Health Organization. The uses of epidemiology in the study of the elderly. *Tech Rep Ser* 1984;706.
4 World Health Organization. Health of the elderly. *Tech Rep Ser* 1989;779.
5 World Health Organization. *Protecting the health of the elderly. A review of WHO activities.* WHO, Copenhagen: 1983, (Public Health in Europe 18.)
6 World Health Organization. *Health policy aspects of aging.* World Assembly on Ageing; 1982; Vienna. Geneva: WHO. (A/CONF. 113/19.)

Editorial preface

The progressive greying of populations that has occurred in the twentieth century is undoubtedly a collective triumph for the human species. It demonstrates the capacity of the species not only to use its ingenuity to secure its perpetuation but also to enable a substantial proportion of its members to achieve what is usually reckoned to be about the natural life span for members of the species in optimal circumstances.

And yet, as the chapters in this volume amply demonstrate, the achievements must not lead to complacency. Preventable morbidity and physical and mental chronic disabilities marr the lives of many survivors into old age, both in countries that have already achieved a substantial demographic transition and in countries where that transition is just beginning. Moreover, as recent trends in mortality in some of the countries of eastern Europe have shown, the gains in longevity of the twentieth century are not themselves inviolate; they can be reversed.

The progress we look for in enhancing the opportunities of all human beings to fulfil their innate potential throughout their lives wherever they live depends on many factors. Above all it rests on our capacity to establish viable institutions, at local, national, and international levels, that will work together to pursue collective global health objectives. This is not an easy task in a world characterised by ruthless competition at all levels for the power to dominate others for narrow individualistic reasons.

The role of epidemiologists now and in the foreseeable future is basically to inform those who allocate or control resources, as well as the population in general, on how to identify health risks and their magnitude, how to examine causal pathways, how to assess the effectiveness and efficiency of intervention options, and how to set new realistic targets. It must also be, with others, to establish and sustain the objective of equity in opportunities for health for all, irrespective of age, race, and religion.

This book, with its international orientation and emphasis on current dilemmas and opportunities as well as on predictable future problems, is a brave attempt to fulfil these tasks. It should become a standard reference work for those who have the responsibility for the health of older people everywhere.

Margot Jefferys
Visiting Professor,
Centre of Medical Law and Ethics,
King's College,
London

Preface

Population ageing is a major phenomenon that has been quietly ignored for generations in the developed world and is now having profound impacts on health care and social systems in poorer, developing countries. Policy makers, funding bodies, and development agencies are apparently indifferent to the challenges presented by the ageing of populations and the implications for each of us as individuals.

The accelerated pattern of ageing in many poor countries is a direct result of implementation of public health measures of clean water and sanitation, maternal and child health services including immunisation, and family planning; however, there is as yet little interest among international and national agencies in facing up to the epidemiological transition that occurs in tandem with demographic transition. The new public policies—internal markets, public and private sector pluralism, reduction in public spending—on health and social care, now widely adopted throughout the world, are set to exacerbate the universally disadvantaged position of many elderly people.

Research and education are two means by which accepted ideas may be challenged and innovations made. Application of epidemiological methods in the areas of needs assessment, service evaluation, and public health policy are necessary but are often conducted with little appreciation of the potential pitfalls specific to old age.

Our sense of outrage and indignation—shared with many of our coauthors—about the predicament faced by elderly people worldwide has prompted our desire to produce a book on epidemiology in old age. We hope the book will provide information, help, and guidance for all who seek to change the current complacency surrounding ageing as a health policy issue.

The text starts with an introduction to biological mechanisms of ageing; this is followed by an examination of methodological issues in carrying out studies involving older people. Chapters on health care, focusing on utilisation and evaluation, end the first part of the book. The second part is concerned with risk factors and health status assessment in old age, in particular the reasons why some risk factors appear to operate differently and the ways in which health status may be defined and measured. The third and final part of the book provides up to date reviews of the relevant epidemiology and health policy implications of a wide range of common diseases and problems that affect older people. It is not possible to be comprehensive in our coverage: we have chosen to focus on those areas where issues associated with old age are of importance. We hope the book will be of value to public health consultants and trainees, health service researchers, social gerontologists, and epidemiologists new to the field.

Our coauthors of this volume have been selected as experts in their fields and have contributed to the scientific study of elderly people. They come from Europe, North America, and other countries, reflecting the international nature and interest in epidemiology of old age. We are indebted to them for the time and care they have taken to write concise, up to date, and informative contributions. Finally, we wish to thank Mrs Julia Mathews for her care in dealing with the manuscript through all its stages.

Shah Ebrahim
Alex Kalache
January 1996

Part I
Ageing and health care

1 Mechanisms of ageing

TOM KIRKWOOD

It is sometimes said that there are more than 300 different theories of ageing.[1] This is misleading because many of the so called theories are unrealistically narrow and can be subsumed into a smaller number of primary theories. Nevertheless, ageing is a highly diverse phenomenon and there are several distinct kinds of mechanism that have been suggested as causing it.

A significant advance in recent years has been the growing recognition that it is necessary to understand the evolutionary factors that lie behind the ageing process, if we are to understand ageing itself.[2] The evolutionary approach addresses the important "Why?" questions about ageing: why does ageing occur? why do different species have the life spans they do?

The other important questions are the "How?" questions that are concerned with mechanisms and causes. How many factors contribute to the ageing process? How many genes determine longevity? How important are non-genetic factors like lifestyle and environment? How do we distinguish primary and secondary factors? And so on.

At present, the answers to many of the "how?" questions are not yet available, but we can expect rapid progress in the coming years owing to a combination of two developments. Firstly, the evolutionary theories have given us a clearer idea of the kinds of answers we should be seeking. Secondly, advances in molecular and cell biology have provided powerful new techniques for analysing the mechanisms of ageing.

Ageing populations, organisms, and cells

Ageing occurs in a wide range of species. Human ageing needs to be understood as part of a general biological phenomenon. We therefore require a definition of ageing that transcends species' boundaries.

Ageing is usually defined as a progressive, generalised impairment of function resulting in a loss of adaptive response to stress and in a growing risk of age associated disease. The overall effect of these changes is seen in the increase in the probability of dying, or age specific death rate, that occurs among the older age groups in the population (fig 1.1).

With this population based definition it is possible to ask whether or not a particular species exhibits ageing by examining the pattern of age associated mortality.

3

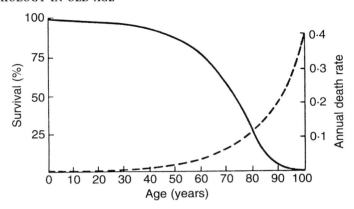

Fig 1.1 Age specific patterns of survival (continuous curve) and death rate (dashed curve) for a population that exhibits ageing. The example is of a human population. (Reproduced from Kirkwood TBL, Holliday R. Ageing as a consequence of natural selection. In Bittles AH, Collins KJ, editors. The biology of human ageing. Cambridge: Cambridge University Press, 1986: 1–16.)

It is thought that all mammals, birds, reptiles, and fish undergo ageing, although in the wild this is masked by the high level of extrinsic mortality (fig 1.2). Many invertebrate species—for example, insects—also age. Some simple animals such as coelenterates (for example, sea anemones, hydra) do not, however, show an age associated increase in death rate; it is thought that these animals do not age.

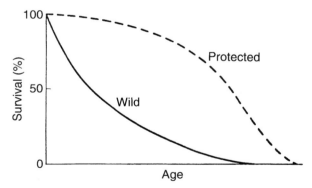

Fig 1.2 The survival curve in a wild population is influenced mainly by the high level of extrinsic mortality. This tends to mask the age associated increase in intrinsic mortality that is seen in protected conditions (Reproduced from Kirkwood TBL. Biological origins of ageing. In Evans JG, Williams TF, editors. Oxford textbook of geriatric medicine. Oxford: Oxford University Press, 1992: 35–40.)

Where ageing does take place, it is broadly reproducible within a species. Some alterations, such as changes in skin elasticity, affect all individuals. The rate of development of these alterations can, however, vary considerably. Even within genetically homogeneous populations (for example, inbred rodent strains), individuals vary both in age associated pathology and in life span.

Close examination of ageing individuals reveals an extremely broad array of functional changes. It may be hard to distinguish which of these changes are the secondary consequences of some underlying cause—for example, changes in the functions of tissues and organs are likely to result from changes at the cell level. There is the potential for feedback between different levels—for example, altered function of a gland that produces a circulating hormone or growth factor will in turn influence the behaviour of the cells that respond to this signal.

Intrinsic age changes occur in many types of cells. One of the best studied models of ageing at the cell level is the cultured fibroblast. These cells have finite proliferative life spans, dividing as many as 50 or more times in cell cultures before ceasing to divide and eventually dying. This phenomenon is often called the "Hayflick limit" and its relevance to ageing of the body as a whole is supported by the observations that cells from old donors manage fewer divisions in culture than cells from young donors.[3 4]

Dividing cells are widely studied for the ease with which they can be grown and manipulated. However, non-dividing (post-mitotic) cells, such as neurones, may be just as important in the ageing process.[5]

Theories of ageing: wear and tear versus programming

An old idea is that ageing is simply the result of unavoidable biological wear and tear. We know that organisms are continually damaged in ways that range from major wounds through to changes in single molecules. Many of the observable features of the ageing process can be accounted for as wear and tear. There is a ready parallel with inanimate objects, which do age through wear and tear.

Living systems differ, however, from inanimate objects in their ability to repair themselves. In thermodynamic terms an organism is an "open system" and it is not therefore condemned to undergo progressive increase in disorder. As an open system, organisms utilise resources from their environment to fuel their vital processes, and there is no fundamental reason why these resources cannot be used to sustain life indefinitely.

Non-ageing species provide the counterargument to the wear and tear hypothesis. These organisms must be endowed with sufficient powers of renewal and regeneration to combat wear and tear. Similarly, the "germ line" (reproductive cells) of all extant species must be able to avoid wear and tear or life could not continue.

An alternative is the "programme" theory of ageing. This suggests that the ageing process is under active genetic control because ageing is somehow beneficial or necessary—for example, to prevent overcrowding.

5

There are major arguments against the programme theory. In most animal species ageing is not normally seen in the wild environment (fig 1.2). This means that ageing cannot be serving any direct role, such as population control. It also means that there is a severe limit to the extent that natural selection can operate actively to programme a process that is so rarely seen. Natural selection should in any case act to increase the Darwinian fitness of the individual organism, and this cannot generally be achieved by killing it.

Disposable soma theory

We have just seen that evolutionary arguments cannot sustain the idea of an active programme for ageing, and it is important to develop the evolutionary approach further, for it can provide powerful insights into the mechanisms of ageing.

A direct link from evolutionary theory to the physiological study of ageing is the "disposable soma" theory.[6-8]

The disposable soma theory explains ageing by asking how best an organism should allocate its metabolic resources (primarily energy) between *maintenance* to keep itself going from one day to the next and *reproduction* to secure the continuance of its genes when it itself has died.

No species is immune to extrinsic hazards (for example, predation, starvation, infection). All that is necessary by way of maintenance is that the body has the ability to remain in sound condition long enough for most individuals to have died from extrinsic, accidental causes before intrinsic failure becomes apparent. In fact a greater investment in maintenance is a disadvantage because it uses resources that in terms of natural selection are better used for reproduction.

The disposable soma theory leads to several useful inferences. Firstly, ageing is due to an accumulation of unrepaired somatic damage. This is similar to the wear and tear theory but with one essential difference: damage accumulates not because wear and tear is inevitable but because organisms are tuned to put insufficient resources into maintenance of the somatic (that is, non-reproductive) parts of the body. (Non-ageing species are, without known exception, capable of reproducing by vegetative growth and so do not have a true soma.)

We can also see in broad terms how the genetic control of life span is organised and why it is that different species have the life spans they do. If we recall that it is the presence of extrinsic mortality that makes it not worthwhile to invest in better maintenance than is necessary to preserve somatic functions through the normal expectation of life in the wild, we can see that it is the level of environmental mortality that imposes the selection for a longer or shorter life span. A species subject to a high level of environmental mortality (for example, a mouse) will do better not to invest a lot in somatic maintenance but should concentrate instead on more rapid and prolific reproduction. On the other hand, a species with a low level of environmental mortality (for example, an elephant) will tend to do the opposite.

The disposable soma theory predicts that the mechanisms responsible for ageing are those types of damage for which maintenance and repair processes are metabolically costly. These include many very basic functions, such as DNA repair, antioxidant defences, and so on. Because the theory applies with equal force to each of these mechanisms, we must relinquish any idea of a single mechanism of ageing and must instead expect to find a number of interacting, possibly synergistic mechanisms at work. The next section examines some of the major processes likely to contribute to ageing.

Molecular mechanisms

DNA damage and mutations

Damage to DNA results from a wide variety of causes and ranges in severity from large scale (chromosomal type) mutations to fine scale alterations in the individual nucleotides that make up the DNA sequence. Damage to DNA is a natural candidate for a primary mechanism of ageing because, once an alteration to the DNA sequence has occurred, the altered sequence is preserved as faithfully as the original. This means that damage accumulates progressively over time. Because DNA specifies the information for all metabolic processes, the accumulation of damage becomes ever more disruptive.

Although damage to DNA must in the long run lead to loss of function, it is not known if this occurs at a fast enough rate to explain ageing.[9] All organisms possess a powerful range of DNA repair systems whose function is to correct most of the damage that arises in DNA. The upshot is that damage to DNA accumulates only slowly.

Damage to DNA is known to be an important contributor to one important age associated kind of disease, namely cancer. It also appears that progressive loss of special DNA sequences (telomeres) from the ends of chromosomes is associated with the finite division of human cells in culture.[10] It is, however, not yet clear if DNA damage contributes significantly to the overall ageing process.

Free radicals

Free radicals are highly reactive molecules that are produced as byproducts of cell metabolism, particularly the pathways that utilise oxygen. Radicals can cause oxidative damage to almost any component in the cell, including proteins, nucleic acids, and membranes. Protection against the damaging actions of radicals is provided by vitamins A and C and by enzymes like superoxide dismutase, catalase, glutathione peroxidase, and

7

glutathione reductase. The fact that organisms have evolved potent antioxidant defences is evidence of the threat posed by free radicals.

Because free radicals can produce such an extensive range of cellular damage, it has been proposed that they play an important role in the ageing process. This is supported by a range of experimental observations[11]—for example, it is estimated that one third of the protein molecules in an old animal may be damaged by oxidation. Transgenic fruitflies with elevated levels of the enzymes superoxide dismutase and catalase show increased life spans.[12]

Aberrant proteins

Accumulation of normal proteins in an aberrant form is a prominent feature in several important diseases of ageing[13]—for example, in Alzheimer's disease there is an accumulation of the β amyloid fragment of the amyloid precursor protein within the neuritic plaques, and of the tandem repeat region of the tau protein in the paired helical filaments. In the course of normal ageing there is accumulation of altered forms of several proteins, such as the deposition of lipofuscin that occurs in many different types of cell.

Aberrant proteins can arise as a consequence of errors in the original synthesis (translation) of the protein from the genetic message or of abnormalities of post-translational processing, such as misfolding of the protein chain, abnormal phosphorylation, and covalent or non-covalent polymerisation.

The cell enjoys significant protection from accumulation of aberrant proteins because of the action of its proteolytic scavenging pathways that are mediated by the so called stress proteins. The aberrant proteins that accumulate during ageing are, however, highly resistant to proteolysis.

Defective mitochondria

All eukaryotic cells rely on mitochondria (subcellular organelles containing their own DNA) as their major source of metabolic energy. The mitochondria are, however, also the main cellular source of free radicals, and the mutation rate of mitochondrial DNA (mtDNA) is much higher than for the chromosomal DNA contained in the cell nucleus. Damage to the mtDNA is of great importance because it will often impair cellular energy production. Damaged mitochondria can, however, still replicate because the enzymes required for mitochondrial replication are encoded entirely in the cell nucleus. For these reasons it has been suggested that accumulation of defective mitochondria may be an important cause of ageing.[14]

Mathematical modelling of the accumulation of defective mitochondria has shown that the collapse of cellular energy production is delayed and may be postponed indefinitely only if the rate of turnover and renewal of mitochondria is high enough.[15]

There is growing evidence for declines in cell energy production with age in mammals, including humans, and for age associated accumulation of mtDNA mutations in tissues, especially those comprised mostly of post-mitotic cells, such as brain and muscle. In the mitochondria of the fungal genera *Podospora* and *Neurospora* the mtDNA undergoes rearrangements and deletions that have been directly linked to the occurrence of an ageing process in these species.[16] This process in fungi depends, however, on the release and amplification of a specific genetic element, not found in mammalian mtDNA, and it is not clear if the process has general relevance to ageing.

Longevity, genes, and environment

Heritability of life span

There is clear evidence in human populations that longevity tends to run in families, although estimates of the coefficient of heritability are low.[17 18] The disposable soma theory indicates that the genetic factors affecting longevity are likely to influence a number of distinct maintenance processes. Thus the theory points firmly to a polygenic control of life span.

On the average within the population the period of longevity assured by each specific maintenance system is expected to be similar, but genetic variance within the population will mean that individuals tend to vary in the exact levels of different maintenance systems—for example, in one family there may be a gene conferring an above average level of a particular DNA repair function, whereas in another family the same function may operate below the average level.

Certain genes predispose to risk factors that may shorten life. Recently, it has been shown that the ε4 allele of the gene for apolipoprotein E is associated with an elevated risk for Alzheimer's disease and, perhaps not surprisingly, this allele is less frequent among centenarians than among the general population.[19]

Progeria

Some rare disorders appear to accelerate the ageing process itself.[20] An example is Werner's syndrome. This is a rare recessive genetic disorder affecting around 10 in a million people. The first clinical evidence of abnormality is a failure to undergo the usual adolescent growth spurt. This is soon followed by premature greying of the hair, bilateral cataracts, skin changes, diabetes, osteoporosis, atherosclerosis, neoplasms, and other diseases characteristic of the elderly. Neurones appear unaffected, however, and Alzheimer's disease is rare. Life span is much reduced—to around 45 years—and Werner's syndrome is studied as a model of some aspects of human ageing.

Environment, lifestyle and nutrition

Non-genetic factors, such as environment, lifestyle, and nutrition, probably influence the ageing process in important ways—for instance, monozygotic twins can age differently even though their life spans tend to be more similar than those of dizygotic twins. This can be readily understood in terms of the picture developed above of how genes cause ageing.

If, as the disposable soma theory suggests, ageing is due to accumulation of unrepaired somatic damage, non-genetic factors can alter both the degree of exposure to damaging agents and the potential for intrinsic maintenance processes to operate. For example, poor nutrition can both introduce toxic factors and fail to provide necessary vitamins, and so on. Early nutrition has been shown to have important effects on late life diseases.[21] Similarly, exercise can be an important modulator of ageing processes.

In the final analysis the picture now emerging of the mechanisms of human ageing suggests that this complex process derives from the underlying genetic limitation of somatic maintenance systems. The upshot is that the lifelong trajectory of health and disease for an individual is the result of a combination of genetics, environment, lifestyle, nutrition, and, to an important extent, chance.

1 Medvedev ZA. An attempt at a rational classification of theories of ageing. *Biol Rev* 1990; **65**:375–98.
2 Kirkwood TBL, Franceschi C. Is aging as complex as it would appear? *Ann N Y Acad Sci* 1992;**663**:412–7.
3 Hayflick L. The cell biology of human aging. *Sci Am* 1980;**242**:58–66.
4 Martin GM, Sprague CA, Epstein CJ. Replicative life-span of cultivated human cells: effect of donor's age, tissue and genotype. *Lab Invest* 1970;**23**:86–92.
5 Martin GM. Cellular aging—postreplicative cells. A review (Part II). *Am J Pathol* 1977; **89**:513–30.
6 Kirkwood TBL. Evolution of ageing. *Nature* 1977; **270**:301–4.
7 Kirkwood TBL. Repair and its evolution: survival versus reproduction. In: Townsend CR, Calow P, editors. *Physiological ecology: an evolutionary approach to resource use.* Oxford: Blackwell, 1981:165–89.
8 Kirkwood TBL, Holliday R. The evolution of ageing and longevity. *Proc R Soc Lond [Biol]* 1979;**205**:531–46.
9 Vijg J. DNA sequence changes in aging: how frequent? How important? *Aging Clin Exp Res* 1990;2:105–23.
10 Harley CB, Futcher AB, Greider CW. Telomeres shorten during ageing of human fibroblasts. *Nature* 1990;**346**:866–8.
11 Sohal RS. The free radical hypothesis of aging: an appraisal of the current status. *Aging Clin Exp Res* 1993;5:3–17.
12 Orr WC, Sohal RS. Extension of life-span by overexpression of superoxide dismutase and catalase in Drosophila melanogaster. *Science* 1994;**263**:1128–30.
13 Rosenberger RF. Senescence and the accumulation of abnormal proteins. *Mutat Res* 1991; **256**:255–62.
14 Linnane AW, Marzuki S, Ozawa T, Tanaka M. Mitochondrial DNA mutations as an important contributor to ageing and degenerative diseases. *Lancet* 1989;i:642–5.

15 Kowald A, Kirkwood TBL. Mitochondrial mutations, cellular instability and ageing: modelling the population dynamics of mitochondria. *Mutat Res* 1993;**295**:93–103.

16 Osiewacz HD, Hermanns J. The role of mitochondrial-DNA rearrangements in aging and human diseases. *Aging Clin Exp Res* 1992;**4**:273–86.

17 Schächter F, Cohen D, Kirkwood TBL. Prospects for the genetics of human longevity. *Hum Genet* 1993;**91**:519–26.

18 McGue M, Vaupel JW, Holm N, Harvald B. Longevity is moderately heritable in a sample of Danish twins born 1870–1880. *J Gerontol* 1993;**48**:B237–44.

19 Schächter F, Faure-Delanef L, Guénot F, *et al.* Genetic associations with human longevity at the APOE and ACE loci. *Nature Genet* 1994;**6**:29–32.

20 Martin GM. Genetic syndromes in man with potential relevance to the pathobiology of ageing. *Birth Defects* 1978;**14**:5–39.

21 Barker DJP, editor. *Fetal and infant origins of adult disease*. London: BMJ Publishing Group, 1992.

2 Principles of epidemiology in old age

SHAH EBRAHIM

Epidemiology is concerned with the description of the distribution and determinants of disease in defined populations. The International Epidemiology Association has widened this definition to include the use of epidemiological methods to provide data for the evaluation of health services for the prevention, control, and treatment of disease and for deciding on service priorities.[1]

Epidemiological investigation among older people has focused on three main areas: the investigation of the determinants of longevity and demographic and epidemiological transitions; the evaluation of health care; and the aetiology and natural history of diseases (and problems) common in old age. While the basic principles of epidemiology do not differ, whether the population of interest is children or elderly people, there are special considerations that require additional caution in the conduct and interpretation of epidemiological work involving predominantly older people. This chapter aims to highlight some of the methodological issues of epidemiological studies in old age.

Population at risk

Defining a population for study appears to be straightforward but may present serious problems in the very old because of institutionalization. Levels of institutionalization rise dramatically with age (see chapter 13) and vary depending on the availability of places, which may differ markedly between and within countries. Inclusion or exclusion of institutional residents will have effects on the rates of disease or problems observed.

Table 2.1 shows data from the British disability survey[2] and demonstrates that the most severe levels of disability among residents in private households are about half the levels found in the total population including institutional residents. This effect is particularly evident above the age of 70 years because of the increased likelihood of institutional rather than home care in the face of severe disability at older ages. The effect is not apparent when all severities of disability are considered, as the milder disability swamps the effects of institutionalization for more severe disabilities.

12

Table 2.1 *Disability prevalence rates per 1000 residents in private households and in the total population including institutional establishments*

Age (years)	Private households		Total population	
	Disability level		Disability level	
	Most severe	All	Most severe	All
50–59	1	131	2	133
60–69	3	236	4	240
70–79	6	395	11	408
80+	25	674	55	714

Migration of older people to seaside towns is also a phenomenon that may result in biased estimates of the levels of disease or problem. In the United Kingdom migration to coastal resorts is common among wealthier elderly people and a similar phenomenon exists in Florida, USA. Migration requires a reasonable level of health, so, initially at least, older migrants are likely to be healthier than long term residents.

Sampling frames that include information about age are relatively uncommon and consequently studies of elderly people may entail an initial phase of determining where they live. In the United Kingdom family doctor lists are age stratified (65 + and 75 + years) and are often used as sampling frames. Sometimes it is necessary to use electoral registers to identify populations and this requires an initial contact to define older people living at a particular address.[3] Telephone contact may lead to exclusion from the sampling frame of poorer, older people who do not possess a telephone. In inner city areas accuracy of family doctor lists is often low and a combination of methods is required to achieve adequate accuracy.[4]

In developing countries it is usually necessary to compile sampling frames from household registers or to conduct a local census. It may be feasible to use existing "population laboratories" established for maternal and child health services evaluation or other research programmes.

Response rates will determine who is actually included in a study. There is evidence to suggest that older people may be less likely to respond to interview surveys: at ages 25–34 response rates of 71–77% were reported compared with rates of 49–54% at ages over 85 years.[5] The predominant reason for non-response is ill health, which may be transitory, so repeat contact may be rewarded by a higher response rate. Response may be higher if the topic is of interest to the participants. A survey in London[6] found that the proportion of disabled people fell from 16·6% at the first mailing of a disability questionnaire, to 15·8% at the second mailing, and 11·5% at the third mailing, suggesting that those with disability had been more likely to respond to the first mailing.

Case ascertainment

Epidemiological investigation often requires decisions to be made about the classification of individuals as cases or non-cases. At younger

13

ages the focus of interest is usually a disease that may be diagnosed with accuracy in clinical settings; screening tests are then used in population settings to categorise people into diseased and healthy groups. The performance of such screening tests is compared with more accurate methods of diagnosis and is described by the test's sensitivity and specificity.

Lack of gold standard

Many of the major diseases in old age defy accurate diagnosis and consequently an ideal standard is not available. Examples include Alzheimer's disease, and depressive illness where comparisons of screening tests with clinical assessment is the best that can be done. An additional difficulty is when problems of old age (for example, falls, immobility, incontinence) are the topic of interest. Since these problems are not clear cut or well defined syndromes but comprise several different causes and natural histories, ascertainment by questioning may prove more or less accurate for different types of problem.

Multiple pathology and altered presentation of disease

These are the hallmarks of medicine of old age and lead to major challenges in epidemiological studies. Multiple pathology may result in modification of risk factor status—for example, a previous myocardial infarction may result in a lower blood pressure; dietary changes due to a coexisting malignancy may lead to lower blood cholesterol levels. Multiple pathology is increasingly common at older ages and may modify the expression of diseases or problems under study. High levels of comorbidity are associated with increased risk of mortality[7]—for example, depressive illness may lead to reduced activity and consequent muscle weakness, which may then lead to increased joint pain and a diagnosis of osteoarthritis. The same underlying disease may result in immobility, falls, or even incontinence of urine. Comorbidity also leads to treatment that may modify risk factors or the natural history of the disease or problems under study. Careful assessment is required to detect and distinguish the common causes of disease that may be present in a single individual. It must be accepted that unlike at younger ages, it is impossible to examine the effects of risk factors on single diseases or end points.

Altered presentation of disease may give rise to serious under-ascertainment of even common diseases. Myocardial infarction in old age may present without classical symptoms of pain and consequently may be misdiagnosed. Such problems may contribute to the attenuation of risk of mortality associated with hypertension found at older ages.[8]

14

Use of health service records

At younger ages it is common to use hospital or primary care records to identify cases of disease. At older ages this becomes more inaccurate, as older people are less likely to present their symptoms and are more likely to remain undiagnosed. For example, in primary care the identification, diagnosis, and treatment of hypertension is heavily biased towards younger people despite the true prevalence of the condition being greater among older people.[9]

Measurement of health status

There is a widespread consensus that disease status is less relevant at older ages than assessment of global "health" status.[10] Many surveys of older people include questions about general health status but the understanding of such questions may vary between age groups and between countries, and thus inferences about true differences in health status are difficult to make. Table 2.2 shows some data from a World Health Organization study of 11 countries.[11]

Table 2.2   Percentages of women in different countries who thought their health was bad or fairly bad and who had some chronic disease affecting their daily living

	Health bad or fairly bad			Chronic disease affecting daily life		
	70–74 years	75–79 years	80–84 years	70–74 years	75–79 years	80–84 years
Brussels	28	31	12	52	41	41
Leuven	21	6	0	83	68	69
Berlin	16	25	26	62	64	73
Tampere	23	29	29	68	79	77
Midi-Pyrénées	23	24	21	57	71	71
Upper Normandy	27	21	25	74	71	84
Greece	35	40	43	90	90	86
Florence	15	18	21	58	63	58

The gradient from highest to lowest in defining health as bad or fairly bad is almost sevenfold (Leuven v Greece, age 75–79), whereas the gradient in chronic disease is much less extreme at twofold (Brussels v Greece). It is very unlikely that the large differences in health status reflect differences in disease prevalence or in need for health care. It is much more likely that these differences reflect differences in sampling, in interviewers used, and in cultural perceptions of the questions asked.[12]

Such problems are even more apparent in studies carried out in developing countries, where large variations in responses to a study of ageing, using the same protocol and the same question about difficulty walking 300 metres, were obtained (fig 2.1).[13] Such findings should lead to refinements in the methods of asking about health status so that they are culturally relevant and appropriate to the purpose of investigation. For example, an activities of daily living index has been produced[14] that appears to perform well in Thailand, together with a behavioural index that has a higher predictive value than tests of cognition for the detection of dementia.[15]

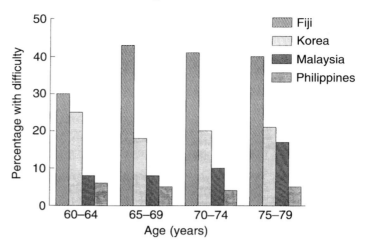

Fig. 2.1   *Percentage of women with difficulty walking 300 m.*
(Reproduced from Andrews et al.[13])

There is increased interest in the application of more appropriate models of disease consequences in old age derived from the International Classification of Impairments, Disabilities, and Handicaps.[16] Methods of measurement of disability[2] and handicap[17] have been developed from the classification, which may have wider application in understanding the social, environmental, and disease interactions that result in loss of health and autonomy in old age.

Causes of death

At older ages it is more common for multiple causes of death to be recorded on certificates, and the trend is increasing.[18] At very old ages (85+ years) it has been reported that in about a quarter of deaths no acceptable cause of death can be found.[19] The majority of certificates do, however, record a cause of death, and a remarkably small proportion of deaths are classified to ill defined causes (see chapter 44—Dying). In developing countries the proportion of death certificates without any cause of death attributed increases with age, making this routine source of information much less useful.

Multiple cause of death data are now widely available from national mortality registries and it makes sense to examine risk factor associations with multiple cause classifications of specific diseases rather than underlying causes. The differences between multiple and underlying cause classifications may be quite large—for example, in the United States (1979) the percentage

16

distribution of causes of death showed that 38·3% of deaths were due to heart disease using underlying cause of death but this rose to 54·6% when multiple causes were included.[20] In Alzheimer's disease use of multiple cause data increases the number of deaths identified by a factor of 2·5.[21]

Measurement and bias

Errors will occur when measurements are made of the presence or absence of disease or of risk factors. These errors may be random in nature or they may be systematic, occurring more often in one particular group than another. Random error contributes to the imprecision of a measurement, assessed by the standard error, and may be reduced by increasing sample size. Systematic errors, or biases, cannot be reduced by this means but require attention to aspects of study design and analysis. Many different types of bias have been described[22] but the most important are due to selection and confounding.

Selection bias occurs when a factor is associated not only with an adverse exposure or disease but also with the probability of being included in a study. Recruitment of cases from hospitals is prone to selection bias because the factors that lead to hospital admission, such as disease severity, smoking behaviour, and older age, are also associated with many risk factors and will thereby distort relationships found in hospital case series.

Confounding occurs when two variables are associated but part (or all) of the association is due to independent associations with a third, confounding, variable—for example, falls may be associated with diuretic drug use, suggesting a causal role for diuretics. Heart failure, however, confounds this relationship as it is associated with use of diuretic drugs for treatment and is also an independent cause of falls. This may be overcome by examining the relationship between drug use and falls among those subjects with and without evidence of heart failure.

Age is a potential confounder of many relationships because it is so frequently associated with both exposure variables and outcomes. The effects of age may be controlled in study design by age matching of comparison groups, or more often by means of age standardisation of rates used in making comparisons. In studies of very old people it is often better to standardise by single years of age than by broad five or 10 year age groups to ensure that adequate control for age is achieved.

Questionnaires, interviews, and use of proxies

Older people are more likely to have practical problems with the use of self completed questionnaires; visual impairment, the phrasing of questions, literacy, and the duration of recall required may all cause more difficulty than at younger ages.[23] Interviews are frequently longer than with younger subjects and considerable skill and training of interviewers are required to ensure that information of reasonable quality is obtained. These factors all

17

tend to make measurement less precise and may also introduce bias due to selection effects, recall effects, response effects, and observer effects. In a British interview survey of elderly people, considerable between-interviewer effects in the assessment of mood and quality of life were observed despite intensive training and monitoring of interviewers.[24]

Very elderly people may be too cognitively impaired or too ill to take part in either self completion questionnaire or interview surveys. The use of proxy respondents is an option to be considered on the grounds that obtaining some information is better than obtaining none. Proxy derived information may be useful in defining case status but is more commonly used to define exposures in aetiological studies. Proxy information may lead to poor precision or to bias,[25] leading to misclassification of exposure status. Such misclassification may be biased by the presence or absence of disease—for example, in aetiological studies of Alzheimer's disease proxy respondents for cases may report head injury more commonly than control respondents because of recall bias in the face of a disease of the brain.[26] Proxy respondents' agreement with index subjects has been examined: serious medical events, smoking history, and use of medications are reported with high levels of agreement (κ 0·5–0·9), whereas dietary intakes are much less reliable (κ 0·1–0·3).[27]

Risk attenuation and ageing

While many common cardiovascular disease risk factors become more common with increasing age, the relative risk tends to decline. Explanations include survivorship effects (reductions in the susceptible populations), competing causes of death or disease, interactions between the risk factor and age, high absolute levels of mortality at very high ages resulting in a ceiling effect, and changes in the biological importance of a risk factor in disease initiation and progression at different ages.[28] Distinguishing these different reasons for attenuation is not usually possible owing to limited information on susceptibility but attempts may be made to examine absolute risk levels and to look for interactions with age. Mathematical modelling of competing causes of disease with time dependent covariates may also be used to make allowance for the interdependence of comorbid states.

Age, period, and cohort effects

Age, period, and cohort effects are intimately related and any relationship observed between a risk factor and an outcome at a particular age may be confounded by cohort or period effects. Disentangling age, period, and cohort effects in large routinely collected data sets may be carried out using mathematical modelling techniques.[29]

Table 2.3 shows the interrelationships between cohort, cross-sectional and cohort sequential study designs. A cohort born in 1920 studied at intervals of five years from 1990 will provide information about the combined effects of ageing and the period influences existing during the 1990–2005 period. For example, the life satisfaction of the cohort might decline during the study. This might be due to a true ageing effect or a period effect (for example, worsening economic conditions for all older people).

Table 2.3 Relationships between different study designs for assessing age, period, and cohort effects

Birth cohort	Age (years) of cohort in the study years				
	1990	1995	2000	2005	
		cohort design			
1920	70	75	80	85	cross-
1925	cohort–	70	75	80	sectional
1930	sequential		70	75	design
1935	design			70	

A cross-sectional study may find an increase in a characteristic, such as blood pressure, with age. This may be because blood pressure really does increase with age, or it may be the effect of the differing experience of cohorts born in 1920, 1930, 1940, etc, leading to those born earlier having higher blood pressures than those born in subsequent cohorts.

A cohort sequential design cannot separate period from cohort effects. For example, a cohort sequential study of blood pressure[30] has shown that the blood pressure of 70 year old individuals belonging to three successive birth cohorts (1901–2, 1906–7, and 1911–12) has fallen (table 2.4). This may be due to a birth cohort effect—perhaps maternal, infant, or childhood nutritional factors changed between 1901–2 and 1911–12 and resulted in differences in blood pressure found in 1971–2, 1976–7, and 1981–2. Alternatively, this may be a period effect; for example, reduction in dietary salt content between 1971 and 1981 may have occurred and might explain lower blood pressures, which would be experienced by all ages.

A complete study of the effects of age on a characteristic requires a series of birth cohorts to be examined repeatedly, allowing cross-sectional, cohort, and cohort sequential analyses.

Heterogeneity in old age and generalisability

Old age is an imprecise term and may mean anything from 60 to 100 years of age. During this phase of the life span people become more heterogeneous. There is greater variation in biological characteristics, such as blood pressure, lung function, and muscle strength, and in health status than at younger ages. This results in large differences in the elderly patients

19

Table 2.4 Cohort sequential data demonstrating the changes in mean systolic blood pressure of females aged 70 years

Birth cohort	Mean systolic blood pressure (mmHg) (Age (years) of cohort in the study years)		
	1971–2	1976–7	1981–2
1901–2	168 (70)		
1906–7		166 (70)	
1911–2			160 (70)

Derived from Svanborg.[30]

who are included in studies recruiting volunteers (for example, fitness class attenders) and those recruiting from family doctor lists. Such differences in population studied, particularly in treatment trials, will have implications for the generalisability of findings derived from fit compared with sick elderly people. For example, trials of antihypertensives have demonstrated benefits in people up to the age of 85 years—but the majority of participants in these trials have been fit elderly people[31] and it would therefore be extremely unwise to apply these trial results to frail elderly people suffering with multiple pathology.

Ageing and disease

Epidemiological methods might be expected to throw light on the distinction between what is disease and what is ageing, on the grounds that ageing is "normal" whereas disease is not and epidemiology is concerned with distinguishing disease from normality. Such a simplistic notion has been vigorously rejected and an alternative model comprising true ageing (with intrinsic and extrinsic factors) and non-ageing (selection effects, cohort effects, and differential challenge) has been proposed.[32] This model has major advantages in defining hypotheses that may be tested, and alerts investigators to the apparent ageing phenomena explained by cohort and other effects. It also avoids the dangers of defining problems as "normal ageing" and thereby irreversible, untreatable, and ultimately of no interest.

1 World Health Organization. *The uses of epidemiology in the study of the elderly.* WHO, Geneva, 1984.

2 Martin J, Meltzer H, Elliot D. *The prevalence of disability among adults.* London: HMSO, 1988. (OPCS surveys of disability in Great Britain. Office of Population Censuses and Surveys, Social Survey Division. Report 1.)

3 Cartwright A, Smith C. Identifying a sample of elderly people by a postal screen. *Age Ageing* 1987;**16**:119–22.

4 Bowling A, Hart D, Silman A. Accuracy of electoral registers and Family Practitioner Committee lists for population studies of the very elderly. *J Epidemiol Community Health* 1989;**43**:391–4.

5 Herzog AR, Rodgers WL. Age and response rates to interview sample surveys. *J Gerontol* 1988;**43**:S200–5.

6 Locker D, Wiggins R, Sittampalam Y, Patrick DL. Estimating the prevalence of disability in the community: the influence of sample design and response bias. *J Epidemiol Community Health* 1981;**35**:208–12.

7 Seeman TE, Guralnik JM, Kaplan GA, Knudsen L, Cohen R. The health consequences of multiple morbidity in the elderly: the Alameda County Study. *J Aging Health* 1989;**1**: 50–66.

8 Glynn RJ, Field TS, Rosner B, Hebert PR, Taylor JO, Hennekens CH. Evidence for a positive linear relation between blood pressure and mortality in elderly people. *Lancet* 1995;**345**:825–9.

9 Dickerson JEC, Brown MJ. Influence of age on general practitioners' definition and treatment of hypertension. *BMJ* 1995;**310**:574.

10 Fried LP, Bush TL. Morbidity as a focus of preventive health care in the elderly. *Epidemiol Rev* 1988;**10**:48–64.

11 Heikkinen E, Waters WA, Brzeninski ZJ. *The elderly in eleven countries. A sociomedical survey.* Copenhagen: WHO, 1983. (Public health in Europe 21.)

12 Ebrahim S. The elderly in different countries. *Lancet* 1984;**i**:1064.

13 Andrews G, Esterman AJ, Braunack-Meyer AJ, Rungie CM. *Aging in the Western Pacific. A four-country study.* Manila: WHO, 1986.

14 Jitapunkul S, Kamolratanakul P, Ebrahim S. The meaning of activities of daily living in a Thai elderly population: development of a new index. *Age Ageing* 1994;**23**:97–101.

15 Phanthumchinda K, Bunnag S, Sitthi-amorn C, Jitapunkel S, Ebrahim S. Prevalence of dementia in an urban slum population in Thailand: validity of screening methods. *Int J Geriatr Psychiatry* 1991;**6**:639–46.

16 World Health Organization. *International classification of impairments, disabilities, and handicaps.* Geneva: WHO, 1980.

17 Harwood RH, Rogers A, Dickinson E, Ebrahim S. The London Handicap Scale: a new outcome measure for chronic disease. *Quality Health Care* 1994;**3**:11–16.

18 Manton KG, Stallard E. *Chronic disease modelling: measurement and evaluation of the risks of chronic disease processes.* Oxford: Oxford University Press, 1988.

19 Kohn RR. Causes of death in very old people. *JAMA* 1982;**247**:2793–7.

20 Israel RA, Rosenberg HM, Curtin LR. Analytical potential for multiple cause-of-death data. *Am J Epidemiol* 1986;**124**:161–79.

21 Havlik RL, Rosenberg HM. The quality and application of death records of older persons. In: Wallace RB, Woolson RF, editors. *The epidemiologic study of the elderly.* Oxford: Oxford University Press, 1992:262–80.

22 Sackett DL. Bias in analytic research. *J Chronic Dis* 1979;**32**:51–63.

23 Kelsey JL, O'Brien LA, Grisso JA, Hoffman S. Issues in carrying out epidemiologic research in the elderly. *Am J Epidemiol* 1989;**130**:857–66.

24 Ebrahim S. Quality of life measurement: clinical and public health perspectives. *Soc Sci Med* 1995 (in press).

25 Magaziner J. The use of proxy respondents in health studies of the aged. In: Wallace RB, Woolson RF, editors. *The epidemiologic study of the elderly.* Oxford: Oxford University Press, 1992:120–9.

26 French LR, Schuman LM, Mortimer JA, *et al.* A case-control study of dementia of the Alzheimer type. *Am J Epidemiol* 1985;**21**:414–21.

27 Nelson LM, Longstreth WT, Koepsell TD, van Belle G. Proxy respondents in epidemiologic research. *Epidemiol Rev* 1990;**12**:71–87.

28 Kaplan GA, Haan MN, Cohen RD. Risk factors and the study of prevention in the elderly: methodological issues. In: Wallace RB, Woolson RF, editors. *The epidemiologic study of the elderly.* Oxford: Oxford University Press, 1992:20–36.

29 Osmond C, Gardner MJ. Age, period and cohort models applied to cancer mortality rates. *Stat Med* 1982;**1**:245–59.

30 Svanborg A. The health of the elderly population: results from longitudinal studies with age-cohort comparisons. *Ciba Found Symp* 1988;**134**:3–11.

31 Mulrow CD, Cornell JA, Herrera CR, *et al.* Hypertension in the elderly: implications and generalisability of randomized trials. *JAMA* 1995;**272**:1932–8.

32 Evans JG. Ageing and disease. *Ciba Found Symp* 1988;**134**:38–57.

3 Ageing worldwide

ALEX KALACHE

Unprecedented declines in mortality and fertility rates in most of the developing world over the last few years have led to a rapid population ageing process. These trends are likely to continue and are often not fully appreciated by the governments concerned, the health and social professionals in those countries, and, more broadly, development and international agencies. In the developed world the ageing process will continue further: in these already aged societies it will be the age group of the very old (80 years and over) that will grow the fastest. This chapter outlines the main features of the ageing process that will occur worldwide within the next three decades, describes some of the challenges to be faced, and introduces the newly established World Health Organization programme on ageing and health.

Ageing in the developing world

By the beginning of the twenty first century, of the 11 largest elderly populations in the world, eight will be in the developing world (China, India, Brazil, Indonesia, Pakistan, Mexico, Bangladesh, Nigeria). From 1985 to 2025 the rate of increase of the elderly population in developing countries will be up to 15 times higher in countries such as Colombia, the Philippines, Kenya, and Thailand, compared, for example, with the United Kingdom and Sweden.[1] With few exceptions the elderly are now the fastest growing segment of the population in the developing world. Most of the world's elderly population (200 million of a total of 356 million) are already in the developing regions; by the year 2020 the proportion will increase to three quarters of the predicted 650 million total.

Demographic transition

Such a fast ageing process is the result of demographic transition—a concept, developed in the early part of the twentieth century, that refers to the effect of birth and death rates on the size and age distribution of populations. The classical exposition of this process was based on the experience of northern Europe[2] and its stages can be summarised as follows: (a) mortality concentrated in early life—most of the population is very

22

young; (b) mortality falls, growth rates rise—proportion in the younger ages increases further; (c) fertility rates decline, mortality continues to fall—proportion of adult population increases; (d) further decline in mortality in all age groups, fertility rates remain low—ageing process is completed. The demographic transition process can be summarised as a shift from high mortality/high fertility to low mortality/low fertility—and consequently from a low to a high proportion of elderly people in the population.

Different pace of the demographic transition today

The pace of the demographic transition varies from country to country—and within the same country overlapping of its stages can be detected when regions and/or population groups are compared. Such differences are dictated by a complex set of socioeconomic factors. The reasons for the evolution of the demographic transition in the countries that first experienced it and the current situation in developing countries differ. Western European countries experienced the transition over a relatively long period of time. After the industrial revolution there was a steady but slow decline in mortality that preceded by many decades the decline in fertility rates, whereas in the developing world the process started not only much later but is also being compressed into a few decades. It has, for instance, taken 115 years (1865–1980) for the share of the elderly population in France to increase from 7 to 14%. The equivalent time for the same doubling to happen in China is expected to be 27 years (2000–27).[3]

By and large the transition in the countries first to experience it resulted from improved living standards, which gradually benefited most of the population. Consequently there was a relatively slow decline in mortality as more and more people enjoyed better housing, working conditions, safer environments, and improved nutrition. Raised educational standards gradually allowed women to exercise more control over the number of children they would have. By contrast, in most of the countries in the developing world that are experiencing the demographic transition it has been triggered by different factors. Mortality has fallen, largely as a consequence of "external" interventions that have little relation to the conditions people lived in. Diseases previously responsible for high premature mortality, such as measles, tuberculosis, and gastroenteritis, can now be effectively treated or prevented, regardless of how poor people are. Conversely, powerful and effective methods of birth control no longer require relatively high educational levels for their successful use. Thus population ageing was largely the result of socioeconomic development in the developed countries of the North, while in the developing countries of the South it is being achieved through the adoption of new technologies, irrespective of the living standards of large segments of the population.

23

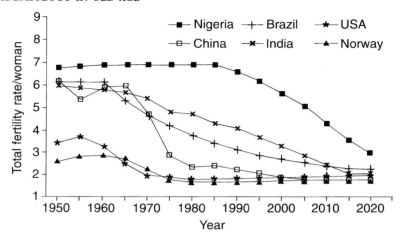

Fig 3.1   Secular trends and projections of total fertility rates in selected countries, 1950–2020.

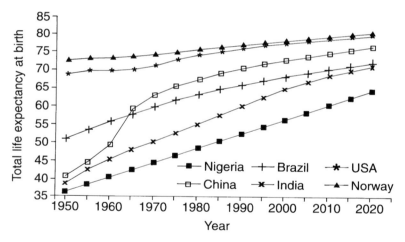

Fig 3.2   Secular trends and projections of life expectancy at birth in selected countries, 1950–2020.

Figures 3.1 and 3.2 illustrate the sharp changes in fertility rates and life expectancy in a range of countries that are illustrative of their respective regions.

The large differentials that characterised the world in respect of these variables until as recently as the 1970s are already much narrower and will tend to disappear within the next few decades. By the year 2025 not only will life expectancies at birth be much closer together (reflecting the declining mortality rates) but the proportion of elderly people in the developing countries will have risen sharply. Indeed, within the next three decades the proportion for most of the developing world (exceptions will be largely confined to sub-Saharan countries) will be higher than that currently exhibited by the already aged societies of the industrialised world.[4]

Resulting epidemiological transition

As populations age the main causes of death previously associated with premature death in childhood lose their pre-eminence and are gradually replaced by causes of death more typically associated with the developed world. For instance, in 1970 in Latin America the proportional contribution of the four most common causes of death were infectious diseases (33·4%), circulatory diseases (21·7%), injuries (8·9%), and neoplasms (7·2%). By the year 2015 the respective figures are expected to be 9·3, 42·4, 10·8, and 16·9. Adults constituted 51·5% of the South American population in 1970; the figure projected for 2015 is 64·2%.[5]

By 1990, in countries such as Uruguay, Puerto Rico, and Cuba, fewer than 5% of deaths occurred in individuals under 16—while three decades earlier the share was close to one third. In the developing world most deaths now occur in old age; for example, in countries such as Argentina, Uruguay, Chile, Costa Rica, Puerto Rico, Cuba, and Trinidad and Tobago, 60% or more deaths currently occur in individuals aged 65 years or over.[6] As in the developed world, the vast majority of these deaths in old age are caused by ischaemic heart and cerebrovascular diseases, followed by neoplasms and respiratory diseases (largely pneumonias). It is important to note that often cause specific, age standardised mortality in developing countries is higher than that experienced by countries in the developed world. For instance, in the late 1980s age specific death rates per 100 000 for cerebrovascular diseases for males aged 55–64 in China (292), in Argentina (189), and in Trinidad and Tobago (242) far exceeded the rate (167) for Canadian males aged 65–74.[7]

Mortality figures are, however, deceptive. They may give a false perception that the "diseases of the past" no longer prevail. Thus morbidity figures are much more important and indicate that many diseases "no longer kill but neither do they die." Consequently, developing countries already face—and will continue to face for the foreseeable future—the challenge of coping with both high morbidity and disability rates for infectious diseases and equally high rates for the superimposed emerging chronic diseases characteristic of ageing societies. In addition, there are the epidemic level of injuries: in Canada, for instance, 7·2% of deaths were caused by "external" causes in 1990, while in Mexico the equivalent figure was 16% in the same year.[8] As the countries of the developing South age, their scarce resources will have to be further stretched to provide for all these multiple demands—something that the much richer societies of the North did not have to cope with at the time they themselves were ageing.

Resource implications

The persistent problem of poverty combined with ageing, while still tackling basic problems of development, has no precedent in the history of mankind.[9 10] Even though by the year 2030 most of the developing world will have an age structure resembling that of developed countries today, the resources and infrastructure needed to provide for such rapidly ageing societies will not on the whole be in place. Figure 3.3 gives the current gross national product (GNP) per capita for a range of countries. The gap is considerable, and according to World Bank projections it is going to grow much bigger. By the year 2030 it is expected that the countries of the Organisation for Economic Cooperation and Development will enjoy a GNP per capita of around $43 000—a growth of $27 000 from the 1990 level of $16 000. In the meantime the GNP per capita in sub-Saharan Africa will not increase from the current $300; it will reach $4000 in North Africa, $6000 in Latin America, and a quarter of that amount in South Asia.

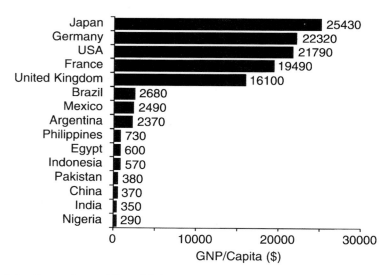

Fig 3.3   Comparisons of Gross National Product (GNP) for selected countries, 1992. Source: World Development Report 1993, Washington, World Bank.

Currently aged societies not only have had a relatively much longer period of time to adapt to their ageing process but also have available considerably more resources than do developing countries that are to grow older within persistent poverty. If ageing is perceived as a major societal problem in the rich countries[11] that have had many decades and plenty of resources to face the challenge, it can only be deduced that the challenge will be even more formidable in the South.

A further point to be considered is the rapidly changing sociocultural ethos within which care of dependent elderly people is to be provided. Traditional intergenerational relationships are fast disappearing. Urbanisation particularly results in social dislocation of young and old, without adequate social security measures being in place. In many developing countries the great majority of the younger generation will lack the material resources to offer any significant support to the older generations. The potential for intergenerational tension will be considerable unless immediate action is taken.

Need for affordable policies

In the absence of appropriate policies to deal with population ageing, resources are often ill spent. A study by the World Bank in 1989 indicated that the social benefits paid by the Brazilian government to those over the age of 55 in the mid-1980s (when they represented only 9% of the population) amounted to 46% of total social expenditure. By the year 2010 the proportion of adults over 55 will have doubled. Policies adopted in the recent past by countries such as Brazil generate disproportionate expenditure between the generations and will not be sustainable in the twenty first century. Such imbalances will significantly determine the resources available for the health sector. As developing countries age, demands on scarce resources by adult and elderly populations will continuously grow. The strain placed on very limited health care resources by infectious diseases yet to be conquered will be compounded by growing levels of non-communicable diseases and related disability.[12]

For all these reasons it can be said that ageing is largely a neglected development issue. Only by the development and careful evaluation of culturally appropriate, effective, and realistic policies will developing countries be able to release resources to tackle other pressing demands.[13] How will the young in a poor country like Brazil be educated and have their health needs cared for if virtually all the social benefits (assuming current policies remain unchecked) are to be absorbed by older adults? And even so, the needs of the elderly poor are not the target of such policies. The richest quintile of the older Brazilian population in the mid-1980s received eight times more benefits than the poorest quintile.

Further ageing of the developed world

A particularly important feature of the future demographic changes in the developed world is the ageing of the elderly population. In most of these countries the oldest old (those 80 years and older) are the fastest growing part of the elderly population.[14] In 1992 they constituted 22% of the elderly population; by the year 2025 the proportion is expected to increase to, for example, 35% in Japan and 32% in Sweden.[15] In the United

Kingdom in 1961 there were about 300 000 people aged 85 and over; by 1991 the total was close to 800 000; and by the year 2021 it is expected that the very old will reach over 1·5 million.[16]

The increase in absolute numbers combined with the increasing heterogeneity (in no other age group are individuals so unlike each other, reflecting their longer lives and accumulated different experiences) represent a challenge to social and health care planners.[17] The oldest old consume disproportionate amounts of health and long term care services.[18] Most of them are women (reflecting the average six years longer life expectancy at birth for women in developed countries), often frail, living alone (the majority are widows), and in poverty (for the current cohort of the very old only a small minority of women ever participated in the paid workforce/ contributed to pension schemes). Recognition of their special needs will require specific policies throughout both the developed and the developing worlds.

Ageing in eastern Europe and the former Soviet Union

Most of the newly independent countries of the former Soviet Union and eastern Europe face similar patterns and trends of ageing populations without the political stability and economic resources available in the West.[19]

The current cohort of elderly people in this region reflects the catastrophic impact of the second world war. Figure 3.4 shows the pyramid for Russia in 1990; among Russian elderly people there are only 36 men for every 100 women—and female advantage in life expectancy at birth is amongst the highest in the world: 10·4 years in 1990. This is in part due to a rise in male mortality caused by circulatory diseases—from the mid-1960s to the mid-1980s in Russia, as well as in the majority of the countries in the region.[20] In Bulgaria, for instance, the increase would have reduced male life expectancy at birth by four years if all other cause specific mortality had remained the same.

Fertility rates, which affect both present and future population ageing, vary widely in the region. In certain traditionally Islamic republics of the former Soviet Union total fertility rates are still higher than five children per woman, while in others—as in parts of eastern Europe—fertility is below the replacement level of 2·1 children per woman.[21]

The political, social, and economic transitions underway in the region have greatly affected the coping mechanisms of the current cohorts of elderly people. World Bank figures indicate that poverty has sharply increased throughout the region in the last few years. For example, in Bulgaria the proportion of the population below the poverty line in 1989 was 12·1%; by 1993 the proportion had increased to 57%. The respective figures for Poland are 24·7 and 43·7%, for Romania 33·9 and 51·5%, and for Russia

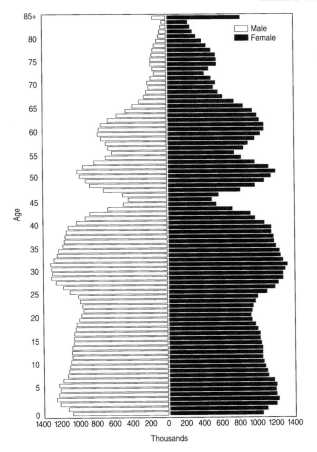

Fig 3.4 Single year age pyramid for Russia, former USSR, 1990.
Source: Velkoff A, Kinsella K. Aging in eastern Europe and the former Soviet Union.
Washington, US Department of Commerce, 1993.

15·8 and 61·3%. It is in this context of increasing poverty and eroded social security mechanisms that the European countries in transition will age further and fast.

WHO programme on ageing and health

As a response to the wordwide ageing process outlined in this chapter, WHO launched (in April 1995) a new programme on ageing and health. It builds on achievements of its previous programme on health of the elderly and incorporates the following perspectives: *life course* (elderly people not compartmentalised but inserted into the life cycle); *health promotion* (with a focus on healthy ageing/ageing well); *cultural* (the settings in which individuals' age will determine their health status in older age); *gender* (differences in both health and ways of living); *intergenerational* (with emphasis on strategies to maintain cohesion between generations); and *ethical* (multiple considerations emerge as populations age—for example, undue hastening or delaying of death, human rights, long term care, abuse).

This new programme requires WHO to provide worldwide leadership on the health dimension of what is to become a dominant societal issue in the year 2000 and beyond. Ageing and health is to be a horizontal programme, acting as a catalyst for action in WHO divisions, regional offices, and member states, and other agencies. Collaborative work with academic institutions and non-governmental organisations is to be firmly established. Its key programme components are *information base strengthening, policy development, advocacy, community based programmes, training*, and *research*. A WHO global media strategy on healthy ageing is to be created.

The full background paper on which the programme on ageing and health is based and further information on its activities can be obtained from WHO, 1211 Geneva 27, Switzerland.

1 United Nations. *Population aging and the situation of elderly persons*. New York: UN Department for Economic and Social Information and Political Analysis, Statistical Division, 1993.
2 Stolnitz GJ. *Demographic causes and economic consequences of population aging*. New York: UN Economics Commission For Europe and UN Population Fund, 1992. (Economic studies, No 3.)
3 Ikels C. Aging and disability in China: cultural issues in measurement and interpretation. *Soc Sci Med* 1991;**32**:649–65.
4 Torrey BB, Kinsella KG, Taeuber CM. *An aging world*. Washington: US Department of Commerce, 1987.
5 Feachem RGA, Kjellstrom T, Murray CJL, Over M, Phillips MA. *The health of adults in the developing world*. Washington: World Bank, 1993.
6 World Health Organisation. *World health statistics*. Geneva: WHO, 1990.
7 Kalache A, Aboderin I. Stroke: the global burden. *Health Policy Plann* 1995;**10**:1–21.
8 Kalache A. Recent trends in mortality rates among the elderly in selected low mortality developing populations. Proceedings of a conference; 1993 Jun 21–25; Sendai City, Japan. Liege: International Union for the Scientific Study of Population, 1993.
9 World Bank. *Investing in health: world development indicators*. New York: Oxford University Press, 1993. (World development report.)
10 World Bank. *Development and the environment: world development indicators*. New York: Oxford University Press, 1992. (World development report.)
11 Suzman R, Kinsella KG, Myers GC. Demography of older populations in developed countries. In: Grimley Evans F, editor. *Oxford textbook of geriatric medicine*. Oxford: Oxford University Press, 1993.
12 Restrepo HE, Rozental M. The social impact of aging populations: some major issues. *Soc Sci Med* 1994;**39**:1323–38.
13 United Nations. *Profiles of national coordinating mechanisms on ageing*. New York: UN Centre for Social Development and Humanitarian Affairs, 1991.
14 Dooghe G. *The ageing of the population in Europe; socio-economic characteristics of the elderly population*. Brussels: Galant, 1992.
15 United Nations. *The world ageing situation 1991*. New York: UN Centre for Social Development and Humanitarian Affairs, 1991.
16 Coombes Y, Kalache A. Demographic characteristics. In: Shukla RB, Brooks D, editors. *A guide to the care of the elderly*. London: HMSO, 1995 (in press).

17 Cliquet RL, Vanden Boer L, editors. *Economic and social implications of aging in the ECE region*. Brussels: NIDI-CBGS, 1989. (Interdisciplinary Demographic Institute and the Population and Family Studies Centre Series, No 19.)

18 Leidl R. Health economic issues relevant to countries with aging populations. *World Health Stat Q* 1992;**45**:95–108.

19 Stolnitz GJ. *Social aspects and country reviews of population aging*. New York: UN Economic Commission for Europe and UN Nations Population Fund, 1994. (Economic studies, No 6.)

20 Kingkade WW, Torrey BB. The evolving demography of aging in the United States of America and the former USSR. *World Health Stat Q* 1992;**45**:15–28.

21 Velkoff VA, Kinsella K. *Aging in Eastern Europe and the former Soviet Union*. Washington: US Department of Commerce, 1993.

4 Demographic aspects

KEVIN KINSELLA

Patterns of ageing in the world

Human population ageing refers most commonly to an increase in the percentage of all extant persons who have lived to or beyond a certain chronological age, herein age 65. While the size of the world's elderly population has been growing for centuries, it is only in recent decades that the proportion has caught the attention of researchers and policy makers.

The global population aged 65 and over is estimated to be 368 million persons in 1995, 6·4% of the world total. This represents an increase of 48 million since 1990. In the mid-1990s the net balance of the world's elderly increases by more than 800 000 persons each month. Projections to the year 2010 suggest the net monthly gain will then be in excess of 1·1 million elderly. In 1990, 26 nations had more than 2 million elderly citizens; by 2025, an additional 33 countries are likely to join the list.[1]

Industrialised countries

Sweden, as of 1995, was the demographically oldest of the world's nations, with 18% of its population aged 65 and over. Other notably high levels are seen in Norway, the United Kingdom, Italy, and Belgium (16% each). The percentage elderly will increase modestly in most industrialised nations between 1995 and 2010, and may even dip slightly as a function of the relatively small cohorts born before and during the second world war (fig 4.1). After 2010, numbers and percentages of elderly should increase rapidly in many countries as the large post-war birth cohorts (the baby boom) begin to reach the age of 65.

As a result of past trends in fertility and current trends in mortality, age categories within the elderly aggregate may grow at different rates. An increasingly important feature of societal ageing is the progressive ageing of the elderly population itself. The fastest growing age segment in many countries is the "oldest old", defined here as persons aged 80 and over. This group constitutes more than 20% of the aggregate elderly population in industrialised countries (table 4.1) and represents approximately 4% of the total population in Scandinavia, France, and Switzerland. In 1995 nine

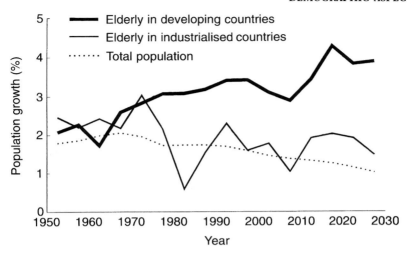

Fig 4.1   Annual percentage growth of total and elderly population (1950–2025).

Table 4.1   Dimensions of elderly and oldest old population in selected countries: 1965–2025

	Elderly (65 +) population (in thousands)			Elderly as % of total population			Oldest old (80 +) as % of all elderly		
	1965	1995	2025	1965	1995	2025	1965	1995	2025
All industrialised countries	90 595	164 633	281 052	9·0	13·2	20·2	15·3	22·8	26·8
All developing countries	87 229	202 903	567 008	3·7	4·5	8·2	9·3	12·5	16·3
Australia	966	2 161	4 407	8·5	11·8	18·8	15·8	21·1	24·5
Brazil	2 667	7 359	21 945	3·2	4·6	10·7	9·6	12·7	17·8
China	32 057	73 574	198 343	4·4	6·1	13·7	9·7	12·7	17·1
France	5 904	9 079	13 982	12·1	15·6	22·6	17·6	28·1	27·7
Germany	9 522	12 664	19 979	12·5	15·6	24·4	14·1	26·6	31·7
India	17 518	37 561	107 713	3·5	4·0	7·8	7·1	11·1	14·5
Indonesia	3 313	7 241	24 816	3·1	3·6	8·6	9·6	9·0	14·8
Italy	5 196	9 463	13 766	10·0	16·2	24·1	15·8	24·3	31·2
Japan	6 179	17 787	32 164	6·2	14·2	26·1	12·6	21·2	32·8
Mexico	1 682	4 030	12 829	3·9	4·3	8·9	15·0	19·0	22·1
Nigeria	1 133	2 918	9 115	2·3	2·9	3·7	7·1	7·8	13·5
Russia	8 591	17 958	30 153	6·9	12·0	18·8	15·0	18·8	21·6
South Africa	761	1 827	5 172	3·8	4·1	5·7	12·7	15·3	17·4
United Kingdom	6 526	9 220	12 912	12·0	15·8	21·5	16·9	25·8	29·1
United States	18 406	33 594	62 423	9·5	12·8	18·4	16·5	23·8	23·9

industrialised nations had oldest old populations in excess of 1 million. The importance of the oldest old with regard to policy making will increase markedly in the twenty first century as a result of levels of morbidity and disability that are much higher than in other population groups, and the fact that the oldest old consume health and social services and benefits far out of proportion to their numbers.[2]

Developing countries

Sometimes lost amid the attention given to population ageing in Europe and North America is the fact that older populations in developing countries are typically growing faster than their industrialised counterparts. Of the net monthly gain exceeding 800 000 elderly mentioned above, 70% occurs in the developing world. Between 1990 and 2025, numerous developing countries (for example, Indonesia, Colombia, Kenya, and Malaysia) may expect a tripling or quadrupling of their elderly populations. Projections for China suggest that it will take only 27 years (beginning in the year 2000) for the percentage of population aged 65 and over to increase from 7 to 14%. The same increase in France occurred over a period of 115 years.

Another way to look at population ageing is to consider a society's median age—the age that divides a population into numerically equal parts of younger and older persons. While the median ages of nearly all industrialised countries are above the 31 year level, most developing nations have median ages under 25. In some African and Asian countries (in the mid-1990s) half of the entire population is younger than 15. In developing countries where fertility rates have fallen dramatically, however—for example, Korea, Cuba, and Singapore—median ages are rising rapidly and should exceed 40 by the year 2025.

Demographic transition

Changes in population age structure result from changes over time in fertility, mortality, and international migration, although the last of these has only a minor effect in a majority of countries. Historically, most societies have had high levels of both fertility and mortality. As major infectious diseases are eradicated and public health measures proliferate, overall mortality levels decline and life expectancy at birth rises, while fertility tends to remain high. Much of the initial improvement in mortality occurs among infants, meaning that more babies survive. Consequently, younger age cohorts grow in size relative to older cohorts, and the percentage of children and young adults in the population is relatively high. This is the situation today in many of the world's developing nations.

Populations begin to age only when fertility falls and mortality rates continue to improve or remain at low levels. Successive birth cohorts may eventually become smaller and smaller, although some nations experience a "baby boom echo" as women from large birth cohorts reach childbearing age. Countries that have both low fertility and low mortality have completed what demographers call the demographic transition, as illustrated by data for the United Kingdom in fig 4.2. The United Kingdom's population age structure in 1920 shows a pyramidal shape common to societies with relatively high fertility and mortality, although a decline in fertility is evident from the size of the cohorts aged 0–4 and 5–9. By 1970 the age structure's centre of gravity had shifted upward. Life expectancy had increased and persons aged 45–64 formed a much greater share of the total. As the population of United Kingdom ages into the twenty first century, the "pyramid" will evolve into a rectangle. By the year 2020 nearly half of the population is likely to be aged 45 or more and the ranks of the oldest old will continue to swell.

Reasons for declining mortality and fertility

Throughout most of its existence, *Homo sapiens* experienced little if any change in life expectancy. Until the last century, the shape of the human age structure was relatively constant. The species was continuously threatened by predators, climate, disease, and lack of food, and survived only because its number of births more than compensated for deaths. High birth rates were one component of a successful survival pattern of favourable evolutionary adaptations.[3]

The spectacular increases in human life expectancy (see table 4.2) that began in the 1800s and continued during the following century are often attributed to the beneficent role of medicine. The major impact of improvements in medicine and sanitation did not, however, occur until the late nineteenth century. Prior, more important factors in lowering mortality were innovations in industrial and agricultural production and distribution that enabled nutritional diversity and consistency for large numbers of people.[4] A growing research consensus attributes the gain in human longevity to a complex interplay of advancements in public health medicine and sanitation coupled with new modes of familial, social, and political organisation.[5]

One correlate of this interplay has been an epidemiological transition that is related to but has lagged behind the demographic transition. The initial mortality declines that characterise the demographic transition result largely from reductions of infectious diseases at young ages. As children survive and age they are increasingly exposed to risk factors linked with chronic disease and accidents. And when fertility declines induce population ageing, growing numbers of older persons shift national morbidity profiles toward a greater incidence of continuous and degenerative ailments.[67]

Exceptions abound to any generalisation about the causal chain of factors resulting in fertility decline. On a broad level it is safe to say that urbanisation, industrialisation, and social mobility have altered family structures and interacted with rising levels of education and female social status to exert downward pressures on fertility levels. Later marriages and

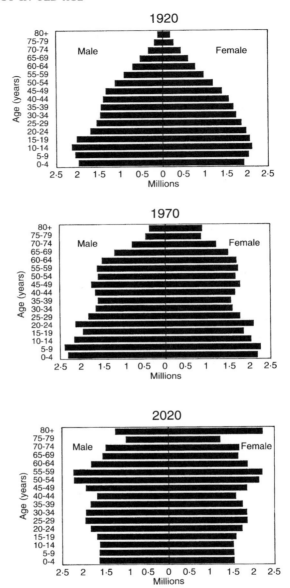

Fig 4.2 Population age structure of the United Kingdom (1920–2020).

desires for viable household formation have been linked to fertility decline in Europe.[8] The availability of contraceptives is arguably the primary enabling factor in fertility decline in many developing countries.[9] Causality aside, nearly all nations have now experienced reductions in fertility levels, usually after their mortality levels had declined. In Europe, where fertility decline started around 1870, most countries now have fertility levels below the replacement rate of 2·1 children per woman. As of 1994 more than 20 developing countries had achieved similarly low levels. These nations with low fertility rates are together home to nearly half of the world's population.[10]

Increased life expectancy and the role of health services

Japan had the highest overall life expectancy (more than 79 years) in the mid-1990s, while the level in various European nations approached or exceeded 78 years. Industrialised countries have made enormous strides in extending life expectancy at birth since the beginning of the twentieth century (table 4.2). Several general observations can be made concerning the trend. (1) The relative difference among countries has narrowed with time. (2) The pace of improvement has not been linear, especially for males—from the early 1950s to the early 1970s, for example, there was little or no change in male life expectancy in Australia, the Netherlands, Norway, and the United States, while in eastern Europe and much of the former Soviet Union male life expectancy declined in the 1970s and early 1980s. (3) The difference in female versus male longevity, which universally has been in favour of women in the twentieth century, widened with time.

Table 4.2 Years of life expectancy at birth in 15 industrialised countries: 1900–1990

	Circa 1900		Circa 1950		Circa 1990	
	Male	Female	Male	Female	Male	Female
Austria	37·8	39·9	62·0	67·0	73·5	80·4
Belgium	45·4	48·9	62·1	67·4	73·4	80·4
Former Czechoslovakia	38·9	41·7	60·9	65·5	68·7	76·5
Denmark	51·6	54·8	68·9	71·5	72·6	78·8
England and Wales	46·4	50·1	66·2	71·1	73·3	79·2
France	45·3	48·7	63·7	69·4	73·4	81·9
Greece	38·1	39·7	63·4	66·7	75·0	80·2
Hungary	36·6	38·2	59·3	63·4	67·2	75·4
Italy	42·9	43·2	63·7	67·2	74·5	81·4
Japan	42·8	44·3	59·6	63·1	76·4	82·1
Netherlands	48·6	51·2	70·3	72·6	74·2	81·1
Norway	52·3	55·8	70·3	73·8	73·3	80·8
Spain	33·9	35·7	59·8	64·3	74·8	81·6
Sweden	52·8	55·3	69·9	72·6	74·7	80·7
United States	48·3	51·1	66·0	71·7	72·1	79·0

Changes in life expectancy in developing regions of the world have been more uniform, with practically all nations showing continued improvement. The most dramatic gains have been achieved in east Asia, where regional life expectancy at birth increased from less than 45 years in 1950 to more than 71 years in 1990. Extreme variations exist, however, throughout the developing world. While Costa Rica, Hong Kong, and numerous Caribbean island nations enjoy levels that match or exceed those in a majority of

European nations, the normal lifetime in some other developing countries, particularly in sub-Saharan Africa, spans fewer than 50 years. Aggregate life expectancy at birth in Latin America (68 years) is 17 years higher than in sub-Saharan Africa. On average, individuals born in an industrialised country in the mid-1990s can expect to outlive their counterparts in the developing world by 13 years.

The major worldwide impetus for the increase in life expectancy since the mid-1800s has been the decline in mortality from respiratory diseases, primarily tuberculosis and pneumonia (although tuberculosis still accounts for roughly one third of an estimated 7 million avoidable adult deaths in developing countries annually).[11] Most of the improvement can be attributed to changes in natural human resistance rather than to medical interventions and vaccinations. Concurrently, however, public health interventions (including sanitation) were effective in reducing mortality from cholera and other intestinal and infectious diseases.[12] Safe water, sanitation, and immunisation initiatives have been especially potent in improving late twentieth century life expectancy in developing countries, where population coverage for adequate excreta disposal increased from 46% in 1985 to 71% in 1991. Immunisation programmes in 1990 prevented an estimated 3·2 million deaths from measles, neonatal tetanus, and pertussis alone, largely in developing countries.[13]

The HIV–AIDS epidemic threatens to reverse life expectancy gains, particularly in the developing world. The impact of the epidemic on life expectancy at birth may be considerable, given that AIDS deaths are concentrated in the childhood and middle adult (30–45) ages. Projections to the year 2010 suggest that AIDS may reduce average life expectancy by more than 25 years from otherwise expected levels in countries such as Thailand, Uganda, and Zimbabwe. The impact on future population age structure is less striking insofar as the effects of a protracted epidemic become more evenly distributed across age groups.[14]

Is mortality being compressed?

Where infant mortality rates are still relatively high but declining, as is typical in developing countries, most of the improvement in life expectancy at birth results from infants surviving the high risk initial years of life. After infant and childhood mortality reach low levels, as in industrialised countries, longevity gains are greatest among the older segments of the population. Under the mortality conditions of 1990, the average Japanese woman aged 65 years could expect to live an additional 20 years, and the average Japanese man more than 16 years. Japanese life expectancy at age 65 increased by 30% between 1970 and 1990, compared with an overall increase in life expectancy at birth of less than 10%.

As mortality rates at older ages decline, ever greater proportions of persons survive to older ages (fig 4.3). Medical screening and educational

38

campaigns can delay the onset and progression of fatal disease, while therapeutic interventions allow persons with diseases to live longer than in previous eras. A growing body of evidence suggests that many physiological functions decline much more slowly with age than was previously estimated.[15] Research has increasingly focused on whether older age morbidity is proportionally more extensive than in earlier eras, or whether it is being compressed into a relatively shorter and later period of life.[16 17]

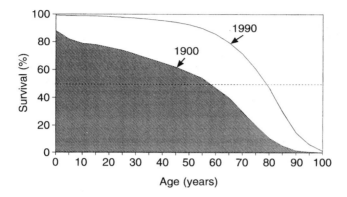

Fig 4.3   Survival curves for the United States (1900 and 1990).

As science reconsiders the biological limits to human life, a related question is whether we are living healthier as well as longer lives, or spending an increasing portion of our older years with physical and/or mental disabilities (see chapter 5). The measurement of health expectancy partitions overall life expectancy into components such as active life expectancy, disabled life expectancy, and institutionalised life expectancy.[18] Cross national problems of comparability notwithstanding, available data suggest that there is a greater range in healthy life expectancy than in remaining life expectancy for persons reaching age 65.[19] Women can expect to spend a greater proportion of their lives in a disabled state compared with men, thus negating some of the benefit of greater female longevity.

1 Kinsella K, Taeuber C. *An aging world II*. Washington: US Government Printing Office, 1993.
2 Suzman RM, Willis DP, Manton KG, editors. *The oldest old*. New York: Oxford University Press, 1992.
3 Olshansky SJ, Carnes BA, Cassel CK. The aging of the human species. *Sci Am* 1993; **268**:46–52.
4 Thomlinson R. *Population dynamics. Causes and consequences of world demographic change*. New York: Random House, 1976.
5 Moore TJ. *Lifespan*. New York: Simon and Schuster, 1993.
6 Breslow L. The future of public health: prospects in the United States for the 1990s. *Annu Rev Public Health* 1990;**2**:1–28.
7 Frenk J, Bobadilla JL, Stern C, Frejka T, Lozano R. Elements for a theory of the health transition. *Health Transit Rev* 1991;**1**:21–38.
8 Coale AJ, Watkins SC, editors. *The decline of fertility in Europe*. Princeton: Princeton University Press, 1986.

9 Ross JA, Frankenberg E. *Findings from two decades of family planning research*. New York: Population Council, 1993.
10 Jamison E, Hobbs F. *World population profile: 1994*. Washington: US Government Printing Office, 1994.
11 Jamison DT, Mosley WH. Disease control priorities in developing countries: health policy responses to epidemiological change. *Am J Public Health* 1991;**81**:15–22.
12 McLeroy KR, Crump CE. Health promotion and disease prevention: a historical perspective. *Generations* 1994;**28**:9–17.
13 World Health Organisation. *World health statistics annual*. Geneva: WHO, 1992, 1993.
14 Way P, Stanecki K. *The impact of HIV/AIDS on world population*. Washington: US Government Printing Office, 1994.
15 Manton KG. Mortality and life expectancy changes among the oldest old. In: Suzman RM, Willis DP, Manton KG, editors. *The oldest old*. New York: Oxford University Press, 1992:157–82.
16 Fries JF. The compression of morbidity: near or far? *Milbank Q* 1990;**67**:208–32.
17 Manton KG, Stallard E, Tolley HD. Limits to human life expectancy: evidence, prospects, and implications. *Popul Dev Rev* 1991;**17**:603–37.
18 Manton KG, Stallard E, Liu K. Forecasts of active life expectancy: policy and fiscal implications. *J Gerontol* 1993;**48**:11–26.
19 Robine JM, Romieu I. *Statistical world yearbook on health expectancy*. Montpellier: Laboratoire d'Epidémiologie et d'Economie de la Santé, 1993.

5 Disability free life expectancy

ALAIN COLVEZ

Disability free life expectancy: current thinking

Disability free life expectancy (DFLE) is a health indicator that aggregates in a single index the mortality and the morbidity state of a population; it was first defined in the 1960s.[1] In the 70s the US National Center for Health Statistics published the first calculation procedure, using disability data issued from the US national health interview survey.[2] At that time a working group of the Organisation for Economic Cooperation and Development discussed the use of such an index to assess the effect of social inequalities on the health of different populations, but finally dropped it.[3]

Later in the 80s DFLE was promoted again, probably because of the growing necessity of evaluating the health of ageing populations. Mortality data on their own are not sufficient to assess the health status of these populations; furthermore, the high prevalence of associated diseases requires an additional evaluation of their consequences in terms of disability. For these reasons DFLE appears particularly useful for defining health objectives in the elderly.[4][5]

There is nowadays a tendency to generalise the procedure of calculation based on DFLE to other dimensions of health, such as the handicap and its components (life expectancy free of handicap, or free of mobility restriction, or free of physical dependency, etc), or life in nursing homes (life expectancy out of nursing homes). The same procedure may be applied to mental health (life expectancy free of dementia) or to the subjective expression of health. All these indices represent what are called "health expectancies". Within this context DFLE is one particular indicator in the family of health expectancies.[6]

Conceptual basis and calculation principles

DFLE is defined as the average number of years that a person of a given age may expect to live free of disability. The calculation is made from a

41

life table used to compute current life expectancy. It provides the number of years lived between each age interval (x and $x+a$) by the subjects of a cohort experiencing the mortality rates of the current year. The average number of years lived from age x up to the age of death of the last survivor of the cohort represents the *life expectancy at age x*. For each age interval (x, $x+a$) in the table it is necessary to estimate the proportion of years lived in a disabled state, using disability prevalence data from a population survey. The average number of years lived is calculated again, excluding the years lived in the state of disability. The mean of the years lived free of disability from age x, up to the extinction of the cohort, represents the *DFLE at age x*. An example is given in table 5.1.

Table 5.1   Example of DFLE calculation at age 65 in an elderly population

Age (years)	Survival S_x	Years lived $(x, x+5)$	Disability rate	Disability free years $(x, x+5)$
65–69	100 000	463 715	0·078	427 545
70–74	85 486	376 533	0·137	324 948
75–79	65 127	266 085	0·243	201 426
80–84	41 307	145 690	0·310	101 906
85–89	17 769	59 025	0·615	22 725
90 and over	5 841	19 043	0·522	9 103

Life expectancy at 65:
LE 65 = years lived/100 000 = 1 330 091/100 000 = 13·3 years

Disability free life expectancy at 65:
DFLE 65 = years lived/100 000 = 1 087 653/100 000 = 10·9 years

From Robine et al.[6]

Cross-sectional versus longitudinal estimates

The method described above is that of Sullivan,[2] which uses vital statistics and disability data from current life tables and cross-sectional population surveys. Up to now most calculations are made using Sullivan's method because the only available disability data are provided by cross-sectional health interview surveys. DFLEs obtained from prevalence of disability data are, however, only crude estimations. Cross-sectional disability data are not comparable with mortality rates. In a life table the force of mortality is expressed by the probability of dying between age x and $x+a$ calculated from the vital statistics of a given year. It is based on the flow of death for each age interval of year studied. These mortality data relate to the current conditions of a given year.

Unlike the probability of dying displayed in a life table, prevalences of disability derived from cross-sectional surveys are not probabilities of becoming disabled in the current year. They do not represent the *flow* but the *stock* of people living in a state of disability at the exact time of observation. This stock is not only the result of the current year conditions but also the result of the whole cohort history. Considering the importance of generation (cohort) effects, especially in elderly populations, a significant error could be induced. Thus it is extremely difficult to interpret DFLE time variations and to distinguish between generation and period effects.

In order to compute methodologically more accurate DFLE, incidence—rather than prevalence—data on disability are necessary, but this requires longitudinal surveys, which are more difficult to organise. Several methods were proposed to improve the calculation of DFLE, taking into account disability incidence as well as possibilities of reversibility of disability. The "double extinction calculation" and the "multistage method" are two examples among others.[7] Some disability incidence data from longitudinal surveys are available but no nationally representative series is available to examine secular trends in DFLE. Some countries are planning specific longitudinal surveys or longitudinal supplements to existing national health surveys in order to assess incidence of disability (for instance, the "longitudinal supplement on ageing" (LSOA) of the US health interview survey).

Criteria for disability

The level of DFLE is mainly determined by the definition of disability and by the threshold chosen to separate persons in a state of disability from those who are not. Thus it is important to know the conceptual basis chosen and the procedure of construction of the disability indicators. Sullivan's first calculations relied on the disability indicators defined by the National Center for Health Statistics for the national health interview survey.[8] They were based on short term and long term limitations of the major activity. Similar conceptual models have been implemented in several surveys in Canada[9] and Australia.[10] In other countries calculations of DFLE used a range of disability concepts. Some results are given in table 5.2. No common conceptual basis has yet been agreed and comparisons remain difficult. The International Classification of Impairment, Disability, and Handicap developed by the World Health Organization[12] is, however, frequently proposed as a common basis for international comparisons, but a large amount of work will be necessary to agree on standardised indicators of disability.

Variations

Age

The proportion of disability years to the total number of years lived increases consistently with age. From birth the disability years measured

Table 5.2   Calculation of DFLE at birth and at 65: some results from different countries

Country (year)	Sex	Life expectancy at birth (years)	Disabled life (years)	DFLE
Canada	M	70·8	11·6	59·2
(1978)	F	78·3	15·5	62·8
France	M	70·7	8·8	61·9
(1982)	F	78·9	11·7	67·2
United Kingdom	M	71·8	13·1	58·7
(1985)	F	77·8	16·3	61·5
Quebec	M	71·9	9·5	62·4
(1986)	F	79·5	13·2	66·3

Country (year)	Sex	Life expectancy at 65 (years)	Disabled life (years)	DFLE
United States	M	14·6	4·1	10·5
(1985)	F	18·6	5·2	13·4
United Kingdom	M	13·4	5·7	7·7
(1985)	F	17·5	8·6	8·9
Australia	M	14·8	8·1	6·7
(1988)	F	18·7	10·1	8·6

From Robine et al[6] and Strohmenger and Peron.[11]

by the restriction of major activities represent about 10% of life expectancy. After the age of 65 this proportion is about 30%. It varies with the type and severity of the disability considered.

Gender: excess disability in women after 60 years of age

Most of the surveys performed on the prevalence of disabilities in old age show that women are more affected than men. When calculating DFLE the number of disability years is higher in females. Thus the difference in DFLE between males and females is in general less than the difference observed for life expectancy.

Secular trends: three theories to be tested

DFLE and its components are relevant to three current theories on the evolution of the population's health status: (a) "compression of morbidity", (b) "disabling chronic conditions pandemy", (c) "balance" between mortality amd morbidity.

According to the compression of morbidity theory,[13 14] increases in life expectancy will reach a limit but morbidity and related disabilities will continue to decrease. In these circumstances the gain in DFLE results from a shorter lifetime with disability, and morbidity is compressed.

The theory of disabling chronic conditions pandemy is presented by Kramer.[15] Increased longevity, particularly due to falling mortality rates at older ages, is associated with an additional period of ill health marked by "end of life" chronic conditions. According to this theory each year of life expectancy gained is a year of disability. Life expectancy increases but DFLE remains stable.

Manton developed another theory,[16] stating that a balance exists between mortality and disability so DFLE increases as fast as life expectancy. Therefore, the burden of chronic health problems will depend on this balance over time.

The different possibilities are summarised in table 5.3. In order to test these proposed theories it would be necessary to know the concomitant variations of DFLE components, mortality and disability. Mortality data are readily available but in general disability data are too recent to provide reliable evidence of the secular trends in DFLE. The scarce data available suggest that secular trends in disability vary according to the level of severity.[17] Some analyses conducted on light or moderate levels of disability showed that prevalence increases with time, supporting the theory of a disabling chronic conditions pandemy. On the other hand, other analyses conducted on more severe disabilities showed a slight decrease of disabilities with time, giving support to the compression of morbidity and balance theories.

Table 5.3   Possible trends in DFLE according to different theories of population transition

Situation	Life expectancy	Disabled life	DFLE
Compression of morbidity (Fries[13 14])	Stable	Decrease	Increase
Pandemy of chronic disease (Kramer[15])	Increase	Increase	Decrease
Equilibrium (Manton[16])	Increase	Increase or decrease	Stable

Geographical trends

DFLE represents a statistical tool of interest for comparing different geographical areas. It summarises mortality amd morbidity in a single tool and, like life expectancy, yields results independent of the population age structure.

Recently, exhaustive health expectancy calculations—including DFLE—available from different countries all around the world were collected in a directory.[18] At the present time, however, geographical comparisons are very difficult to interpret because of a lack of common definition of disability and of differences in measurement techniques for disability indicators.

Social variations

It is of interest to examine the impact of social inequalities on DFLE. The few analyses conducted in this field show that social inequalities observed with DFLE are similar to those observed for mortality but stronger. In Canada,[9] the difference in life expectancy between rich and poor areas was 6·3 years in males and 2·8 years in females; in the same areas the differences in DFLE were 14·3 years in males and 7·6 years in females (table 5.4).

Table 5.4 *Differences in life expectancy and DFLE according to social class (Canada 1978)*

	Life expectancy	DFLE	
		Years	%
Male			
Poorest areas	67·1	50·0	74·5
Richest areas	73·4	64·3	87·6
Difference	6·3	14·3	
Female			
Poorest areas	76·6	59·5	77·7
Richest areas	79·4	67·5	85·0
Difference	2·8	7·6	

From Wilkins and Adams.[9]

Contribution of specific diseases

DFLE is a global index of health and is independent of underlying medical causes. It is, however, interesting to assess the impact of the different medical causes on mortality and disability. To do this the method of "potential gains" in life expectancy is extended to DFLE.[19] The potential gain in life expectancy that could be expected by eliminating all deaths due to a specific medical cause is added to the potential gain in DFLE that could be expected by eliminating disabilities due to this same cause. With this method the order of importance of specific medical causes differs from that observed for mortality alone.[20] Cardiovascular diseases, for instance, account for the most frequent cause of death and are also a very important cause of disability. Their first rank in health priorities is confirmed when using the potential gain in DFLE method. On the other hand, impairments and diseases related to musculoskeletal causes have no influence on mortality, although they contribute greatly to disability. They achieve a high priority rank by this method, whereas they have no priority when mortality only is considered (table 5.5).

Conclusion

"Add years to life and add life to years." This general formula, largely spread by WHO, gained, with the concept of DFLE, a quantifiable explicit means of measurement. DFLE was proposed 30 years ago and is now gaining ground as a useful policy tool. Considering the large increase in

Table 5.5   Years of life gained by elimination of each disease group*

	Men		Women	
	LE (years)	DFLE (years)	LE (years)	DFLE (years)
Circulatory	7·4 (1)	5·7 (1)	8·3 (1)	5·6 (1)
Neoplasms	3·3 (2)	2·0 (2)	3·6 (2)	2·1 (3)
Respiratory	1·2 (3)	1·6 (3)	1·1 (3)	1·1 (4)
Injury	1·0 (4)	1·3 (5)	0·5 (4)	0·8 (6)
Mental	0·1 (5)	0·7 (6)	0·2 (5)	1·0 (5)
Locomotor	0·04 (6)	1·5 (4)	0·1 (6)	3·5 (2)

LE, life expectancy.
Values in parentheses are rank order of importance.
* For example, avoidance of all circulatory disease would gain men an extra 7·4 years of LE from birth.
Data from M Bone and A Bebbington, personal communication.

the elderly population, DFLE is particularly useful for defining relevant objectives for the health care system[11] and monitoring the effects of policy. At a national level it is necessary to set up surveys to derive disability prevalence and incidence rates. At the international level the priority is to agree on the conceptual basis of disability and the standardisation of instruments for measurement of disability components.

I wish to thank Mrs Annie Lacroux for the help she gave in the elaboration of this chapter.

1 Sanders BS. Measuring community health levels. *Am J Public Health* 1964;**54**:1063–70.
2 Sullivan DF. A single index of mortality and morbidity. *HSMHA Health Rep* 1971;**86**: 347–54.
3 Organisation de Coopération et de Développement Economique. *Mesure du Bien-être Social: progrès accomplis dans l'élaboration d'indicateurs sociaux. Programme d'élaboration des indicateurs sociaux de l'OCDE.* Paris: OECD, 1976.
4 Davis M. Epidemiology and the challenge of ageing. *Int J Epidemiol* 1985;**14**:9–21.
5 World Health Organization. The uses of epidemiology in the study of the elderly: report of a WHO scientific group on the epidemiology of ageing. *WHO Tech Rep Ser* 1984;**706**.
6 Robine JM, Blanchet M, Dowd JE. *Health expectancy.* London: HMSO, 1992.
7 Rogers A, Rogers RG, Branch LG. A multistate analysis of active life expectancy. *Public Health Rep* 1989;**104**:222–5.
8 Sullivan DF. Disability components for an index of health. *Vital Health Stat* 1971;**2**:35.
9 Wilkins R, Adams OB. Health expectancy in Canada late 1970s: demographic, regional and social dimensions. *Am J Public Health* 1983;**73**:1073–80.
10 Mathers CD. *Health expectancies in Australia, 1981 and 1988.* Canberra: ACT, Australian Institute of Health, 1991. (Health differentials Series, No 1.)
11 Strohmenger C, Peron Y. *L'espérance de vie en santé. Cah Québecois Démogr* 1991;**20**.
12 World Health Organization. *Classification of impairment, disabilities and handicap. A manual of classification relating to the consequences of diseases.* Geneva: WHO, 1980.
13 Fries JF. The compression of morbidity. *Milbank Q* 1983;**61**:397–419.
14 Fries JF. Aging, natural death, and the compression of morbidity. *N Engl J Med* 1980; **313**:407–28.
15 Kramer M. The rising pandemic of mental disorders and associated chronic diseases and disabilities. *Acta Psychiatr Scand* 1980;**62**(suppl 285):382–97.
16 Manton KG. Changing concepts of morbidity and mortality in the elderly population. *Milbank Mem Fund Q* 1980;**60**:183–244.

17 Robine JM, Bucquet D, Ritchie K. L'espérance de vie sans incapacité, un indicateur de l'évolution des conditions de santé au cours du temps: vingt ans de calculs. *Cah Québecois Démogr* 1991;**20**:205–35.

18 Réseau REVES. *Health expectancy. Statistical world yearbook.* Montpellier: Laboratoire d'Epidémiologie et d'Economie de la Santé, 1991. (Supplement to bibliography series, No 2.)

19 Colvez A, Blanchet M. Potential gains in life expectancy free of disability: a tool for health planning. *Int J Epidemiol* 1983;**12**:86–91.

20 Dillard S. *Durée ou qualité de la vie?* Quebec: Editeur Officiel, 1983.

6 Ageing in developing countries: a case study of Brazil

RENATO P VERAS

The importance of the theme of "the elderly population" is of increasing interest in many developing countries because of its repercussions for health and social policy.[1] Scientific research, particularly in the area of health and health services for elderly people in developing countries, has, however, been very limited. This may be attributed to a lack of knowledge of the large field of investigation available, low investment, and government agencies' lack of priority in relation to this topic. The lack of investment may simply be a reflection of the economic situation. In countries that have faced decades of economic crisis, research may be viewed as a luxury and reliance may be placed on research conducted in richer Western countries for the development of health and social policy in poorer countries. Furthermore, the prediction of overwhelming demographic burdens, with their implications for state pension funds and health services, may end up paralysing rather than galvanising action.

These points of view must be contested. Demographic growth in different developing countries has its own patterns and social, political, and economic contexts, which lead to particular characteristics that must be captured by investigative studies and designs that take into account the circumstances in each country. Research must be upgraded in status from dispensable luxury to essential prerequisite for decision making. This will require a reorientation of current models of scientific research in many developing countries from the borrowed western style "ivory tower" researcher to the needs related, community orientated researcher who is willing to talk to policy makers—both local and national.

Countries in a transitional phase of development from high to low levels of mortality and fertility are undergoing dramatic changes at present. In Brazil there will be a *fivefold* expansion in the whole population between 1950 and 2025 (75 years—about three generations), while the number of those in the 60 + age group will increase *15-fold*. In comparison, over the same period the elderly (60 +) populations of post-industrialised countries, such as the United Kingdom and Japan, will only increase by factors of 3·5 and 5 respectively.[2] The trends in Brazil, shown in fig 6.1, have been more dramatic since 1970 and are the result of a reduction in the younger age groups.

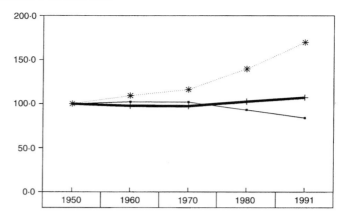

Fig 6.1   Relative variations in population age structure between censuses: Brazil 1950–91 (1950 = 100). (From Instituto Brasileiro de Geografia e Estatistica, IBGE.)

It must be emphasised that population ageing is a new and unprecedented phenomenon all over the world, even in developed countries. With these demographic trends come changes in patterns of disease—the epidemiological transition (see chapter 4). In Brazil various factors have contributed to both demographic and epidemiological transition: the industrialisation process and growing urbanisation since 1930 have changed the organisation of production and the geographic distribution of the population. Reduction of the family size, and consequently of the number of children, is also a new phenomenon, reducing both the role of grandparents and provoking concern about family care of older, dependent relatives. Industrialisation and urbanisation induced the government to implement population policies of water supply and sanitation systems that have undoubtedly had the effect of improving the health of the population and have contributed to the epidemiological transition. The patterns of disease are shown in fig 6.2. Deaths from infectious diseases have declined, while mortality caused by chronic degenerative diseases, such as neoplasms and circulatory disorders, has increased.

Life expectancy has increased dramatically. In 1870, in England, life expectancy was only 26 years and almost half the population were under 20 years old.[3] In the United States, from the beginning of the twentieth century up to 1980, life expectancy at birth rose from 47·0 to 73·6 years.[4] In Brazil changes are even more impressive, as the life expectancy of the Brazilian population has doubled during the century (fig 6.3).

Life expectancy reflects inequalities between different social groups but the patterns may differ with life expectancy at older ages.[5] Greece, though not the richest country in Europe, has the highest life expectancy at 60.[6] In North America, surprisingly enough, Mexican women aged 65 live on average three years longer than neighbouring American women.[7] Similarly, when compared to the British, Brazilians have a higher life expectancy at

50

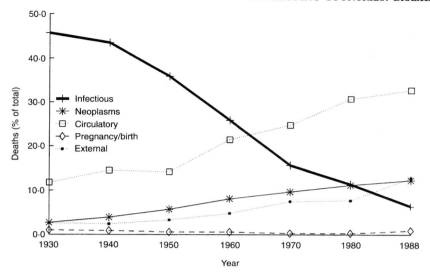

Fig 6.2   Proportional mortality from some causes of death (1930–88).

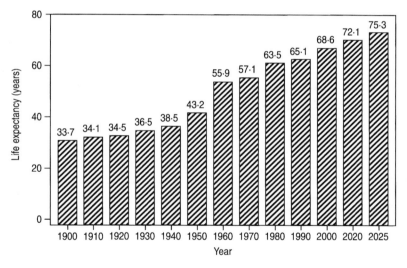

Fig 6.3   Life expectancy at birth: Brazil 1900–2025. (From Santos, Demografia: estimativas e projeçóes. São Paulo, 1978 (1990–1950); UNO, DIESA, Periodical on Ageing. New York, 1985 (1960–2025).)

60.[8] The reason for these apparent contradictions may be that the "poor" who live beyond 60 years of age form a very select group of survivors in developing countries and may be biologically more resilient. Yet such extended longevity does not mean that they are free from infirmities.

In Brazil, according to the 1991 demographic census, the largest proportions of elderly are found in some states of the southeast (Rio de Janeiro, São Paulo, and Minas Gerais), south (Rio Grande do Sul), and northeast (Paraíba, Rio Grande do Norte, Pernambuco, and Ceará) regions. These states have quite different characteristics from the political, economic, and social points of view, which may directly influence the population age structure. In general, northeastern states, the south, and Minas Gerais have suffered greater emigration of young people, which has resulted in ageing of the population, even in the northeast where fertility rates are relatively high. In Rio de Janeiro, a state which attracts younger work-seeking migrants, there has been a tendency for the population to be less aged. As the immigration process is, however, long standing, many migrant communities are now ageing themselves. Declines in fertility, at an advanced stage and accelerated by economic considerations, also contribute to the increased proportion of aged people in these immigrant states. Rural–urban differences in the age structure of the population have also occurred. Rural areas of northeastern states are most aged, while the southeast has the largest proportion of aged populations in urban areas. These differential demographic trends reflect migration and fertility patterns of the young, who tend to move from rural to urban zones and from the northeast to the southeast.[9]

These analyses of a single country show how country-wide statistics mask the subtle differences that are explained by disparities of income, education, housing, transportation, health services, and so forth. The elderly population is concentrated in the most economically developed areas, with better provision of health services and better living conditions, and where expectation of life is higher.

Ageing research in developing countries

Brazil, in common with many developing countries, presents many contrasts and deep inequalities that must be considered when posing research questions, developing study designs, and interpreting findings. The ways in which social and economic factors tend to cluster together present particular challenges in attempting to disentangle, for example, the relative importance of income from access to health care. Richer strata of the population have access to health services comparable to any developed country and often provide relatively easy and accessible populations for ageing research but findings from such populations are of little relevance to the aged in other settings. The socioeconomic gradients that exist between rich populations and the poorest are huge and it may be that it is the relative steepness of the gradients, rather than absolute levels of poverty and disadvantage, that are most important in determining both quality of life and life expectancy.

The United Nations Development Programme built up the human development index (HDI) for the purpose of measuring and comparing aspects of social reality that the United Nations consider relevant and essential to human development. The index combines life expectancy, education, and income indicators in a range between 0 and 1, and is a synthetic device that measures the level of social development of countries for international comparisons.[10] Based on the 1980 demographic census, this index has been applied to Brazilian states and shows sharp regional differences.[11] The northeastern region has the lowest HDI rate, followed by the north, mid-west, south and southeast. The gradient of disadvantage is much greater using HDI comparisons than it is using individual indicators or life expectancy (table 6.1).

Table 6.1   Indicators used for calculating the human development index by regions of Brazil

Region	Mean population completing primary education (%)	Mean monthly income (US $)	Mean life expectation at birth (years)	Human development index
Northwest	59	206	65·6	0·542
Northeast	46	123	50·9	0·161
Southeast	75	254	64·3	0·709
South	79	226	67·3	0·742
Mid-West	64	209	65·1	0·667
Gradient: high to low	1·73	2·07	1·32	4·61

From Brazilian Demography Census of 1980, made by the Instituto Brasileiro de Geografia e Estatistica (IBGE Brazilian Census Bureau).

It must be pointed out that the states of Rio de Janeiro and Paraíba, which have the largest proportions of elderly in the country, presented quite different HDIs, 0·81 and 0·05 (the lowest rate of all) respectively. In Paraíba population ageing is mainly a result of migration away from the wretched living conditions and lack of work. Mortality rates among the young remain high and there has been a dramatic decrease in fertility as a result of massive sterilisation programmes in these poor areas. In Rio de Janeiro the situation is quite different. Its population is more stable and the fertility and mortality rates have already been decreasing for several years. Thus despite the apparently similar proportions of the population aged 60+ years, about 9% in both states, the determinants are quite different, as are the social and health consequences and possible policies required.

Considering social, economic, and demographic structures as uniform, either in the design of social–medical research projects or in examination of routinely collected data, is therefore a methodological error that brings serious consequences to planning because it distorts reality, preventing its

53

correct understanding. Study designs must consider the heterogeneity of populations in order to capture correctly the real needs and demands of different social groups. This is a major challenge and is often associated with increased costs and difficulty of research.

The elderly: a heterogeneous group

In the design of projects the importance of socioeconomic factors exerting strong confounding effects on relationships must always be borne in mind and allowed for in either design or analysis. For example, among older people lack of regular income may be a confounding factor explaining relationships between health status and use of health services. In order to emphasise the importance of such factors and to provide practical examples, some findings from a study carried out in selected districts of Rio de Janeiro, chosen to represent distinct socioeconomic segments, will be presented.[12]

Household sampling was carried out and elderly people aged 60 + were interviewed about their health, from their own point of view. Interestingly, a majority (83%) of elderly from all socioeconomic groups reported their health as good and did not report any physical health problem; this is in agreement with other studies.[13] The remaining fifth of elderly people were, however, extremely high users of health services.

Of those who reported health problems, 64% had one or more complaints, predominantly arthritis, cardiopathies, hypertension, sight and hearing impairments, digestive diseases, respiratory problems, and diabetes. Frequent use of health services was considered normal among aged people: 35% of the interviewees had used a health service at least once in the three months preceding the interview. The majority (59%) returned once or more often for further consultation. The consultation rate was 1·51 per elderly person over three months, which is high (considering the short time) and equates to six consultations per year—comparable with the rate in Britain where there is much easier and free at the point of use access to primary care.[14]

Women used health services more often than men in all three areas investigated. The percentage of women who reported use of a health service was particularly high in the area of higher purchasing power (40%) compared with the poorest area of the city (20%). No more than 4·8% of the elderly had been hospitalised within the three month period before the interview. Rate of hospitalisation among men was higher than among women, which may result from men not seeking medical care until late in the course of disease or when serious symptoms occur.

Although fewer than 20% of those sampled reported health problems, 80% regularly used drugs prescribed by doctors. This consumption was higher among women in the three districts. The use of drugs was even higher in those aged over 70 years in all three districts. Interestingly, use of drugs not prescribed by a doctor was more common among residents of the poorest area. One hypothesis to explain this finding may be the poor access to doctors in this area, leading to an informal culture of "borrowing" prescriptions from other people, which could involve dangers to health.

Most of the common health problems of aged people were seen more frequently among the poorest in the worst parts of the city; however, the relationship between need for services and use of services followed the classical inverse care law,[15] with greatest need being associated with least service provision. In the case of impairment of sight the highest levels of impairment were in Santa Cruz area but the number of elderly with sight problems who wore glasses was highest in Copacabana, a district of higher purchasing power. Clearly, if a question on visual impairment was expressed in terms of "Do you wear glasses to read or watch television?" (a frequently used question in Western surveys), the need would appear highest in the wealthiest area.

Cognitive impairment appeared to be extremely common in all areas but showed marked variation: lower in Copacabana (6%), above average in Méier (10%), and much higher in Santa Cruz (30%). Although the same methods were used in all three areas it is likely that this does not represent true differences in cognitive impairment but is the result of poorer educational attainment in the poorer areas with resultant worse performance on tests of cognitive impairment—a widely recognised phenomenon.[16-18] None the less, the levels of poor performance on cognitive impairment tests are a cause for concern. Other studies using less education dependent tests have found high levels of dementia[19] and other mental health problems.[20]

Conclusion

The continued lack of information about health and social circumstances of older people reduces the pressure to implement relevant public policies. Research that acknowledges the complexity of the experience of ageing in different social and economic contexts is needed. Researchers must be more willing to consider the public policy implications of their work, collaborate with policy makers in formulating research questions, and disseminate their findings. Collaboration between researchers, policy makers, and health managers should ensure that scarce health care resources are put to best use and that accurate information about the impact of policies is available.

1 World Bank. *Averting the old age crisis. Policies to protect the old and promote growth*. Oxford: Oxford University Press, 1994.
2 Veras RP, Dutra S. Envelhecimento da população brasileira: reflexões e aspectos a considerar quando da definição de desenhos de pesquisa para estudos populacionais. *Physis Rev Saúde Coletiva* 1993;3:107–26.
3 Midwinter E. An ageing world: the equivocal response. *Ageing Soc* 1990;10:221–8.

4 Olshansky SJ, Ault B. The fourth stage of the epidemiologic transition: the age of delayed degenerative diseases. *Milbank Mem Fund Q* 1986;**64**:355–91.

5 Siegel JS, Hoover SL. Demographic aspects of the health of the elderly to the year 2000 and beyond. *World Health Stat Q* 1982;**32**:133–202.

6 World Health Organization. The uses of epidemiology in the study of the elderly: report of a WHO scientific group on the epidemiology of ageing. *WHO Tech Rep Ser* 1984;706.

7 Kalache A, Veras RP, Ramos LR. O envelhecimento da população mundial; um desafio novo. *Rev Saúde Pública* 1987;**21**:200–10.

8 Ramos LR, Veras RP, Kalache A. Envelhecimento populacional: uma realidade brasileira. *Rev Saúde Pública* 1987;**21**:211–24.

9 Bercovich AM. *Características Regionais da População Idosa no Brasil* – Contribuições para o Seminário de Dinâmica Demográfica e Desenvolvimento. Rio de Janeiro: Instituto Brasileiro de Geografia e Estatistica (IBGE), 1993.

10 United Nations Development Programme. *Human development report,* New York: UN, 1990.

11 Carvalho AF, Alves MIC. *O Índice De Desenvolvimento Humano Para os Estados Brasileiros.* Rio de Janeiro: IBGE/DEISO/PNUD, 1992. (mimeo)

12 Veras RP. *A survey of the health of the elderly people in Rio de Janeiro, Brazil.* PhD thesis, University of London, 1992.

13 Veras RP. Prevalência da síndrome cerebral orgânica em população de idosos da área metropolitana da região sudeste do Brasil. *Rev Saúde Pública* 1994;**28**(1):26–37.

14 McCormick A, Fleming D, Charlton J. *Morbidity statistics from general practice. Fourth national study 1991–2.* London: HMSO, 1995.

15 Hart JT. The inverse care law. *Lancet* 1971;**i**:405–12.

16 Cooper B, Bickel H. Population screening and the early detection of dementing disorders in old age: a review. *Psychol Med* 1984;**14**:81–95.

17 Gurland B, Copeland JRM, Kelleher MJ, *et al. The mind and mood of aging: mental health problems of the community elderly in New York and London.* New York: Haworth Press, 1983.

18 Weissman MM, Myers JK, Tischler GL. Psychiatric disorders (DSM-III) and cognitive impairment among the elderly in a US urban community. *Acta Psychiatr Scand* 1985;**71**: 366–79.

19 Blay SL, Mari JJ, Ramos LR. The use of the face–hand test to screen for organic brain syndromes. A pilot study. *Rev Saúde Pública* 1989;**23**:395–400.

20 Almeida Filho N, Santana VS, Pinho AR. Estudo epidemiológico dos transtornos mentais em uma população de idosos—área urbana de Salvador—BA. *J Bras Psiq* 1984;**33**:114–20.

7 Conduct of long term cohort sequential studies

ALVAR SVANBORG

It might sound paradoxical to assert that a detailed understanding of the manifestations of ageing is especially limited in the last decades of life when the biological, functional, and social consequences are most pronounced. The main reason is the simultaneously occurring increase in the incidence and prevalence of morbidity. At ages 80–85 the proportion of persons without symptoms that can be referred to definable abnormal conditions is low, and the possibilities of studying ageing separately from disease are therefore even more complex. A better understanding not only of the old person's health problems but also of ageing itself is urgently needed at these very old ages. The main objective of this chapter is to illustrate, using experiences from the cohort sequential studies of 70 year old people in Gothenburg, Sweden, the opportunities for detailed study of ageing, health, and age related change in need of care by a combination of longitudinal population studies, age cohort comparison, and intervention programmes.

Longitudinal studies are necessary because a clear differentiation between manifestations of ageing and symptoms of definable diseases or other disorders is often impossible without follow up over shorter or longer periods, thus allowing a retrospective evaluation of both ageing and health. In general this evaluation becomes increasingly accurate with increasing follow up time: "One must wait until the evening to see how good the day has been" (Sophocles).

Age cohort comparisons are essential for understanding variations between generations. In many situations, observed differences between age cohorts have been greater than the age related changes measured longitudinally in the same cohorts over the same time, which makes cross-sectional comparison of ageing invalid.

In order to improve understanding of both longitudinally registered decline and differences between age cohorts, intervention studies may be helpful in illustrating causative relationships. This chapter will also show how previously performed longitudinal cohort sequential studies have contributed knowledge essential for an understanding of: (a) the rate and functional consequences of ageing and the possibilities of postponing certain of its negative consequences; (b) age associated morbidity unrelated to the ageing process, and therefore possibly preventable; (c) morbidity/multimorbidity obviously related to ageing and being old; (d) met and unmet needs for care in old age; and (e) possible measures for prevention of disease and postponement of the negative consequences of ageing in old age.

Methodological aspects

Many of the challenges and problems of conducting long term sequential studies of ageing and real health of older people may be illustrated through experiences in the longitudinal study of 70 year old people in Gothenburg, Sweden. At the present time more than 200 reports from that study are available in international journals. For more general descriptions of design, methodology, and procedures the reader is referred to articles by Rinder,[1] Svanborg,[2-4] and Eriksson et al.[5] The study originally included one cohort born in 1901–2, which has now been followed for more than 20 years. When results from the study showed obvious impacts of environmental factors not only on health but also on the rate and functional consequences of ageing, two more cohorts (born five and 10 years after the first cohort) were added. In order to test hypotheses of how lifestyle, environmental factors, and availability of medical care exerted influences on ageing and health, a broad sociomedical intervention was added to the third age cohort. The general design of these parts of the Gothenburg study of ageing is illustrated in table 7.1. Later extensions of this study have been described.[6]

Table 7.1   Design of the longitudinal study of 70 year old people in Gothenburg (H 70) and the added intervention programme (IVEG)

Year of investigation	Year of birth		
	1901–02 H 70	1906–07 H 70	1911–12 IVEG
1971–72	70 years		
1976–77	75 years	70 years	
1980–81	79 years		
1981–82		75 years	70 years
1982–83	81 years		70 years
1983–84	82 years		72 years
1984–85	83 years		72 years
1985–86		79 years	
1986–87	85 years		
1987–88			76 years

During the long period these studies have been going on, resources in the form of new non-invasive methods for identification, definition, and quantification of ageing and health have markedly improved, allowing morphological, functional, and sometimes metabolic organ studies to be conducted in broad population studies. A common and important methodological problem is the challenge of anchoring the new measurements to those already performed in order to allow at least some form of indirect comparison over time.

When our study started we were aware that our detailed medical examination and recommendations were a form of intervention. A control group was therefore sampled in an identical manner and registered for future comparisons—a similar system was used in the intervention study. The combination of challenges and problems caused by medical developments means, however, that medical advantages originally considered to be available only at the level of research, and for our longitudinally followed groups, in the meantime became routine and also used for the control groups, limiting the possibilities for adequate comparisons. This phenomenon, caused by the current dynamic developments of medical resources as well as factors changing the prerequisites for our lives in general, makes age cohort comparison even more important. The faster changes occur, the more urgent are comparisons not only of longitudinal ageing related changes but also of age cohorts who have experienced different life situations.

In the Gothenburg study we added historians to the team, hoping to be able to identify retrospectively differences that might be causatively related to present vitality and health. Because of the multifactorial nature of factors influencing lifestyle, such as social circumstances, educational level, and professional activities, the possibilities for identifying causative relationships were found to be limited. This illustrates the need for the combination of longitudinal studies with not only age cohort comparisons but also with intervention projects where hypotheses of causative relationship can be tested. In the Gothenburg study three age cohorts were thus followed longitudinally and included a socioeconomic intervention in the third cohort, allowing comparison between two non-intervened age cohorts and one intervention cohort over the age interval 70–75 years.

The importance of adequate sampling for population and of obtaining a sample that is representative of a defined population, or at least for a clearly definable part of a subpopulation, is obvious. The need for well defined and identified population samples is paramount, particularly when age cohort comparisons are involved. Even minor variations in the representativeness of samples can cause differences that jeopardise age cohort comparisons.

The characterisation of representativeness is complex and can vary depending on the variables studied. The variables we compared between responders and non-responders for the longitudinal studies of 70 year olds in Gothenburg[1] are illustrated in box 7.1; however, other variables had to be considered when, for example, clinical reference values for different biochemical components were calculated.[78]

Box 7.1—Variables compared between participants and non-participants in the longitudinal study of 70 year old people in Gothenburg, Sweden

- Sex
- Marital status
- Registration of alcohol abuse with the temperance board
- Income and community rent allowances
- Somatic inpatient care and psychiatric inpatient and outpatient care during 1966 to the date of sampling in 1971–72
- Mortality in the age interval 70–81

The importance of using age samples that are as homogeneous as possible should also be emphasised. In the Gothenburg study the goal was to avoid variations greater than age in years plus three months. Furthermore, the first week after the celebration of the birthday was avoided as it presumably did not reflect the ordinary living habits of the participant. Grouping of age cohorts into, for example, those of 70–75 or 70–80 should be avoided. The mean age can vary markedly in such groups, both in comparisons within the same population and even more so between different populations, limiting the possibility for reliable comparison.

Ageing and health of older people varies markedly from country to country; this is reflected, for example, in the marked variations in longevity between different populations. The reasons for differences in longevity between developing and developed countries are understood to a certain extent. Figure 7.1 illustrates, however, that such differences are found in comparisons not only of developing and developed countries but also of countries with a smaller socioeconomic structure and similar availability of medical service and care—for example, in the Nordic countries of Denmark, Finland, Iceland, Norway, and Sweden. Marked variations also occur within different socioeconomic groups in a given country. This can be the case in populations with a generally good socioeconomic standard, as illustrated by differences in the prevalence of hip fractures among older people in urban and rural areas of Sweden[9] and variations in longevity of males (up to seven years) in different areas of a city such as Gothenburg.

In developing countries the main determinant of change in total longevity is reduction in mortality during childhood and the middle part of life. In contrast, in highly developed countries the main reason for the current increases in life expectancy is a reduction in death rates at ages above 65–70. Such trends are likely to occur in the future in the presently less developed countries. It is also important to know that further life expectancy does not vary very much between the relatively few and probably strong individuals who have survived up to age 65–70 in developing countries, and the higher proportion of survivors, many of them frail, in developed

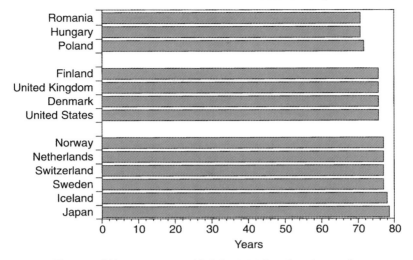

Fig 7.1   Life expectancy at birth in 1990 for selected countries.

countries. When research using cohort sequential study designs is planned, factors related to lifestyle and environment, as well as selective mortality before old age is reached, have to be taken into consideration at the initial planning stage. Furthermore, there are several observations indicating that survivors to very old age show qualitatively and quantitatively different manifestations of ageing over time compared with those who do not survive as long.

At any age the size of the sample studied needs to be related to the type of study; for example, if the goal of the study is to analyse a phenomenon existing or expected to occur in a higher or lower proportion of the sample or to vary more or less over the follow up periods, sample size requirements will vary accordingly. Furthermore, the prediction of the sample size needed in studies of older people is complicated not only by marked changes in vitality and health status over short periods but also by loss of participants as a result of selective mortality, migration caused by change in health status, and other circumstances related to vitality, function, and need for care. For adequate planning of long term sequential studies, many of these factors have to be predicted before the start of the study.

A special and challenging problem to consider is selective mortality. Some individuals in a birth cohort will have died at an early age, before the study is set up, and this "earlier" mortality differs between populations and between age cohorts within the same population. From a biological, physiological, and often also social perspective, there are certain special people who survive to very old age; for example, we observed that those who survived more than nine years from age 70 had better cognitive performance at age 70 than those who died before age 79.[10] There are also observations indicating that the rate of functional decline—for example, of

61

the kidney's excreting function—is faster in those of 70–75 than it is in representative samples of those still alive beyond 75.[11]

A methodological problem that is much more common than generally realised is that dates of birth are not known and/or adequately registered in many populations. A study of 70 year old people in Jerusalem showed that in a country of high immigration such as Israel, with many migrants coming from developing countries, no less than 15% of the inhabitants were not sure of their exact birth date (J Stessman, personal communication). Such a lack of knowledge, problematic in itself, can also be expected to be associated with variations in the degree of education and other socioeconomically influenced variables, thereby further complicating, or even hindering, true population based studies of ageing.

On the other hand, advances in demographic statistics have greatly improved the possibilities for identification of relatively small population samples, which can not only evaluate political ideology and predictions of election outcomes but are also of value for the study of vitality, health, and needs of care in the older and frailer members of a population.

Outcome aspects

As a result of longitudinal studies of ageing related decline in organ function, initially performed in the United States[11] and later on also in, for example, Finland,[12] and of cohort sequential studies (for example, Framingham, USA, and Gothenburg, Sweden), knowledge on ageing itself has accumulated, mainly through studies of "younger olds". Even up to ages around 80, a significant proportion of the population has been found to be "healthy", that is, without symptoms that can be referred to definable diseases or other abnormal conditions; consequently, studies of younger olds are valuable in studying ageing. Normative values for many biochemical variables, blood pressure, cardiac morphology and function, hormone production, and target organ effects have been produced from such studies. In clinical psychology[10 13 14] ageing related changes in certain cognitive parameters and personality traits have been studied, allowing a better definition of when impaired cognition and personality changes are related to abnormal conditions. Morphological changes in height, weight, and body composition[15] have been reported and related to nutritional requirements and physical activity level.[11] We were astonished to find marked differences between age cohorts born at only five year intervals. The practical consequences are that normative value limits may have to be revised over short intervals. What are known to be upper and lower limits of normative criteria in the present cohort might not be applicable, even for the generation of older people born five years later. Future needs for long term sequential studies on ageing might never end!

These attempts to identify ageing separately from disease have demonstrated the influence of lifestyle and environmental factors on ageing.

Tobacco smoking is not only a risk factor for lung and certain other forms of cancer but also accelerates the rate of decline of bone density during ageing. Smokers have—for example, at age 70—less bone and a higher risk of fractures than non-smokers.[9][15] Thus epidemiological results of cohort sequential studies are accumulating indirect evidence that interventions aimed not only at improving the state of health but also at postponing at least some of the negative consequences of ageing might be realistic.

Would it really be possible to postpone the functional decline caused by ageing itself? Several studies have shown that muscular strength in old age can be influenced to a greater extent than has previously been considered possible.[16][17] The proportional increase in muscle strength with training has been reported to be of a similar order as that seen in young individuals,[18][19] although old people will not reach the same level of strength. These findings imply that different populations and cohorts within populations vary in old age because of variations in their level of physical activity over their life span and also in relation to their activity level when they are old.

It might be too generalised a statement to say that organ systems, organs, and cells are meant to be used and might survive fitter (and longer?) if adequately used. Muscle strength, bone density, and balance are examples of organs and functions that are shown to be positively influenced by systematic activity and reasonable loading. On the other hand, there is no clear evidence that, for example, tissue elasticity/distensibility/compliance, which is of central importance for the function of the ageing heart, blood vessels, and lungs, can be trained to the same extent. Knowledge about the physiology of inactivity, a situation unwillingly imposed on many older persons, is even more limited and needs to be studied in more detail. Results from longitudinal studies show that older persons who experience loneliness as a common problem are more tired, have a less positive evaluation of their state of health, visit physicians more often, and consume more drugs than active persons of the same age, even if their general health is similar. In general more research on both muscle tissue and connective tissue, their functional decline, and possibilities of preserving their function is urgently needed. This is also the case for the cardiovascular and respiratory systems. Such studies have to be based on well defined subsamples of representative populations of older persons.

Possibilities of preventing or postponing diseases common in old age by avoiding or eliminating risk factors have been extensively discussed and to a certain extent tested. Two of the most common reasons for dying in old age are arteriosclerosis related disorders and malignant disorders. Recent longitudinal epidemiological studies—for example, within the Framingham study—have demonstrated relationships between lifestyle at younger ages and cardiovascular manifestations later in life. Recent reports also indicate that vascular dementia at age 85 is at least as common as Alzheimer's dementia, which is considered to become more and more dominant with increasing age.[20] The possibility of prevention of vascular dementia therefore has to be given more intense consideration. We can also hope that ongoing improvements in diagnostic and treatment criteria in older people will produce positive benefits for future age cohorts.

The fact that the incidence of most malignant neoplasms increases rapidly, especially in men (fig 7.2), at ages above 60–70 has fostered statements that we would die of malignant disorders if cardiovascular disease could be avoided. Recent epidemiological observations indicate, however, that for several common cancer locations (for example, lung cancer and gastric cancer) time exposed to carcinogenic compounds plays a greater role than ageing itself. Improved knowledge of the nature of carcinogenic exposition and of anticarcinogenic compounds and their mechanisms might therefore imply a base for a more optimistic view of age and ageing related mortality from malignant disorders in future age cohorts.

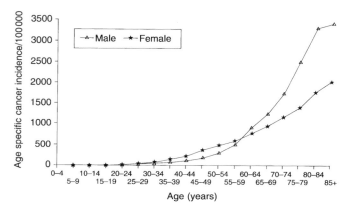

Fig 7.2   Age specific incidence of all cancers in Sweden in 1982. In the age groups from 20–24 to 55–59 years the higher incidence in women is mainly because of the predominance of breast and genital cancer.

The occurrence of disability increases markedly with age. Disability, especially at ages above 75–80 years, is a reflection not only of morbidity and multimorbidity but also of the fact that the reserve capacity declines in old age. Too many older persons will never be able to regain previous levels of functional performance even after a full recovery from curable conditions. They will instead experience a series of stepwise declines, sooner or later leading to a state of disability and helplessness that might have been prevented or postponed if help with rehabilitation and reactivation had been available. A decline in functional performance often occurs after episodes of curable disorders. This illustrates that the reserves of old and frail people trying to re-establish functional performance levels by themselves are very often insufficient and the individuals need help to regain their premorbid functional performance level; and they need qualified help, often over a period longer than many societal insurance systems will pay for, in order to regain their performance level. They need more help with "reactivation"! Unfortunately, the reduction of length of stay in hospitals and earlier discharge too often implies discharging patients "quicker and sicker".[21] This might produce a negative trend for future age cohorts.

Combinations of cohort sequential studies with systematic epidemiologically based intervention programmes are required to understand ageing and ageing related change in vitality and health. They also provide a means of examining the impact of reactivation and rehabilitation. To understand ageing itself also means to understand the ability to *regain* functional performance after events threatening vitality, whether curable disease or other incidents. This is one reason why a broad medical–social intervention study was added to the third age cohort included in the Gothenburg study. In general it seems to be difficult to convince generations of older people, who have been living with the idea that ageing cannot be influenced, that some efforts to do so might be not only realistic and truly meaningful but also stimulating and pleasant.

The more the present trends of ever increasing life expectancy at older ages influence future cohorts, the more urgent it is, and will be, to broaden the understanding of different reasons for terminal decline in vitality and/ or health and when death and dying is "natural". "Overmedicalisaton" of terminal care programmes might have unwanted effects on the care of such patients, for whom other forms of service and support should be made available.

Both positive and negative ongoing trends are occurring in the present generation of older persons. Examples of positive trends are improving cognitive test results between generations of the same age[13 14] and the decline in blood pressure already described (table 7.2).[22] Unfortunately, negative trends are also occurring with, for example, decline in bone density and stability, leading to increasing risk of hip fractures.[9 16] A general conclusion might be that the functional consequences of ageing for the generation reaching, for example, 70 today are different from those for the generation that reached that age 10–20 years ago. The necessity for further age cohort comparison, which it is hoped will contribute results that will

Table 7.2   Arterial blood pressure (mm Hg) in three age cohorts of 70 year old people

	1	2	3	p
Women				
Systolic	168	166	160	<0·000
Diastolic	93	90	85	<0·000
Men				
Systolic	159	160	157	<0·361
Diastolic	96	92	84	0·000

From Svanborg.[22]

make predictions of societal planning for the future more reliable, are obvious.

1 Rinder L, Roupe S, Steen B, Svanborg A. Seventy-year-old people in Gothenburg. A population study in an industrialized Swedish city. General design of the study. *Acta Med Scand* 1975;**198**:397–407.

2 Svanborg A. Seventy-year-old people in Gothenburg. A population study in an industrialized Swedish city. General presentation of social and medical conditions. *Acta Med Scand* 1977;**611**(suppl):5–37.

3 Svanborg A. The health of the elderly population: results from longitudinal studies with age-cohort comparisons. *Ciba Found Symp* 1988;**134**:3–16.

4 Svanborg A. A medical–social intervention in a 70-year-old Swedish population: is it possible to postpone functional decline in aging? *J Gerontol* 1993;**48**(special issue):84–8.

5 Eriksson BG, Mellström D, Svanborg A. A medical–social intervention in a 70-year-old Swedish population. *Compr Gerontol [C]* 1987;**1**:49–56.

6 Steen B, Djurfeldt H. The gerontological and geriatric population studies in Gothenburg, Sweden. *J Gerontol* 1993;**26**:163–9.

7 Nilsson-Ehle H, Jagenburg R, Landahl S, Svanborg A, Westin J. Haematological abnormalities and reference intervals in the elderly. A cross-sectional comparative study of three urban Swedish population samples aged 70, 75 and 81 years. *Acta Med Scand* 1988;**1224**:595–604.

8 Landahl S, Jagenburg R, Svanborg A. Blood components in a 70-year-old population. *Clin Chim Acta* 1981;**112**:301–4.

9 Mannius S, Mellström D, Oden A, Rundgren Å, Zetterberg C. Incidence of hip fracture in Western Sweden 1974–1982. Comparison of rural and urban populations. *Acta Orthop Scand* 1987;**58**:38–42.

10 Berg S, Nilsson L, Svanborg A. Behavioural and clinical aspects: longitudinal studies. In: Wattis JP, Hindmarch I, editors. *Psychological assessment of the elderly.* New York: Churchill Livingstone, 1988:47–60.

11 Shock NW, Greulich RC, Andres R, *et al*, editors. *Normal human aging. The Baltimore longitudinal study.* Springfield, VA: NTIS, 1984. (National Institutes of Health Publication No. 84–2450.)

12 Heikkinen E, Arajärvi R-L, Era P, *et al*. Functional capacity of men born in 1906–10, 1926–30 and 1946–50: a basic report. *Scand J Soc Med* 1984;**337**(suppl).

13 Schai KW, Parham IA. Cohort-sequential analyses of adult intellectual development. *Dev Psychol* 1977;**13**:649–53.

14 Berg S. Psychological functioning in 70- and 75-year-old people. A study in an industrialized city. *Acta Psychiatr Scand* 1980;**62**(suppl):288.

15 Steen B. Body composition in 70-year-old males and females in Gothenburg, Sweden. A population study. *Acta Med Scand* 1977;**611**(suppl):87–112.

16 Mellström D, Rundgren Å, Jagenburg R, Steen B, Svanborg A. Tobacco smoking, aging and health among the elderly. A longitudinal population study of 70-year olds and an age cohort comparison. *Age Aging* 1982;**11**:45–58.

17 Aniansson A, Gustafsson E. Physical training in elderly men with special reference to quadriceps muscle strength and morphology. *Clin Psychol* 1981;**1**:87–98.

18 Fiatarone M, Marks EC, Meridith CN, Lipsitz LA, Evans WJ. High intensity strength training in nonagenarians: effects of skeletal muscle [abstract]. *Clin Res* 1989;**37**:330.

19 Grimby G. Physical activity and muscle training in the elderly. *Acta Med Scand* 1986; **711**(suppl):233–7.

20 Skoog I, Nilsson L, Palmertz B, Andreasson L-A, Svanborg A. A population-based study of dementia in 85-year olds. *N Engl J Med* 1993;**328**:153–8.

21 American Medical Association. *White paper on elderly health: report of the Council on Scientific Affairs* [special article]. *Arch Intern Med* 1990;**150**:2459–72.

22 Svanborg A. Blood pressure changes with aging: the search for normality. In: Cuervo CA, Robinson BE, Sheppard HL, editors. *Geriatric hypertension.* University of South Florida, Tampa: International Exchange Center on Gerontology, 1989:5–17.

8 Clinical trials and meta-analysis

NAWAB QIZILBASH

Bradford Hill defined the clinical trial as "a carefully and ethically designed experiment with the aim of answering some precisely framed question".[1] A clinical trial may be more specifically defined as a (randomised) prospective study comparing the effect of intervention(s) against a control in human subjects. Prospective allocation of the individuals to intervention(s) or control groups by a process of randomisation are now considered to be essential ingredients of a modern clinical trial. The randomised trial is the best method for evaluating the efficacy and effectiveness of an intervention—medical treatment, changes in human behaviour, or the delivery of care.

The lack of evidence for many interventions in the elderly is a consequence of considering the elderly to be so different that they should be excluded from trials. Although there are important differences between the elderly and the middle aged with respect to interventions, recent large trials have shown the similarity of relative benefits between the elderly and the middle aged.[2] For trials the similarities between these age groups are likely to be greater than any differences. Thus the elderly should form part of all trials which involve middle aged individuals unless compelling reasons exist to do otherwise. Although the principles of clinical trials in the elderly are the same as in middle aged,[3] the differences will be highlighted in this chapter.

Selection criteria

Defining the study population is an integral part of specifying the primary objectives of the trial. This ensures that the trial patients are identified as "representative" of a future class of person to which the trial findings will be applied. There is a balance to be struck between homogeneity and heterogeneity of the selected individuals. In the quest to find those individuals most likely to benefit from the intervention, entry criteria may be so restrictive that the findings lack general applicability. The major aspects of selection to consider are (a) source of patient recruitment, (b) problem under investigation—disease, impairment, disability, or handicap, and (c) patient exclusion criteria.

67

Inclusion of older people

The principal advantage is generalisability of the results to elderly people, therefore avoiding the potential danger of age discrimination should an intervention prove to be efficacious. It is particularly important to study both older and middle aged people if the intervention turns out to produce different results at different ages.

There are disadvantages of including elderly people in trials. Polypharmacy is common and such ancillary treatments, together with associated multiple pathology, may exclude elderly subjects from being eligible. These problems may also make assessment of trial end points more difficult and add increased variability in patient characteristics, which may mitigate against detecting treatment effects. The greater inability of some older people (for example, very frail residents in institutions) to comply with procedures may result in poor treatment adherence, missing data, and greater attrition due to losses to follow up.

Diagnosis is more difficult in elderly people because the greater biological variability of many physiological and pathological variables, both within and between individuals, makes identification of the problem under investigation more difficult. This also applies to the assessment of disability and handicap. Concomitant drug therapy may alter the variables under investigation, both diagnostic and end points. Multiple conditions make assessment of the problem under investigation more elusive.

Diagnostic criteria therefore need to be validated in elderly people and not simply extrapolated from younger age groups. Possible methods of improving diagnostic criteria are validation in the type of population from which the trial will recruit subjects; use of standard methods where possible; repeat measurement to allow for mismeasurement error; use of more than one observer with quality control checks; and use of panels of two or three independent (blind) observers.

Consent and mental competence

As clinical judgment on treatment by the doctor is suspended in a trial and treatment is allocated at random, consent from the patient is required. Ideally this consent should be fully informed and written. As few patients can be expected to understand fully all the complex issues related to a trial, an ethics committee must act on behalf of the patient. It assumes responsibility for examining the objectives, the study design, the procedures, the expertise of the investigators, and any other points deemed to be of importance in protecting the patient.

A guiding ethical (and useful practical) principle of trials is that the design of trials should in general be governed by the "uncertainty principle".[4] Patients can only be enrolled if the responsible doctor is substantially uncertain as to which of the interventions would be most appropriate for the particular patient. Likewise, patients should not remain on their allocated intervention if the responsible doctor and/or patient become reasonably certain that to do so would be inappropriate.

Unfortunately many frail elderly patients have sufficient impairment of their mental faculties that consent (if obtained) can in no way be considered to be informed. In such cases the investigator should seek the consent of a third party, such as a relative, guardian, or friend.[5] It is this proxy who should weigh the benefits and risks of the intervention and decide whether the patient should be entered into the trial. If the proxy and patient had discussed participation in research in a general or specific way while the patient was still mentally competent, the proxy's task may be simple. More often the proxy must decide without the benefit of knowledge of the patient's wishes. The relevant issues are the definition and determination of mental competence, selection of an appropriate proxy, instructions to be given to the proxy, and the degree of ethical and legal oversight needed. The legality of proxy consent, should harm arise as a direct result of involvement in a trial, is not clear and varies from country to country.[6]

If no proxy is available most trialists would not enrol such a patient into a trial. The degree of concern also depends on the type, duration, risks, and benefits of the intervention. If the treatment is not new but well established for another disease, with a well documented side effect profile, the risk–benefit assessment becomes easier for doctor and proxy. If a treatment has greater potential risk, rigorous monitoring of toxicity and side effects is a particular ethical imperative. Doctors also have the responsibility to withdraw patients from trials if they consider that patients do not wish to proceed with the trial, although this may be difficult to identify.

Stratification

Stratification at randomisation by variables can be seen as an insurance policy in the unlikely event that there is a major imbalance in patient characteristics between the intervention groups. Stratification therefore becomes less relevant if the trial is very large and there is proper randomisation, if there is uncertainty about which patient characteristics may influence the response to treatment, and if the relevant information cannot be easily or reliably obtained.

Variables that are likely to have an important impact on outcome (prognostic variables) should be considered for stratification. All trials, irrespective of size, should stratify by age and sex. Additional variables to consider are place of residence, comorbidity, disability, handicap, and level of care and social support in trials involving elderly people. In general, however, the procedure adds little to the effective power of a trial, while increasing its complexity. If the units to be randomised are groups (for example, institutions, general practices, or villages) rather than individuals, stratification may be easy to perform as the relevant information may be easily obtained. Institutions may be considered as another important stratifying variable, especially in trials with old people.

Randomisation

The process of random allocation assigns individuals (or groups of individuals) to the intervention groups purely by the play of chance and removes the conscious or subconscious bias of the investigator. Its advantage lies not in producing study groups comparable for known prognostic factors but in producing study groups comparable for unknown prognostic factors. Several methods are available for randomly allocating individuals to the intervention groups.

Simple randomisation is equivalent to repeated tossing of an unbiased coin but in small trials, commonly carried out in health services research involving elderly people, serious imbalances between intervention and control groups may arise. A method that solves this problem is block randomisation, which ensures that there will be equal numbers of treated and control subjects at predetermined points in the sequence of randomisation. Alternatively a "biased coin" method may be used, which gives a higher probability of assignment of each participant to the group with the least number of subjects. Minimisation techniques assign individuals to intervention and control groups in a fashion that will tend to correct any existing imbalance or cause the least imbalance in prespecified prognostic factors. This requires continual monitoring of group assignments by these prognostic factors.

The timing of randomisation is important if it is likely that losses may result before intervention starts. In trials of treatment for acute medical problems in elderly people who have a high case fatality rate, for example, randomisation in the emergency department with treatment administered on another ward might be associated with a high death rate before the start of treatment, which might seriously imbalance intervention and control groups. Ideally randomisation should be as close as possible to the introduction of the interventions.

Interventions

Polypharmacy—Trials involving older people frequently involve the assessment of complex interventions, for example, physical exercise and rehabilitation programmes rather than simple drug treatments. The appraisal of complex interventions is made even more difficult by potential interactions between concomitant drug therapy, which may be given to the intervention group more often than to the control group because the former are receiving greater attention. Even in simple drug treatment trials, polypharmacy may lead to problems because of interactions with

70

intervention medication and adverse side effects. Problems with side effects may result in higher than expected proportions of older participants leaving and rejoining trials, which makes analysis difficult. Starting new medication may even result in post-randomisation exclusion as a consequence of fulfilment of an exclusion criterion.

Co-morbidity is common in elderly people and if it occurs during a trial may pose problems by confounding the relationship between treatment and outcome, fulfilling an exclusion criteria and requiring withdrawal, causing interactions with the intervention, and reducing ability to comply with trial procedures. Standardising treatments (especially complex interventions and delivery of health services) may be made more difficult by the presence of other conditions.

Compliance—Poor compliance results in underestimation of the size of a treatment effect. If the degree of compliance can be measured, inferences can be made about the size of the true treatment effect. Comorbidity and adverse social support may reduce the ability of individuals to adhere to procedures. Measures of compliance are therefore particularly important in trials involving elderly people.

Methods of improving drug compliance include excluding non-compliers in the "run in" period before randomisation, adequate explanation, including explanatory pamphlets, reinforcement at each visit of the need for compliance, enlisting the help of relatives or main carers, legible and large labelling, and decreasing the interval between visits. Drug compliance may be assessed by pill counts and measurement of variables influenced by therapy (for example, blood pressure, cholesterol level).

Comparability of intervention and control groups

If a trial has reliable random allocation of individuals and is large, the intervention(s) and control groups should be comparable for age, sex, disease severity, living alone, disability, comorbidity, handicap, level of care, and so on. If a trial is small, there is a greater chance that comparability may be poor. It is not possible to show that the intervention group is identical to the control group but that baseline characteristics differ by no more than chance. At the $p = 0.05$ level of significance 5% of the comparisons would be expected to show "significant" differences by the play of chance alone. If imbalances appear, the data need to be examined to discover a possible cause, for example, by examining study centres or institutions in multicentre trials. If there is imbalance in a key prognostic factor (for example, disease severity), stratification by this factor can be carried out in the analysis of treatment effects.

Variables for comparison should be selected to describe the type of patient in the trial, as an aid to generalisability of the findings to typical

71

patient groups (for example, age range, sex, socioeconomic status, disease severity), and to demonstrate comparability in outcome measures used (for example, level of disability). The measures should be kept to a minimum to avoid too many chance significant differences.

Follow up procedures

Participants in trials are followed up not simply to count trial end points. Other reasons for careful monitoring of progress are to check compliance to the protocol procedures, treatment compliance, reasons for drop out; identify adverse effects of treatment; and maintain interest, morale, and enthusiasm in staff and subjects. The frequency of follow up depends on such factors as provision of adequate care, expected compliance with treatment, degree of inconvenience to patients, and the resources required.

The duration of the study is influenced by two major factors: the latency of effect predicted from a pathophysiological understanding of how treatment works; and the number of end points required to demonstrate benefit or harm and exclude a given size of benefit in the case of a negative (null) trial.

Whether the follow up procedures are carried out by clinic visits, home visits, postal questionnaires, or telephone will vary according to the trial requirements, local circumstances (such as distance from trial centre, availability of transport, etc), and resources. When postal questionnaires and telephone follow up are used they should be validated by comparison with more accurate methods of obtaining data (for example, face to face interviews) before use in the trial setting.

End points

The main criteria indicating response should be listed in relative importance and the one primary measure of response should be selected. This is often difficult in trials of services where treatment may affect a wide range of patient (and carer) characteristics. In general the appropriate end point is determined by an understanding of the mechanisms by which treatment is supposed to work—for example, a trial of the effects of growth hormone on the muscle strength of frail elderly people would examine muscle strength as its primary end point. It would be hoped that improvements in muscle strength would result in faster walking speed, less postural sway, fewer falls, and improved quality of life but all of these other end points should be considered secondary to the primary goal of therapy.

Having decided on the primary end point, independent secondary measures of response should then be chosen. In preliminary trials short term effects, such as toxicity, and side effects are of great importance. Secondary end points should include subject orientated assessment, such as quality of life and disability, especially in elderly people.

72

The numbers of end points required to detect reliably clinically important differences should be calculated in the planning stage. This should be seen to provide a "ball park" figure so that the feasibility of the trial can be assessed. The basic methods used to calculate trial size are given in most standard statistics textbooks. It is always sensible to consult a statistician at the outset of designing a trial. The information required from the clinician by a statistician is the likely frequency of end points (or its mean and standard deviation for continuous variables) in the control group and the clinically important difference to be detected. The former information can often be obtained from published data or from observations carried out routinely. The clinically important difference is much more difficult to determine, depending on clinical judgement and the size of the problem, but has a disproportionate effect on the final sample size arrived at by calculation. Sample size calculations are further complicated by the following: randomisation ratio between intervention groups and control; the variability of the response differs between intervention groups; end point is an ordinal or continuous variable; the response is "time to end point". Increased precision and accuracy of end point measurements result in less random error and will therefore reduce sample size requirements.

Objectivity in end point measurement is important but it is essential to be aware of the possibility of measurement bias. This may be due to an awareness of the type of treatment received on the part of participant or observer. Some of the end points used in trials involving elderly people are particularly prone to measurement bias; assessment of disability, handicap, and level of social support are commonly carried out but may be biased by knowledge of allocation to intervention or control groups. Blinding of observers and participants (so called double blind allocation) is the best means of avoiding measurement bias but can be difficult to maintain in many therapies, particularly those involving complex interventions or overall services. As a minimum standard, attempts should be made to ensure that the observer and therapist (or doctor) are not the same person. Where mortality is the principal end point, blindness is less important but allocation of deaths to specific causes may obviously be biased if done with knowledge of treatment or control status.

Adverse effects—For any intervention, information on safety as well as efficacy is needed. Where side effects are well known, this is straightforward, but it is more difficult with new interventions. It is sensible to make systematic inquiry about known side effects among both intervention and control subjects and also to use open ended questions to identify any unexpected adverse effects experienced. A generic "quality of life" indicator may prove useful in detecting such unexpected effects because a very wide range of domains are covered in an efficient way. Attributing adverse effects to the intervention is most easily done in double blind trials because unbiased estimates of adverse effects experienced by individuals on both

73

active treatment and placebo are obtained. Multiple pathology and polypharmacy in the elderly will increase the range and frequency of adverse effects experienced by both the placebo and intervention groups.

Analysis

All eligible individuals irrespective of compliance with the protocol should be included in the analysis according to the group to which they were randomised. This type of analysis is called an "intention to treat" analysis and is the standard and preferred method. It avoids biased assessment, which can occur when randomised individuals are excluded—for example, those lost to follow up or those who drop out. Often the bias involved in excluding such subjects is of unknown magnitude and direction. The "explanatory approach" confines analysis to only those who complied with the protocol and therefore does not reflect real life situations. Both types of analysis have their place: the former reflects an assessment of the effects of adopting a treatment policy as described by the protocol; the latter gives an assessment of effects of treatment if applied ideally—but may be seriously biased by non-random drop outs.

Lack of compliance with the trial protocol may arise from the following: ineligible individuals being randomised; non-compliance with the intervention; "drop in"—in that the other intervention is adopted in addition to or instead of that originally assigned to the individual; poor quality or missing data. In long term trials individuals may be lost to follow up, although survival status and cause specific mortality may be traced through central registries if the individual has not left the country. If losses to follow up are different in intervention and control groups, bias may be introduced; however, even if losses to follow up are the same in each group there may still be bias if the individuals lost in each group have different prognoses and eventual outcomes. Losses to follow up should therefore be kept to a minimum by high quality trial design and staff training.

Survival analysis methods that involve time from commencement of the intervention to response (for example, achieving independence, death) can use the experience of individuals up to the time of loss to follow up.

Competing events ("non-trial" end point events) are especially common in the elderly and may preclude the assessment of the primary response variable. It is necessary to decide in advance how they will be dealt with as some may require withdrawal from the trial, others may not. They should be foreseen and allowed for in the sample size calculations. They tend to dilute the power of the trial.

Continuous variable end points are a particular problem in trials where substantial losses occur, because the subject is not available to provide an end point and a biased assessment of treatment effects may result from considering only those remaining in the trial. In essence only explanatory analysis may be feasible. Continuous variable end points may be examined in several ways: mean of all scores after starting treatment; mean of last few scores; difference from baseline; difference from baseline in intervention group minus difference from baseline in control group (a net change); and time to minimum/maximum score. Essentially, a simple summary measure of each individual's outcome is required so that only one significance test is necessary.

Subgroup analysis—Subgroup analysis is conducted to answer the question, "for which categories of patient is this treatment helpful?" Unfortunately clinical trials are rarely large enough to be able to provide a reliable demonstration that treatment works in some subgroups but not in others. The one exception to this rule is that low absolute risk may indicate low absolute benefit. This condition will rarely apply to the elderly, who are usually at high absolute risk. In general, therefore, subgroup analyses should be viewed with scepticism; only a priori hypotheses should be examined and post hoc hypotheses posed after examining the data can be considered as hypothesis-generating only and subject to testing in subsequent trials.

Age is such an important variable that analyses of clinical trials are often stratified by age. The "elderly" are a heterogeneous group: people over 85 are very different biologically from people aged between 65 and 74. Hence subgroup analysis by age should band the over 65 age group into 65–74, 75–84, 84–94, and 95+ where possible.

Negative (null) trials

The interpretation of a negative (or null) trial is not as straightforward as is often assumed. The term $p<0.05$ does not mean that the null hypothesis is false. It simply means that if there really is no difference between treatment and control groups, and the trial were to be repeated a large number of times with similar subjects, a difference of the size detected would be found on average 5% of the time. If $p>0.05$ in a trial, this supports the null hypothesis of no difference but it is also possible for a real difference to be missed in an individual trial. A lack of a statistically significant difference does not necessarily mean that there is no real difference between the intervention and control groups. Small trials may be unable to detect real differences that are of clinical importance between treatment and control groups. Appraisal of clinical importance is a subjective matter and requires examination of the confidence intervals of the difference observed to see whether the trial could exclude a clinically useful difference with any certainty; for example, in some very common diseases, such as myocardial infarction, the clinically useful difference may be as small as a 5% reduction in mortality because even such a small treatment effect would produce very useful benefits to the population as a whole. In other circumstances only very large treatment effects are of interest and a small trial may be sufficient to exclude a large treatment effect.

Meta-analysis

Meta-analyses (overviews) use formal statistical techniques to pool or combine the results from all relevant randomised trials.[7] This is now seen as one method of dealing with the detection of clinically small but important treatment effects. As it is seldom possible to mount a single trial sufficiently large to prove whether a treatment is beneficial in a wide range of patients, in different settings, and at different times and places, pooling the results of several smaller trials may be helpful.

Trials using similar interventions in similar groups of patients or diseases and with common end points should be pooled. It is essential to avoid the trap of pooling a series of dissimilar trials or trials of poor quality. Such an approach may result in a seriously spurious result. In general the analysis uses previously published data but often attempts are made to obtain extra unpublished data from original investigators to supplement the published reports. The most common failing of published reports is failure to carry out an intention to treat analysis.

Meta-analysis does not compare individuals in one trial with individuals in another trial but rather examines the effects of each trial and then pools the results of these differences between trials and their variances. This is generally done using the odds ratio together with confidence intervals and significance tests. An odds ratio of 1 implies that bad and good outcomes occur equally often in treatment and control groups. An odds ratio of less than 1 usually indicates that good outcomes predominate and that treatment is beneficial. An odds ratio of greater than 1 indicates that bad outcomes predominate and that treatment is harmful. Again interpretation of null meta-analyses must involve examination of the confidence intervals to determine what size of difference has been excluded.

Several examples of meta-analysis in the field of geriatric medicine have recently been published. The overviews of stroke units[8] and comprehensive geriatric assessment[9] illustrate some of the problems of combining trials where the intervention varied between trials and the outcome considered was not always the most appropriate; however, since individual trials in these areas were all extremely small and unable to rule out clinically important differences, meta-analysis has proved a valuable step forward in aiding decision making. The same is true in other areas of drug therapy[10] where small to moderate effects are important.

Disadvantages of meta-analysis[11] are the heterogeneity of trials due to differences in design and study populations, assuming that point estimates of efficacy apply to all patients, and selection of trials that may bias the findings—for example, only those published in the English language or exclusion of unpublished trials which tend to be negative.

The problem of making decisions on the basis of a meta-analysis of several small trials is a major concern,[12] particularly in evaluation of health service interventions for elderly people where trials tend to be small. As more and more meta-analyses of the same treatments are conducted it is likely that the play of chance will result in some contradictory results, in the same way that an individual trial may yield a false negative or false positive result. Very large multicentre trials using a standard protocol are a useful safeguard against the possibilities of publication bias, selective identification of positive trials, and inadequate handling of event data (especially losses to follow up); however, in many areas of medicine, particularly given the costs and logistic difficulties of mounting large trials of health service interventions, meta-analyses are likely to remain the best means of reducing clinical uncertainty. Further methodological work is required to improve their conduct and better understand their limitations.

1 Bradford Hill A. The clinical trial. *Br Med Bull* 1951;7:278–82.
2 ISIS-2 (Second International Study of Infarct Survival) Collaborative Group. Randomised trial of intravenous streptokinase, oral aspirin, both or neither among 17 187 cases of suspected acute myocardial infarction: ISIS-2. *Lancet* 1988;ii:349–60.
3 Pocock SJ. *Clinical trials: a practical approach.* Chichester: Wiley, 1983.
4 Collins R, Doll R, Peto R. Ethics of clinical trials. In: Williams CJ, editor. *Introducing new treatments for cancer: practical, ethical and legal problems.* London: Wiley, 1992:49–65.
5 Warren JW, Sobal J, Tenney JH, *et al.* Informed consent by proxy. An issue in research with elderly patients. *N Engl J Med* 1986;315:1124–8.
6 High DM. Research with Alzheimer's disease subjects: informed consent and proxy decision making. *J Am Geriatr Soc* 1992;40:950–7.
7 Dickersin K, Berlin JA. Meta-analysis: state-of-the-science. *Epidemiol Rev* 1992;14:154–76.
8 Langhorne P, Williams BO, Gilchrist W, Howie K. Do stroke units save lives? *Lancet* 1993;342:395–8.
9 Stuck AE, Siu AL, Wieland GD, Adams J, Rubenstein LZ. Comprehensive geriatric assessment: a meta-analysis of controlled trials. *Lancet* 1993;342:1032–6.
10 Peto R, Collins R, Gray R. Large-scale randomized evidence: large, simple trials and overviews of trials. *Proc N Y Acad Sci* 1993;703:314–40.
11 Thompson SG, Pocock SJ. Can meta-analyses be trusted? *Lancet* 1991;338:1127–30.
12 Eggar M, Davey Smith G. Misleading meta-analysis. *BMJ* 1995;310:752–4.

9 Health economics

SHELLEY FARRAR, CAM DONALDSON

The aim of this chapter is to provide an introduction to the use of economics in the evaluation of health services for elderly people. In the following section, the basic concepts of economics and their relevance to the health care sector are introduced. The reader is given examples of the application of economic evaluation to care of elderly people. This section identifies some of the issues which have been raised under the heading of "economics and old age" and the following sections discuss each of these in more detail. The issues are whether the growing elderly population represent an increasing burden, whether the application of health economics techniques discriminate against elderly people, and to ensure that evaluations are undertaken from an appropriate perspective, that is, that of society.

Introduction to economics

The underlying premise of economics is that resources are scarce. As a result of this scarcity, decisions have to be made regarding the best use of resources. Thus health economics is about how health care resources are used to produce the greatest benefit to the community.

More formally, the crucial underlying concept of economics is *opportunity cost*. In order to undertake an activity we use resources. The opportunity cost is the benefit that would have been obtained from those resources if they had been used in a different way. This concept of cost can be seen to fit the health care sector very neatly. When we are concerned about the costs of a service it is not parsimony that feeds our interest but the health benefits that could be gained by using those resources in a different way. If health care resources can be reallocated in some way to produce greater overall gain then, other things being equal, some change should be made. Thus health economics, in combination with other disciplines, is concerned with identifying the costs and benefits of possible changes and helping decision makers to weigh whether and what changes should take place. By providing information on *who* accrues the benefits and incurs the costs of resource allocation decisions, health economics is also concerned with equity of health care services. It is only by estimating the costs and benefits of proposed changes of action that decisions can be made to produce an equitable and efficient use of resources.

78

There are a number of studies that have done this, though a comprehensive knowledge of the costs and benefits of different types of care for elderly people is some way off. Much work has, however, been done on the costs of institutional continuing care[1-3] but we have limited evidence on how dependency effects costs within an institution. There is a small body of detailed work published on the costs of community care packages that identifies how costs vary with client characteristics.[4-6] Other studies have looked at the "balance of care" between community and institutional care to help plan a more efficient service.[7]

The costs and benefits of health services can be viewed at two different levels. The first is the macro level. Here the issue which draws the most attention is the total cost of the care of elderly people. Is the ageing population a growing burden that can be afforded? There are two issues within this. Firstly, is an ageing population going to constitute a growing economic burden? Secondly, what do we mean by the "affordability" of health care? We will turn to the economic contribution to these issues in the next section of the chapter.

The second level at which we can examine health care services for elderly people is from a micro perspective. Here we are concerned specifically with the costs and benefits of different ways of caring for elderly people and, therefore, ensuring that we do the best with available resources. This leads to three further issues of importance. The first is whether the outcome measures used in economic evaluations are appropriate and relevant to this sector. Secondly, how to deal with costs and benefits occurring at different points in time; that is, should costs and benefits of health care interventions be discounted? The third issue is how the perspective taken affects the results of the evaluation and why this presents particular problems for care of the elderly. These will be addressed in the following sections.

Caring for elderly people: a growing burden?

There is often much interest in the total cost of a particular group of people to society or a particular kind of disease to the public health services.[8,9] Services for elderly people have been no exception.[10,11] The concerns here have been the trend in the costs of caring for elderly people and whether these are "affordable".

There is a view that the costs of health care will rise at an increasing rate because of the demographic changes (see chapter 4 for a detailed account) that are taking place in both developed and developing countries. The idea is that elderly people consume more health care resources per capita than young people and therefore as they increase in number they will place a growing burden on the health care system. Despite the apparent simplicity of this argument, there has been much debate in the area. Much of the counterargument stems from the theory of "morbidity compression", whereby morbidity will be concentrated into the very later years of life, making up a smaller proportion of length of life[12] (see chapter 5 for a full discussion).

The notion of the health care of elderly people representing a growing burden is supported by evidence that draws on demographic and health care expenditure patterns. Firstly, an association between a high proportion of elderly people and high health care expenditure across countries has been identified and, secondly, a trend of increasing health care expenditures concurrent with expanding elderly populations has been noted[13 14]; however, more robust empirical evidence has found the link between population ageing and health care expenditure to be weak. Getzen in his examination of countries of the Organisation for Economic Cooperation and Development has shown that, once he controlled for other factors such as gross national product (or national income), the correlation between elderly people as a proportion of the population and health care expenditures disappears.[13] In addition, in defence of the compression of morbidity school of thought, Defever, in her European review, notes that, although elderly people consume a higher proportion of health care resources, within a predicted 5% net annual increase in health care expenditures between 1990 and 2015 only 0·3–0·8% is estimated to be attributable to elderly people.[14]

With regard to the question of whether growing health care expenditures are affordable, it is useful to approach this from an economics perspective. When we ask if something is affordable we are asking what has to be given up as a result and whether we want to give the alternative up. So when we ask whether something is affordable, we really mean: is the opportunity cost too high? That is, are we willing to reallocate resources within the health care sector to meet the growing demand? If not, are we willing to take funds from another sector to meet the growing demand? In his study of health care expenditures, Getzen's analysis suggests that an ageing population may affect the allocation of health care resources but not the overall level of expenditure, adding further credence to the suggestion that affordability is a question of willingness to redistribute resources.[13] The reallocation of resources (from other public expenditure budgets or from increases in taxation) should be a policy decision reflecting society's values.

Economic evaluation: a discriminatory practice?

It has been suggested that using economic analysis to evaluate health care services for elderly people discriminates against that group because of the types of outcome measures used and the way in which those outcomes are treated when they occur in the future.

Economic evaluations can use various types of outcome measures, some of which include a dimension of time. For instance, life years saved and days free of pain, measures used in cost effectiveness analysis, assess the outcome of an intervention or programme solely in very simple terms. The use of measures such as life years saved has been criticised as discriminatory against elderly people.[15] The quality adjusted life year (QALY) adds a quality of life dimension to the number of years of life gained but is still open to the same criticism.

Measures that include time as a dimension will tend to register fewer benefits for elderly people than younger people because of the shorter life expectancy of the former. It does appear that if we take into account the costs and benefits of different interventions there will be a systematic bias because the benefits accrued by elderly people are unlikely to continue for as long as those incurred by younger people; however, this is fact, it is not discriminatory. Indeed to ignore this difference in outcomes may be discriminatory *in favour* of elderly people; however, such positive discrimination towards elderly people, that is, for special priority to be given to care of the aged, could well be what people want from their health service. Indeed the publication of policy documents such as SHARPEN[16] suggest that such explicit discrimination in favour of care of elderly people is favoured by the government.

There is even some tentative evidence to show that the assumption about one QALY being of equal value to everyone is erroneous. It has been suggested, on the basis of survey work, that there may be some support amongst the population for discriminating in the distribution of marginal QALY gains in favour of the young, an idea which gained support even from the elderly members of the sample.[17] Of the 10 stages of life at which respondents thought it important to be well which were asked about in this survey, the two stages above (or around) the age of 65 ("just having retired" and "getting very old") were, however, ranked third and fourth in terms of importance.

The second criticism is levelled at the use of generic outcome measures such as the QALY in economic evaluation. The objectives of health care programmes for elderly people are often different from those for other patient groups. Many of the programmes for elderly people are based on care rather than cure.

Health outcome measures such as the QALY are geared more towards outcomes of acute care. It is argued that, consequently, they do not pick up the benefits which are accrued from many health care programmes for elderly people. Donaldson *et al*[18] used the QALY alongside the Modified Crichton Royal Behavioural Rating Scale (CRBRS) and the Life Satisfaction Index (LSI) to measure the change in health status of a group of elderly people in long term care over 15 months. They found the CRBRS and LSI to be more sensitive to changes in distress and general wellbeing than the QALY and suggest that this could be the case for other services for elderly people that have a care rather than cure emphasis.

Using QALY measures to set priorities could therefore put services for elderly people lower down on a priority setting list than they should be. Nevertheless, QALY league tables (though these should be interpreted with a great deal of caution, see Gerard[19]) have ranked hip replacements and chiropody highly.

Thirdly, discounting has been criticised as discriminating against elderly people because it puts a lower weight on future benefits than on present ones.[15] There seems to be an assumption that, because people are going to be older in the future, "old" life years are discounted and therefore discriminated against. However, it is *when* an event occurs *not who* incurs it that determines the extent of discounting. Old years now are equal to young years now and old years in the future are equal to young years in the future.

Who cares?

Care of elderly people is undertaken by a range of agencies and individuals; as such, the financial responsibility is often shared and varies across individual patients and clients. This division and diversity of responsibility makes the issue of what is the appropriate *perspective* to take when evaluating a service particularly pertinent for the case of services for elderly people.

When an economic evaluation is carried out it is normal for the costs and benefits to be looked at from a particular perspective. Table 9.1 shows how the perspective that is taken may affect the costs and benefits included in the evaluation. If we take a societal perspective then all the costs and benefits of the given service will be taken into account. When the costs and benefits are viewed from the perspective of an individual organisation within society the catchment area for costs and benefits may be narrowed. In the United Kingdom, for instance, a health authority or board will have sole responsibility for accident and emergency costs, some responsibility for inpatient referral, primary care, and outpatient costs, but generally no responsibility for social services, patient, and carer costs. Although each organisation might have concerns about other costs, there is little incentive to include the costs incurred by other agencies when evaluating different ways of providing a service. The most immediate and visible effect of this could be cost shifting between agencies whereby, by changing the pattern of a person's care, an agency can reduce its financial contribution to that care. The more serious long term problem could be the inefficient use of resources.

The way to ensure that society's resources are used efficiently would be to include costs and benefits incurred by all the organisations and individuals; however, the demarcation of budgets discourages this approach. A study undertaken in Ireland shows how the perspective taken can affect the results of an evaluation study. O'Shea and Corcoran[20] measured the costs of placing elderly people in domiciliary care and institutional care settings. By using an opportunity cost approach, the authors showed the *societal* cost of caring for the elderly to be similar in the two settings: £Ir222·25 (1987 prices) a week in domiciliary care and £Ir227·67 in institutional care. If, however, they had chosen to look at the costs from the perspective

Table 9.1   Financial responsibility and organisations

Perspective	Financial responsibility					
	Inpatient	Primary care	A & E	Outpatient	Social services	Patient/carer
Society	Yes	Yes	Yes	Yes	Yes	Yes
Public sector	Yes	Yes	Yes	Yes	Yes	No
NHS	Yes	Yes	Yes	Yes	No	No
Health board/ authority	Part	Part	Yes	Part	No	No
GP fundholder	Part	Yes	No	Part	No	No
Social work department	No	No	No	No	Yes	No

GP, general practitioner; A & E, accident and emergency department.

of the NHS, the difference would have been dramatic, with home care costed at £Ir32·90. Donaldson and Gregson[21] have produced findings with similar implications. Although the cost of implementing a family support unit for elderly people with dementia was similar to the cost of a service package without such a unit, the cost to social services of funding the service was greater than the savings made by that particular agency. The important message here is that an option which looks more cost effective from one perspective—for example, from that of the health service—when viewed from a broader perspective, taking into account local authority and carer costs, may look less attractive. Overall, for resources to be used to best effect in caring for elderly people, the broader perspective is the correct one to take.

Conclusion

Economics is useful in setting out who gains and who loses by investing and disinvesting in various types of care for elderly people. There are also techniques that permit estimation of the magnitude of such gains and losses, although these are not perfect. In examining specific issues it has been shown that a growing elderly population does not necessarily represent a growing resource burden on society, that economics methods of evaluation are not necessarily discriminating, and that it is important to devise structures (or legislation) that avoid perverse incentives resulting in inefficient use of resources.

The health economics research unit is funded by the chief scientist's office of the Scottish Home and Health Department (SOHHD). However, the views expressed in this paper are those of the authors, not SOHHD.

1 Wright KG, Cairns J, Snell M. *Costing Care*. Sheffield: University of Sheffield, 1982. (Social services monographs: research in practice.)
2 Wright KG. Long-term care for the elderly: public versus private. *Public Money* 1985;5: 52–4.

3 Donaldson C, Bond J. Cost of continuing-care facilities in the evaluation of experimental NHS nursing homes. *Age Ageing* 1991;**29**:160–8.
4 Challis D, Davies B. *Case management in community care*. Aldershot: Gower, 1986.
5 Challis D, Chessum R, Chesterman J, *et al*. *Case management in social health care: the Gateshead community care scheme*. Canterbury: Personal Social Services Research Unit, University of Kent, 1990.
6 Challis D, Darton R, Johnson L, *et al*. Evaluation of an alternative to long-stay hospital care for frail elderly patients: cost and effectiveness. *Age Ageing* 1991;**20**:245–54.
7 Mooney GH. Planning for balance of care for the elderly. *J Polit Econ* 1978;**25**:149–64.
8 McMurray J, Hart W, Rhodes G. An evaluation of the cost of heart failure to the National Health Service in the UK. *Br J Med Econ* 1993;**9**:99–110.
9 Lindgren B. *Costs of illness in Sweden 1964–1975*. Lund: Liber, 1981. (Swedish Institute for Health Economics.)
10 Bös D, von Wiezsäcker RK. Economic consequences of population aging. *Eur Econ Rev* 1989;**33**:345–54.
11 Schneider EL, Guralnik JM. The aging of America: impact on health care costs. *JAMA* 1990;**263**:2335–40.
12 Fries J. Aging, natural death and the compression of morbidity. *N Engl J Med* 1980;**303**: 130–6.
13 Getzen TE. Population aging and the growth of health expenditures. *J Gerontol* 1992;**47**: S98–104.
14 Defever M. Long term care: the case of the elderly. *Health Policy* 1991;**19**:1–18.
15 Avorn J. Benefit and cost analysis in geriatric care: turning age discrimination into policy. *N Engl J Med* 1984;**31**:1294–1301.
16 Scottish Home and Health Department. *SHARPEN: Scottish health authorities review of priorities for the eighties and nineties*. London: HMSO, 1988.
17 Williams A. Ethics and efficiency in the provision of health care. In: Bell M, Mendus S, editors. *Philosophy and medical welfare*. Cambridge: Cambridge University Press, 1988: 116–26.
18 Donaldson C, Atkinson A, Bond J, Wright K. QALYs and the long-term care for elderly people in the UK: scales for assessment of quality of life. *Age Ageing* 1988;**17**:379–87.
19 Gerard K. Cost-utility in practice: a policy maker's guide to the state of the art. *Health Policy* 1992;**21**:249–79.
20 O'Shea E, Corcoran R. Balance of care considerations for elderly persons: dependency, placement and opportunity costs. *Appl Econ* 1990;**22**:1167–80.
21 Donaldson S, Gregson B. Prolonging life at home: what is the cost? *Community Med* 1989;**2**:200–9.

10 Evaluation of health services

DAVID J HUNTER

Evaluating health services is complex for two principal reasons: firstly, establishing causal connections between inputs, processes, and outcomes is inherently difficult; and secondly, there is a variety of evaluation approaches, research designs, and methods. Each research methodology has its strengths but also its weaknesses; for example, the controlled experiment can test hypotheses and demonstrate causal relationships between variables but the controlled design makes it difficult to estimate whether the responses of the experimental subjects occur in the same way under natural conditions. A multimethod approach to evaluation therefore has attractions.

For these reasons, while recognised as important, and never more so than at a time when efficiency and effectiveness considerations are to the fore, evaluation causes problems. There remain considerable uncertainties with regard to the state of knowledge about effectiveness in health care and how to evaluate effectiveness.

Evaluating health services draws on two research traditions: the biomedical and the social sciences. Both traditions are valid, have different strengths and weaknesses, and are complementary. St Leger *et al* define health services evaluation as "the critical assessment, on as objective a basis as possible, of the degree to which entire services or their component parts (e.g. diagnostic tests, caring procedures) fulfil stated goals".[1] The social sciences have much to contribute to an understanding of health services. They often focus on organisational and sociocultural issues relating to health; for example, the shift in current British health policy of resources and people from hospital to primary care and community based provision needs to be assessed in order to identify optimal service configurations and to ascertain whether such a shift does in fact lead to improvement in health service practice and quality of life of users and providers of that service.

An important issue in evaluative research aimed at identifying the congruence or dissonance between stated goals and what actually happens in practice is that multiple perspectives exist among different groups within a service or organisation as to what constitutes success. Smith and Cantley refer to the importance of pluralistic evaluation as a method aimed at capturing these different notions and perceptions.[2] Such multiple perspectives are all part of the complexity with which evaluative research seeks to come to terms.

The points noted above are all evident to some degree in services for older people and their evaluation. By definition, the needs of older people are inescapably multiple and complex and require investigation from a diverse range of service inputs embracing primary health care, secondary care, and community care. Evaluating health services for older people therefore poses a number of challenges. It is important that these are acknowledged and confronted by both the research community and the users of research.

Evaluating health services for older people is necessary because the costs of an elderly population stem in part from its need for, and demand on, health and social services. These costs are higher in older age. Also to be considered are the costs to carers. Advancing age above 50 years results in a striking increase in admission rates to a range of specialties. Patients' lengths of stay for admission also increase with advancing years, as do consultations with general practitioners. Contact with a wide range of health and social services, notably doctors, district nurses, and home helps, increases with age.

A factor pervading services for older people is the negative stereotyping of old age, which is far from absent in our society. The NHS changes pose particular dangers if elderly people are denied services and treatments on grounds of age. Fiscal pressures can all too easily lead to such discrimination, especially given increasing health and increasing health resource consumption among elderly people.

Structure, process, and outcome

There are three different aspects to understanding the organisation and delivery of services: structure, process, and outcome.[3] Distinguishing between these is important. The *structure* of services is fairly self evident and comprises the distribution, qualifications, and organisation of personnel providing a service, their location, and so on. The *process* aspect of health services is how things are organised and done, and also the manner in which activities and personnel interact. Donabedian's definition of process includes a range of other factors, notably the accessibility of care and the behaviour of health care staff towards the individual. *Outcome* is concerned with the impact of health services on individuals and on communities. The concern is over what outputs one can obtain for a given set of inputs and with how these affect outcomes.

It is conceptually important to distinguish between inputs, outputs, and outcomes, although imprecision surrounds the application of these terms. In particular, the distinction between outputs and outcomes is sometimes blurred. Inputs refer to the raw materials used in the provision of care, that is, manpower, capital, and consumables like drugs, fuel, food, and so on. The output of services refers to the large variety of activities that take place through the use of all the different resources available in the system. Outcomes refer to the extent to which the input of resources and the output of services contribute to the maximisation of an individual's health and wellbeing. The measurement of outcomes presents considerable problems, both conceptual and methodological.

Donabedian's structure, process, and outcome typology corresponds closely with the input–output economic model but has the strength of directing attention to the range of processes by which inputs are translated into outputs and outcomes. Much of what happens by way of outputs and even outcomes is a consequence of the processes of care, which entail a series of sometimes imperceptible interactions between professional groups and their standard operating procedures. Processes do not necessarily result from standard professional practice, which may be codified in guidelines, standards, or protocols. They flow from a myriad of inputs and influences—literature, research results, conversations, meetings, interventions—all of which combine or converge to form a policy, which, if widely accepted, becomes standard practice.

Because of the complexity of evaluating services, and the growing recognition that evaluation should incorporate perceptions and values other than those of professionals or "experts" alone, there is an emphasis on the need for multiple dimensions of evaluation, reflecting the perceptions of patients and demonstrating a concern not only with the efficacy of treatments and interventions but also with notions of patient satisfaction, equity, and access and the nature and quality of the encounter between professional and patient. The language of markets and consumerism and quality of the care setting and environment are now seen to be important matters for evaluation. A pluralistic model of evaluation adopting Smith and Cantley's approach would seek to capture these differing, but equally valid, conceptions of success in respect of outcomes of care. After all, what constitutes "good care" in the opinion of patients may not equate with efficacy, as defined by professionals. The notion of consumerism is especially pertinent in respect of elderly people.[4] Among the reasons put forward are:

- The emergence of a broader range of lifestyles among older people
- The development of charters of rights, especially in the field of residential care, which has raised issues about the needs of older people as consumers of services
- The pressures facing informal carers, which have only recently been acknowledged by government
- The 1989 community care reforms with their emphasis on consumerism and user empowerment.

Invariably, the link between inputs and outcomes is left as a "black box", which a description of formal structure only partially fills. This is why Donabedian's second stage—process—is so important but also difficult to measure. Process evaluation demands a methodology that is capable of capturing the dynamic aspects of the organisation. This can only be accomplished from the inside by watching and listening and by studying individuals and their interactions, both formal and informal. The problem for qualitative researchers, as we shall see below, is to achieve this informed understanding by means that command the confidence of the policy audience.[5] All too often qualitative research is dismissed as being little more than story telling or anecdotal evidence packaged as legitimate research. Qualitative data are often criticised for being too subjective in contrast to quantitative data, which are held to be more objective and reliable. Such stereotyping is, however, unhelpful and incorrect. All data, however collected, must be produced in a way that provides valid and reliable information.

Types of evaluation

The current health status of the elderly population and changes in health status are largely unknown. According to a Medical Research Council review, the present data sources (general household survey, Office of Population Censuses and Surveys, and so on) are not adequate for monitoring the health of older people.[6] This is a serious knowledge gap because of the implications for health care policy and resource allocation strategies.

A variety of approaches exists to measuring the health status of elderly people—ranging from morbidity to quality of life measures. Of particular importance is the definition of desirable outcomes of health care and the benefits likely to be achieved.

As a result of the exclusion of older people from a range of epidemiology studies and trials of clinical interventions, there is a dearth of information regarding the incidence, prevalence, and determinants of disease in elderly people and the effects of intervention treatments. Any study of the effectiveness of care for elderly people should be accompanied by an examination of the costs and benefits to inform service delivery and resource allocation.

Clinical trials are seen as essential. There are two broad groups of trials of treatment: the evaluation of treatment packages as a whole; and trials to identify particular components within packages that are effective. The specific context in each case will determine which approach is more feasible or relevant.

Clinical trials are not, however, the only means of establishing effectiveness of treatments. Observational studies that describe health care delivery are now possible with the increasing availability of computerised health care databases. Such studies are able to examine whether variations are seen in the use of a particular intervention across geographical areas. Observational study designs may be either cross-sectional (and provide a snapshot of one period of time) or may describe changes across time.

Longitudinal observational studies can be of particular value in respect of elderly people where there exists a paucity of data; for instance, it is possible to assess the effectiveness of particular interventions among older people and to ascertain the extent to which the diffusion of such interventions is equitable across regions.

In respect of the effectiveness of health care interventions and the age factor, further research is required. Alternative treatments and prevention strategies need to be assessed for their effectiveness. The organisation of care is another area where evaluative research is required to assess the different models of care. In particular, the health and social care interface is of major concern, a matter to which we return below.

The two principal types of evaluation research were referred to earlier: scientific field research and social science research. The scientific aims of evaluation in field settings are alien to the exponents of randomised controlled trials. They are similarly concerned with proof, evidence, reliability, validity, and so on, but in practice they have to adapt to imposed conditions. Evaluation then becomes a methodology for providing the best approximations to the otherwise unknowable relationships between cause and effect, or between input and output. In this endeavour, social science research can make a contribution through analysis of objectives, processes, and outcomes.

Within social science research there are two approaches: the instrumental/ technocratic approach, which is the dominant paradigm in evaluation studies, with its clear assumption of objectives being rationally pursued; and the interpretive approach, which is concerned with subjectivity and the political processes involved in evaluations.

Methods

As mentioned, there are many research designs available. More than one approach may be used in a single study and, indeed, this may be advisable in particular instances. It is, however, rare for such eclecticism to occur in evaluative research. One study investigating the pattern of care for elderly people used a mix of methodologies and techniques, both qualitative and quantitative: interviews, observation, records analyses, and surveys[7]; but the most commonly used methods in health services research are: the experimental approach, observational methods with quantitative data analysis, and qualitative research methods.[8]

Experimental method

The randomised controlled trial is regarded as the yardstick in evaluative research and has the most credibility in medicine. Careful patient selection and controlled conditions of treatment aim to minimise bias and the influence of confounding variables. The strength of the method rests on its claims to internal validity, achieved by devising statistical control over systematic (bias) error and random (chance) error. The rigorous demands of trial designs can, however, be difficult to achieve.

The randomised controlled trial is of undoubted value in assessing the effectiveness of a drug or any other therapeutic intervention because the necessary controls can be instituted, but even where controls are technically feasible, it is not easy to exclude subtle biases of patient selection, such as that of doctors selectively referring or withholding patients from a trial. Problems with the definition of outcomes can also occur. The most important problem, however, is whether the internally valid results are also externally valid—that is, the extent to which findings can be generalised beyond an experiment to the real world. Can laboratory conditions be created in the social world? Limitations arise from an inability to determine goals, to control input, to measure or evaluate output, or a combination of these.[9] In addition, ethical considerations may prohibit a controlled experiment.

Trials have the virtue of high internal reliability and remain the classic method of research for applying hypothesis testing to the assessment of health care interventions; however, the method has its limitations, as noted above. While the randomised controlled trial is without peer for testing a hypothesis, it has only a restricted application because control of variables is often problematic in complex health care contexts. Hence the attraction of mounting multidisciplinary studies that combine the approaches of the randomised controlled trial and qualitative studies. An example of a study adopting a multimethod design is that by Bond and others, which studied the issue of whether frail elderly people should be cared for in a nursing home or retained in a long stay hospital ward.[10] In addition to the randomised controlled trial, methods involved a case study using participant observation and various surveys of key stakeholders. A multimethodological approach of this type is desirable when addressing the broader questions concerning the *process* of health care delivery.

Observational methods with quantitative data analysis

The aims of these methods may be description, explanation, prediction, or a combination of these. Data may be obtained by questionnaire or from existing records from randomised samples to allow generalisability to a wider population. Studies can include simple fact gathering exercises to international registers that can be used to obtain comparative data on the utilisation of health care and its effects on mortality. It is also possible to follow trends over time.

Surveys are particularly popular for data gathering purposes. They are versatile and practical and can generate both explanations or further hypotheses. Problems with them include the imposition of the researcher's assumptions as a consequence of the processes of categorisation and quantification. Observational studies also lack the control that the experimental approach has over internal validity and sample selection. It becomes more difficult to control for age structure of comparison groups, comorbidity, severity of disease, and similar factors. Observational studies have problems in distinguishing cause and effect relationships from covariation and association of variables. The investigator must also judge which are the important variables, thereby potentially distorting what is actually happening. Surveys, like experiments, cannot by their very nature capture the context of social interaction. To achieve this it is necessary to turn to qualitative research methods.

Qualitative research methods

When it is a case of studying dynamic events or processes involving social interactions between individuals or groups, qualitative methods are necessary. They are particularly valuable in enabling an understanding of how patients and practitioners interpret their experience of health care and the significance that this has for the way in which the health care system functions, and of the cultural, historical, and political circumstances that influence health care.

A variety of methods exist for collecting qualitative data when evaluating services or policies. These include interviews (structured, semistructured, or unstructured), observation (usually non-participant), questionnaires, and the scrutiny and content analysis of relevant documents.

In contrast to other research methods, in qualitative research the precise method emerges with the data as these are collected and sifted. The distinguishing mark of a good qualitative analysis is that it accounts successfully for the way in which individuals interact with their social context. For an account of how older people care and receive (or do not receive) particular services see Hunter et al[7]; for an ethnography of the home help service and elderly clients see McKeganey.[11]

Drawbacks with qualitative research include its cost, its labour intensiveness, and the small samples, which make it difficult to generalise the results of a study. Good qualitative research is often so context specific that it is difficult to teach. It is an art and craft as well as a technical skill. Moreover, the variety of social science theories potentially available to researchers can appear bewildering when compared with the more unified approach of the natural sciences.

There is no single preferred research method for the study of health services for older people. The choice of which of the methods briefly described above is most appropriate is contingent upon the purpose of a particular research study. In seeking to find out which of maybe several medical interventions is most effective, a randomised controlled trial, if it can be achieved, is the best method. If the research question is about trying to find out if a particular policy or service has been implemented and is having the desired impact, qualitative methods will be more appropriate.

Outcomes in old age

A variety of approaches to measuring the health status of elderly people exist, ranging from morbidity to health related quality of life. It is crucially important to the efficacious allocation of resources to know the health status and the impact upon it of different health care services, otherwise policy and resource allocation decisions are driven by inputs in the absence of any appreciation of effectiveness of outcomes.

The critical issue for health services for elderly people is to establish whether the gains in years of life as a consequence of a fall in age specific mortality have led to improved health in old age rather than prolongation of disability and ill health. At present it is not possible to determine whether the health status of elderly people has improved, deteriorated, or remained the same during the past decades of increasing longevity.

Improved quality of life (QOL) is more important than its prolongation in old age. A range of methods has been used to access QOL. These include the psychometric approach to examining people's feelings about life, as expressed in concepts like life satisfaction, decision, or utility analysis, which attempts to assess the valuation of life on the assumption that such value will be revealed in hypothetical choices or trade offs between different states of being.

A drawback with QOL assessment techniques is the absence of a common measure. To address this issue, there is interest in active life expectancy (ALE), that is, the expectation of life without disability. Large scale representative longitudinal studies are needed to provide appropriate ALE measures. None exists in Britain.

The healthy ALE (HALE) expresses the average number of years that a fit person of a specified age can be expected to enjoy before suffering disability and is derived from data on age specific prevalence or incidence rates of desirability. The HALE model has insufficient data at present to make it realisable (see chapter 5).

The quality adjusted life year (QALY) sets out to establish a single index to measure quantity and quality of life. The QALY is a combination of life years gained by health care interventions, or remaining life years if the intervention does not add to life years, and some judgement about the quality of these life years.

While QALYs have attracted considerable interest, their applied use in decision making is limited. There are also considerable problems with the QALY when applied to elderly people.[12 13] They are inherently ageist because they attach the same value to each year of life gained. At older ages this may be too insensitive a measure where the later years may be valued more by older people. QALYs require value judgements to be made and the issue then arises of who is responsible for these and how explicit they will be. QALYs have the effect of lending a spurious "scientific" objectivity to value laden processes.

There is an important distinction to be drawn between HALE and QALYs. HALE is a normative public health measure rooted in epidemiological data. The QALY is an economist's tool to aid decision making by focusing on the marginal consequences of interventions (see chapter 9).

There remains much work to be done to establish effective measures of outcome.

Assessing satisfaction

Issues around consumer satisfaction are uppermost in the minds of health service policy makers since the 1991 NHS reforms. A key aspect of the changes has been to shift the mindset of managers and practitioners from producer led to user driven. The most efficient means of obtaining user views is a customer satisfaction survey. Such surveys are attractive to managers because they are capable of studying large groups of people; however, surveys of this type tend to provide less detailed information that may require ethnographic methods to yield the full picture. Surveys will, for instance, be unlikely to provide explanations of the relationships between beliefs, attitudes, social circumstances, and geographical location. A survey tends to yield broad brush information that can usefully provide a menu of issues requiring closer examination using different techniques.

Rehabilitation and community care

In recent years community care has been advocated for many care groups, including elderly people, who do not require acute care. With the 1991 community care reforms, the emphasis is on needs based planning of services in localities but there are few longitudinal data on the changing needs of elderly populations to allow a proper needs based approach. This is a knowledge gap that must be closed before useful evaluative research can be carried out. The move away from institutionalised care towards enhanced home care is giving rise to a variety of innovative models of service provision and case/care management arrangements that need to be evaluated both for their cost effectiveness and impact on individuals using a combination of the approaches and methods described above.

An area of particular concern and in need of evaluative research is the changing health–social care interface. This includes the boundary between acute and long term care, the precise responsibilities of particular agencies, and the incentives operating in respect of particular modes of care. Methods and criteria of assessment and case/care management are especially important and need to be evaluated for their appropriateness. Developments in joint commissioning between health and local authorities also need evaluating.[14]

Conclusion

In evaluating health services for elderly people or any other care group there is no single "best" way and no single criterion against which a policy or programme may be judged. Rather, this chapter has sought to convey the importance of using a range of methods and designs, where appropriate, and of acknowledging that no single method can provide answers to all research questions. Different methods will yield different data to address certain questions.[15]

Smith and Cantley argue that such a pluralistic approach to evaluative research has a number of advantages:

- It provides a complicated but realistic answer to the question of whether a service is successful or not
- It has the potential to explain why "failures" in service provision occur because the evaluation examines *process* as well as *outcome*
- This explanation opens the way for change
- The approach can facilitate the implementation of research results because it is less likely that stakeholders will argue that their interests have not been taken into account.

This last point is most important. Evaluation of health services is of no lasting use if its results are not acted upon. Unless research demonstrably contributes to the design of health services and their delivery, it is to little avail. Evaluative research has a particularly important role to play because it ought to be concerned with translating knowledge acquired from research into action.

1 St Leger AS, Schnieder H, Walsworth-Bell JP. *Evaluating health services' effectiveness.* Milton Keynes: Open University Press, 1992.
2 Smith G, Cantley C. *Assessing health care: a study in organisational evaluation.* Milton Keynes: Open University Press, 1985.
3 Donabedian A. *Explorations in quality assessment and monitoring.* Vol 1. *The definition of quality and approaches to its assessment.* Ann Arbor: Health Administration Press, 1980.
4 Phillips C, Palfrey C, Thomas P. *Evaluating health and social care.* London: Macmillan, 1994.
5 Dingwall R. Don't mind him—he's from Barcelona: qualitative methods in health studies. In: Daly J, McDonald I, Willis E, editors. *Researching health care: designs, dilemmas, disciplines.* London: Tavistock/Routledge, 1992:161–75.
6 Medical Research Council. *The health of the UK's elderly people.* London: MRC, 1994. (MRC topic review.)
7 Hunter DJ, McKeganey NP, MacPherson IA. *Care of the elderly: policy and practice.* Aberdeen: Aberdeen University Press, 1988.
8 Daly J, MacDonald I. Introduction: the problem as we saw it. In: Daly J, McDonald I, Willis E, editors. *Researching health care: designs, dilemmas, disciplines.* London: Tavistock/Routledge, 1992:1–11.
9 Illsley R. *Professional or public health?* London: Nuffield Provincial Hospitals Trust, 1980.
10 Bond J, Gregson BA, Atkinson A, Newell DJ. The implementation of a multi-centred randomised controlled trial in the evaluation of the National Health Service nursing homes. *Age Ageing* 1989;18:96–102.
11 McKeganey NP. The role of home help organisers. *Soc Policy Admin* 1989;23:171–88.
12 Carr-Hill R. Assumptions of the QALY procedure. *Soc Sci Med* 1989;29:469–77.

13 Donaldson C, Atkinson A, Bond J, Wright K. Should QALYs be programme specific? *J Health Econ* 1988;7:47–57.
14 Knapp M, Wistow G. Implementing community care. *Joint commissioning for community care—a slice through time*. London: Department of Health, 1993.
15 Sykes W, Collins M, Hunter DJ, Popay J, Williams G. *Listening to local voices: a guide to research methods*. Leeds: Nuffield Institute for Health Services Studies, 1992.

11 Health service use in mental illness

JAMES LINDESAY

It is the age-associated problem of dementia that distinguishes old age psychiatry from that of younger adults and determines most of its preoccupations and operational styles. The numerous surveys that have been carried out agree that the prevalence of dementia increases exponentially in late life, with a doubling of rates every five years after the age of 65 years. Up to 20% of those aged 85 years and above are affected—the age group that will see the greatest growth in developed societies in the next two decades (see chapter 29). The economic burden imposed by dementia is already substantial; the costs of care for Alzheimer's disease were about £1039 million in the United Kingdom in 1990–1, compared with £791 million for stroke and £623 million for diabetes[1]; the burden in terms of the suffering of patients and their carers is incalculable. The problem of dementia rightly dominates the planning of old age psychiatry services, but it must not be forgotten that all of the psychiatric disorders of adult life also occur to a greater or lesser extent in the elderly population. Clinically significant depressive symptomatology affects 15–30% of the elderly population, although, despite popular assumptions about the inevitable misery of old age, rates of severe depression in late life do not appear to be much greater than in earlier adulthood (see chapter 30). As with younger adults, rates of depression appear to be greater in women than men. In late life the factors most powerfully associated with depression are physical illness and disability, and as a consequence rates of depression are substantially higher in those in hospital and residential care. The economic burden of depression in old age is not known but is likely to be considerable. Similarly the so called minor psychiatric disorders, such as anxiety and other neuroses, also occur in the elderly at rates not much below those found in younger adults[2]; they colour and complicate other physical and psychiatric conditions and impose a significant burden in terms of both cost and suffering; however, they have yet to receive the attention from clinicians and researchers that they deserve.

Despite the growing awareness of and interest in mental health problems in old age, a major issue still facing health and social services is the hidden nature of much of the psychiatric morbidity in the elderly population. This

96

is due in part to the general assumption by patients, families, and the services themselves that problems such as confusion, depression, and fear are normal and natural accompaniments of the ageing process; patients and families don't complain and doctors fail to diagnose, or, if they do, they do not act. The "filters" on the pathway to psychiatric care[3] are particularly impermeable as far as the elderly are concerned. Certain groups, such as the elderly members of ethnic minorities, suffer particularly badly in this respect. This will change as the more demanding cohorts of the currently middle aged enter late life, but for now it is an important defining feature of specialist old age psychiatry services that they seek to counter popular and professional ageism and to ensure that the mental health needs of the elderly population are equitably and efficiently met.

This chapter outlines the approach to old age psychiatry service provision that has developed in the United Kingdom. Service developments are determined not only by the health needs of the population but also by the history, politics, economics, and the specific geographic and demographic characteristics of individual regions and nations. Models of service that work in one context cannot be exported wholesale, although we can all learn from imaginative approaches developed elsewhere. Service planners will find much of interest in published descriptions of old age psychiatry services as they have evolved in Australia, the United States, Europe, and elsewhere.[4-6]

Old age psychiatry in the United Kingdom

There has been considerable development of old age psychiatry services in the United Kingdom since the policy of specialist services in every locality was accepted by government in 1972. Nationwide, development has been patchy,[7] and there is a great diversity of approaches to delivering a specialist old age psychiatry service, depending on the nature of the locality and the resources available[8]; however, all subscribe to the basic principles underlying such a service[9] (box 11.1), and there is good agreement as to the core elements that must be in place for that service to be effective.

Box 11.1—Principles underlying old age psychiatry services

- Community oriented
- Comprehensive
- Available
- Flexible
- Home assessment where possible
- Communication
- Critical thinking

Who are the clients of an old age psychiatry service? Indeed, should there be a separate specialist psychiatric service for elderly people at all? The trend in geriatric medicine in recent years has been for specialist services to integrate back into the body of general medicine on the grounds that chronologically defined services are inherently ageist and that they result in a second class service for elderly patients. The trend within psychiatry has been in the opposite direction, for several reasons: firstly, it is recognised that the integration of services does not of itself abolish ageism and the existence of an identifiable specialty can provide a useful countervailing advocacy of older patients and their needs; secondly, it is important that underdeveloped and potentially vulnerable services should be able to identify clearly and ring fence the resources due to them for service delivery, service development, training, and research. Specialist psychogeriatric services have higher staffing ratios, a higher proportion of acute beds on general hospital sites, and a greater proportion of long term beds within the area served.[10]

Given the current strategic need for an old age psychiatry specialty, it is important that the boundary between this and psychiatric services for younger adults is clearly defined. In the United Kingdom the age of 65 years is usually taken as the cut off between the two. This does not reflect any sudden major change in the mental health needs of people at this age but is chosen because it coincides with the important social boundary of retirement—at least for men. The over 65 population is made up of several generations of individuals with very different characteristics and needs. One problem with using the 65 year cut off as a basis for service definition and resource allocation is that the growing demand is in fact related to the more rapid growth in the number of over 75s, with their higher prevalence of dementia; a needs based approach to service provision must reflect this if underresourcing is to be avoided. Age alone is not sufficient to define who is cared for by which service, and other criteria have been applied by some old age psychiatry services to define their client group. One example is the "dementia service", in which access is restricted to those with a particular diagnosis; however, it is now generally accepted that, in view of the complex and mixed physical and mental problems encountered in elderly patients and their carers, a comprehensive service best meets their needs and provides the best training experiences for those working with the elderly mentally ill. Although comprehensive old age psychiatry services cater for all diagnostic groups, it is usually the case that they will only take on patients presenting after 65 years. This is because many people with chronic or relapsing conditions, such as schizophrenia and affective disorders, who have been looked after by the general adult services for many years will be best served if they remain under their care in old age. There will be some "graduate" patients whose needs will be better met by an old age psychiatry service, and conversely there will be a small number of patients under the age of 65 years who develop dementia and also need this service's particular skills and

98

resources. Each locality needs to establish rules as to which patient groups are the responsibility of which part of the overall service; these may be arbitrary but this does not matter so long as they are clear and there is provision for negotiating individual cases.

In some districts old age psychiatry is provided as part of an integrated health care of the elderly service, with joint assessment units for those with multiple physical and mental health problems.[11][12] This model of service provision has not developed widely in the United Kingdom, probably because of the increasing community focus of old age psychiatry and the increasing hospital focus of geriatric medicine, and the current division of NHS providers into independent trusts does not encourage such developments; however, established services of this type offer a good example of the collaboration that is possible between the two specialties.

Another important boundary of the old age psychiatry service is that with primary care. Historically, the community oriented development of the speciality was to some extent a response to the neglect of the elderly mentally ill by general practitioners; conversely, some general practitioners responded to the lack of specialist old age psychiatry services in their areas by employing their own community psychiatric nurses. Steady improvements in both services mean that the issue now is how best they can work together, with clearly defined roles and responsibilities. Since the beginning of the 1980s there has been a steady growth of formal links between the two services.[13] On the one hand, this involves members of the old age psychiatry team working sessions in primary care health centres, seeing patients, and providing advice and education; on the other, general practitioners are being employed to provide medical support for dispersed long term care and day hospital units for the elderly mentally ill. The experience of practitioners and patients is that good GPs working in partnership with good old age psychiatry services can provide an excellent standard of care, but this is something that has yet to be evaluated. In the United Kingdom, the shape of specialist services is increasingly being determined by the fund-holding practitioners who purchase them, so it is important that they have good information on which to base their decisions.

Box 11.2—Key elements in old age psychiatry services

- Multidisciplinary community outreach team
- Inpatient assessment
- Day care
- Respite care
- Rehabilitation
- Long term care
- Liaison/consultation
- Education
- Research

The principles of old age psychiatry services set out in box 11.1 are reflected in how most modern services are currently organised and operated. There is as yet little in the way of formal evaluation of the effectiveness of any aspect of these services,[14] but a starting point for future developments is provided by the broad clinical consensus as to what the key elements are[15] (box 11.2).

Multidisciplinary community team

At the heart of all developed old age psychiatry services is a multidisciplinary outreach team drawn from the professions of nursing, occupational therapy, physiotherapy, psychology, social work, and psychiatry. These community teams carry out most of the initial home based assessment and management of cases referred to the service and provide the necessary ongoing support to patients and their carers. Not all teams have representatives from every profession, but as a rule the more comprehensive a team is in this respect, the more efficient its case assessment and management is likely to be. Ideally the team should be the focus for all referrals to the service because this makes the referral process much simpler for those using it. Some teams operate an "open access" policy with regard to referrals; others prefer to restrict access to particular groups, such as general practitioners. Some services are anxious about open access policies, in case they encourage large numbers of inappropriate referrals, but there is no evidence that non-practitioner referrals are any more inappropriate than those from general practitioners.[16]

Teams vary in the manner in which they organise and carry out the assessment and management of cases. Some have developed along the lines of general adult psychiatric teams, with the consultant psychogeriatrician as team leader and principal decision maker and with all patients receiving formal psychiatric assessment at some point during their contact with the service.[17 18] In others the task of assessment is shared and not all patients are necessarily seen at any time by a psychiatrist, who can concentrate instead on the more difficult and urgent cases.[19] There is debate as to which model of teamwork is most appropriate in old age psychiatry; the multidisciplinary approach to assessment is not associated with misdiagnosis of psychiatric disorder, and may well result in fuller assessment of the various presenting problems,[20] but there has been no evaluation of outcomes associated with the various approaches to community team functioning.

Community teams have an important educational and preventive role, which many perform through more or less formal links with local primary health care teams, residential and nursing homes, and social services. These links are also important in establishing clear mutual understanding of the roles of the various agencies in relation to patients/clients they have in common, and in maintaining effective communications.

Inpatient assessment/treatment unit

While many of the assessment and treatment tasks of the old age psychiatry service can be carried out by the community team in the patient's home, a minority of complex or severely ill cases require a period of admission to hospital. Patients likely to require admission include those with dementia and/or delirium complicated by disturbed behaviour; and severe depression, mania, and paranoid psychoses associated with significant distress or behaviour disturbance. In a well developed service, crisis admissions following the collapse of informal care should be avoidable. In addition to assessment and the initial treatment and management of physical, mental, and behavioural problems, some patients will also require a period of rehabilitation before they either return home or move to long term care.

Day hospital

Despite the paucity of research into the effectiveness of day hospital services, most clinicians agree that they are a vital element of psychogeriatric service provision.[21] It is said that day hospital assessment and care can reduce admissions to hospital or residential care, but there is not as yet any clear evidence on this either way; they are certainly expensive when compared with other forms of domiciliary and residential care[22] but are probably cheaper than inpatient care. Broadly speaking, the functions of a psychogeriatric day hospital are: "short term social and medical assessment, treatment, rehabilitation and therapy, longer term maintenance and monitoring, and relief for carers."[23] In most districts day care is also provided by other agencies, such as social services and voluntary organisations, and it is important that health service day hospital provision is planned to be complementary to this, which usually means providing a service to those patients who cannot be managed or tolerated in less specialist settings.

Respite care

Periodic respite care in hospital is an important service element that is much in demand from the carers of demented patients,[24] and as a result provision of this by old age psychiatry services is likely to increase. It is argued that it has a preventive role in avoiding acute and long term admissions, although the evidence for this is meagre and it cannot be assumed when planning services.[25] Respite care is primarily a service for the carers, and one from which they derive significant benefit; it may initially cause some disruption to the patient but the concern that it might be associated with increased mortality[26] has not been borne out by subsequent studies of planned respite services.[27]

Respite care needs planning and coordinating as part of a comprehensive package of social care, including day care and home support, if it is to be effective and useful to the carer. A proportion of those requiring regular respite care will need health service levels of nursing care, and the appropriate provision needs to be made. As with day care, health service respite services need planning in collaboration with those provided by other agencies. In some districts the availability of NHS respite care is declining along with that of continuing care beds[28]; however, there is little sign that the independent sector is at present showing much enthusiasm for offering this form of service.

Long term care

There has always been a mixed economy of long term institutional care for the elderly in the United Kingdom. Until relatively recently the main providers were the public health sector and social services, but changes in the benefits system in the early 1980s led to a great expansion of the independent sector, particularly profit making institutions. This growth has been checked by the recent community care reforms, which give social services the responsibility for this budget and for assessing eligibility for independent residential and nursing homes; however, part of this assessment is financial, and those with savings and assets of more than £8000 will not receive any benefit until they have "spent down" to this level. Since long term care in the public sector still remains free at the point of use, there is an inequity in the system that is currently the focus of much grievance and debate.

In stark contrast to the growth of the independent sector, long term care for elderly mentally ill patients within the NHS has declined as a resource in recent years. This form of care has traditionally been provided in the long stay wards of the old mental hospitals; as these are run down and closed many districts have withdrawn from this aspect of service provision. Although the quality of long term psychogeriatric care on the back wards of mental hospitals is generally unacceptably low, the failure to replace this in some districts as these hospitals close has been questioned, in part because of the financial implications for service users (see above) and in part because of the impact on the range and quality of alternative care available. As a result of the decline in NHS provision there has been an increase in the numbers of elderly residents with mental illness being admitted to local authority and independent nursing homes, only some of which are registered for this purpose. Recent draft guidelines from the Department of Health on NHS responsibilities for meeting long term health care needs[29] have made it clear that the purchasers of health services remain responsible for meeting such needs, and that the range of provision should include, where appropriate, continuing care in NHS units for the most severely disturbed. In some districts a number of innovative alternatives to the long stay mental hospital ward have been developed for this group, either within the NHS,[30 31] or in partnership with independent housing associations and charities.[32] Purchasers and providers of long term care

102

need to agree a locally appropriate range of services, with eligibility criteria controlling access to limited, specialist health service units. Another crucial issue for purchasers is to ensure that their decisions are determined not only by the cost but also the quality of care provided, and that systems are in place to ensure this.[33]

Most evaluations of long term care for the elderly mentally ill focus on the quality of care provided. Outcome measures such as mortality and dependency are relatively insensitive to differences in factors such as unit regime and philosophy that are thought to be important determinants of quality of care.[34] More relevant indicators of quality in the process and outcome of long term care for this group include levels of activity, privacy, choice, and satisfaction. Evidence from detailed studies of small numbers of units indicate that the quality of care is related to factors such as unit philosophy and management, the residents' physical and mental disability, staffing levels and attitudes, the physical environment, and opportunities for activity and social interaction.[30 32 35 36] Innovative schemes such as the housing association-managed Domus programme for the elderly mentally ill in south London deliver a much higher quality of care than is provided in mental hospital wards,[32] but the cost per resident is also higher.[37] Further evaluation work is needed to determine what is cost effective long term care for groups with different levels of dependency.

Liaison–consultation

This refers to the activities of psychogeriatric service personnel in non-psychiatric settings, such as the general hospital. The principal aims of liaison–consultation services are diagnosis and treatment of psychiatric disorders, prevention of psychiatric morbidity secondary to physical illness and treatment, education of non-psychiatric health professionals, and the promotion of positive attitudes towards mental illness. In its fully developed form liaison psychiatry is provided by a specialist team with close involvement with other units and shared responsibility for patients; however, only some psychiatric services in the United Kingdom operate such a system, and nowhere is there a specialist psychogeriatric liaison service, despite the fact that a substantial proportion of medical and surgical inpatients are over the age of 65 years. In the absence of a specialist liaison service, a more limited consultation model operates, with psychiatrists assessing referrals and offering advice on management. There has been no systematic evaluation of this aspect of psychogeriatric services in the United Kingdom.

Communications

The old age psychiatry service has interfaces and interactions with numerous other agencies, including social services, primary care, the geriatric medical service, other medical and surgical specialties, and the

103

independent sector. Effective patient care requires communication and collaboration with all of these,[38] and systems are needed to ensure that this occurs. In particular, effective discharge planning is essential, not only for the individual patient but also for the inpatient units, to ensure that patient throughput can be maintained and to prevent unnecessary readmissions.

Priorities for research

It is vital that the limited resources available to old age psychiatry services are used cost effectively. It is apparent from this chapter that our knowledge about the cost effectiveness of these services is still very limited. There is an urgent need for systematic evaluation of the various service elements, such as community teams, day hospitals, inpatient units, and respite care facilities, together with the systems that link them into a coordinated service. Old age psychiatry is still a low tech specialty, although this may change in the future as antidementia drugs become available; for now, the most expensive component of the service is the staff, and it is essential that they are used as efficiently as possible. To what extent are scarce, expensive professionals (doctors, psychologists) currently employed in tasks that can be carried out just as well by other health professionals? How much of the service budget should be invested in "institutional" care (day hospitals, wards, nursing homes), as opposed to assessment, treatment, and care in the community? What do patients and their carers actually want from the service? How should old age psychiatry services manage their relationships with other agencies, such as the primary care sector, other hospital based specialties, social services, and the independent sector? Different services currently operate very different answers to these questions, and these different approaches need to be compared systematically, always bearing in mind that service solutions that work for one locality may not be appropriate for others with different histories and characteristics.

1 Gray A, Fenn P. Alzheimer's disease: the burden of the illness in England. *Health Trends* 1993;**25**:31–7.
2 Eastwood MR, Lindesay J. Epidemiology. In: Lindesay J, editor. *Neurotic disorders in the elderly*. Oxford: Oxford University Press, 1995:12–30.
3 Goldberg D, Huxley P. *Psychiatric illness in general practice*. Oxford: Oxford University Press, 1980.
4 Ames D, Flynn E. Dementia services: an Australian view. In: Levy R, Burns A, editors. *Dementia*. London: Chapman and Hall, 1994.
5 Cohen C. Integrated community services. In: Sadavoy J, Lazarus LW, Jarvik L, editors. *Comprehensive review of geriatric psychiatry*. Washington: American Psychiatric Press, 1991: 613–34.
6 Murphy E, Banerjee S. The organization of old-age psychiatry services. *Rev Clin Gerontol* 1993;**3**:367–78.
7 Wattis J. Geographical variations in the provision of psychiatric services for old people. *Age Ageing* 1988;**17**:171–80.
8 Health Advisory Service. *The rising tide: developing services for mental illness in old age*. Sutton, Surrey: HAS, 1982.
9 Arie T. The first year of the Goodmayes psychiatric service for old people. *Lancet* 1970; **ii**:1175–82.

10 Wattis J. A comparison of "specialised" and non-specialised psychiatric services for old people in the United Kingdom. *Int J Geriatr Psychiatry* 1989;4:59–62.
11 Arie T, Dunn T. A "do-it-yourself" psychiatric–geriatric joint patient unit. *Lancet* 1973; ii:1313–6.
12 Arie T. Combined geriatrics and psychogeriatrics: a new model. *Geriatr Med* 1990;20: 24–7.
13 Banerjee S, Lindesay J, Murphy E. Psychogeriatricians and general practitioners: a national survey. *Psychiatr Bull* 1993;17:592–4.
14 Melzer D, Hopkins S, Pencheon D, Brayne C, Williams R. *Epidemiologically based needs assessment. Report 5: dementia.* London: NHSME, 1992.
15 Shulman K, Arie T. UK survey of psychiatric services for the elderly: direction of developing services. *Can J Psychiatry* 1991;36:169–75.
16 Macdonald A, Goddard C, Poynton A. Impact of "open access" to specialist services—the case of community psychogeriatrics. *Int J Geriatr Psychiatry* 1994;9:709–14.
17 Arie T, Jolley D. Making service work: organisation and style of psychogeriatric services. In: Levy R, Post F, editors. *The psychiatry of late life.* Oxford: Blackwell, 1982:222–51.
18 Jolley D, Arie T. Developments in psychogeriatric services. In: Arie T, editor. *Recent advances in psychogeriatrics.* Vol. 2. London: Churchill Livingstone, 1992:117–35.
19 Coles RJ, von Abendorff R, Herzberg J. The impact of a new community mental health team on an inner city psychogeriatric service. *Int J Geriatr Psychiatry* 1991;6:31–9.
20 Collighan G, Macdonald A, Herzberg J, Philpot M, Lindesay J. An evaluation of the multidisciplinary approach to psychiatric diagnosis in elderly people. *BMJ* 1993;306: 821–4.
21 Beats B, Trimble D, Levy R. Day hospital provision for the elderly mentally ill within the South East Thames Regional Authority. *Int J Geriatr Psychiatry* 1993;8:442–3.
22 National Audit Office. Report by the Comptroller and Auditor General. *National Health Service day hospitals for elderly people in England.* London: HMSO, 1986.
23 Tester S. *Caring by day: a study of day care services for older people.* London: Centre for Policy on Ageing, 1989. (Policy studies in ageing, No 8.)
24 National Carers Association. *Community care: just a fairy tale?* London: NCA, 1994.
25 Melzer D. An evaluation of a respite care unit for elderly people with dementia: framework and some results. *Health Trends* 1990;22:64–9.
26 Rai GS, Bielawska C, Murphy PJ, Wright G. Hazards for elderly people admitted for respite ("holiday admissions") and social care ("social admissions"). *BMJ* 1986;292:240.
27 Selly C, Campbell M. Relief care and risk of death in psychogeriatric patients. *BMJ* 1989; 298:1223.
28 Alzheimer's Disease Society. *NHS continuing care beds—a report.* London: ADS, 1993.
29 National Health Service Executive. *Draft circular: NHS responsibilities for meeting long term health care needs.* London: Department of Health, 1994.
30 Bond S, Bond J. Outcomes of care within a multiple-case study in the evaluation of the experimental National Health Service nursing homes. *Age Ageing* 1990;19:11–8.
31 Pattie A, Moxon S. *Community units for the elderly in York Health District: an evaluation of the first CUE.* York: Clifton Hospital Evaluation and Research Support Unit, 1991.
32 Murphy E, Lindesay J, Dean R. *The Domus project.* London: Sainsbury Centre for Mental Health, 1994.
33 Ebrahim S, Wallis C, Brittis S, Harwood R, Graham N. Long term care for elderly people. *Qual Health Care* 1993;2:198–203.
34 Booth T. *Home truths.* London: Gower, 1985.
35 Godlove C, Richard L, Rodwell G. *Time for action: an observational study of elderly people in four different care environments.* Sheffield: University of Sheffield Joint Unit for Social Services Research, 1982.
36 Willcocks D, Peace S, Kellehar L. *Private lives in public places.* London: Tavistock, 1987.
37 Beecham J, Cambridge P, Hallam A, Knapp M. The costs of domus care. *Int J Geriatr Psychiatry* 1993;8:827–31.
38 Horrocks P. The components of a comprehensive district service for elderly people—a personal view. *Age Ageing* 1985;15:321–42.

12 Health service use in physical illness

LAURENCE Z RUBENSTEIN, SAMER Z NASR

The population aged 65 and over uses a vastly disproportionate amount of health services—typically in developed countries they use most services at a rate three to four times higher than their proportion in the overall population.[1] This primarily reflects the increased prevalence of various diseases and physical disabilities among older persons. Moreover, the continued expansion of the older population segment worldwide has been one of the major factors leading to the dramatic cost inflation of health services. With health care responsible for between 10 and 15% of the gross national product in most developed countries, public resources are having increasing difficulty in sustaining these services. Health care cost containment is now the global order of the day. The difficulty in attaining this objective without sacrificing older persons' needs for adequate care explains why health services utilisation has become a major subject of concern, and research, worldwide.

This chapter gives an overview of current patterns of health service utilisation for older persons in multiple countries, including data on physicians, hospitals, nursing homes, and other extended care services. Where possible, data predicting major outcomes from these services (mortality, discharge home or to nursing homes) are included. Studies examining determinants for use of health services are discussed, indicating how both physical illness and psychosocial factors play important roles. Finally, some of the major international variations in health service use are summarised, newer models of geriatric health care are discussed, and some of the most persistent research questions are presented.

Descriptive aspects

Health services utilisation contains several categories, including physician, hospital, nursing home, and community services utilisation. Each is quantified in several ways. This section examines, for each category, general age trends for utilisation, international comparisons, and main factors that correlate with utilisation, attempting to identify the main determinants of increased use.

Physician utilisation

The category of physician utilisation has two principal dimensions: a "contact" dimension indicating whether a physician visit or consultation has taken place during a certain period of time; and a "volume" dimension that registers the number of visits or consultations made during this period. A consultation may take place in the office, in the hospital, at the patient's home, or simply by telephone. Table 12.1 shows the trends of physician contacts between 1986 and 1991 in the United States.[2] The total number of contacts has increased by about 14% in these five years. In the 65–74 year old group the increase is accounted for by a greater number of office visits, while in the 75 and over group it is mostly due to increased home visits. All other contact sites (for instance, hospital, telephone) have decreased or remained fairly constant in both groups. Reasons for the lower utilisation of most physician services at older ages are unclear. Hypotheses advanced include increased isolation of the older old group with reduced access to care, increased reliance on hospital services, and possibly increased fatalism among the oldest subgroup.

Table 12.1   Physician contacts with the elderly according to place of contact: United States 1986 and 1991

Age (years)	Total contacts*	Place of contact**									
		Doctor's office		Hospital		Telephone		Home		Other	
	1986 1991	1986	1991	1986	1991	1986	1991	1986	1991	1986	1991
Over 65	9·1 10·4	54·2	56·9	11·8	11·5	10·8	8·4	12·9	14·9	10·3	8·3
65–74	8·1 9·2	56·6	61·1	12·9	12·9	11·6	9·2	8·1	7·5	10·8	9·3
Over 75	10·6 12·3	51·2	52·1	10·4	9·8	9·9	7·5	18·8	23·4	9·7	7·2

From US Department of Health and Human Services.[2]
* Number per person
** Per cent distribution

These trends tend to be paralleled in other countries. Table 12.2 shows data for older females by age category and physician utilisation from different areas of the world.[3] Elderly males show a similar pattern in most instances. One can see that in most countries the number of physician office visits decreases with age and that home visits increase with age. In many of these countries there is a small overall trend towards decreased physician utilisation with increased age, although this is variable. The significant variability in physician visits between countries suggests that factors other than age must be playing important roles.

The major factors contributing to the explanation of the volume of visits have been extensively researched. In one study, low perceived health,

Table 12.2   Percentage of the female elderly population that had a physician contact in one year by age and place of contact in selected countries (1980s)

Country	Doctor's office			Home visits		
	65–74 years	75–84 years	85+ years	65–74 years	75–84 years	85+ years
Belgium (Brussels)	59	39	37	58	68	68
Finland (Tampere)	83	78	84	4	8	9
France (Midi-Pyrénées)	59	45	19	48	66	81
Germany (West Berlin)	88	78	67	15	27	36
Greece (rural)	72	67	58	37	39	36
Italy (Florence)	79	57	42	51	67	77
Kuwait	32	46	42	2	4	14
Poland (Bialystok)	71	64		32	48	
Rumania (Bucharest)	85	74	51	26	37	64
Former USSR (Kiev)	65	38	25	62	56	64

From Heikkinen *et al.*[3]

current health problem, physical activity restriction, inability to climb stairs, and having a regular physician were found to be the significant contributors to increased physician utilisation.[4]

Hospital utilisation

The hospital utilisation category also has two dimensions: the first indicating whether a hospitalisation occurred during a certain period of time, and the second the number of nights spent there. Figure 12.1 shows that hospital use in the United States increases steadily with age.[2] This trend is true whether considering admission, total hospital days per year, or per capita expenditures. This clear cut age trend is not, however, universally seen in other countries. Table 12.3 shows the mean length of stay in selected countries over a one year period by age subcategory and gender.[3] Only Belgium, France, and Germany showed similar trends. In the other countries listed there was no obvious relationship between age, sex, and mean length of stay. Rural Greece showed the highest durations of stay for all groups and a steady decline in length of stay by age, which may suggest a deficit in other services such as nursing home availability or social services.

A recent study examining predictors of hospital admission found that a hospitalisation within the previous year was the single most important predictor.[5] Other significant predictors were, in decreasing order of significance, poor perceived health status, over six physicians visits in the past year, increasing age, coronary heart disease, male sex, a nurse visit in the past year, and no informal care giver.

Type of illness and its severity have also been found to be major determinants of hospitalisation, especially of intensive care use. United States data from 1987 showed that cardiovascular disease, neoplasms,

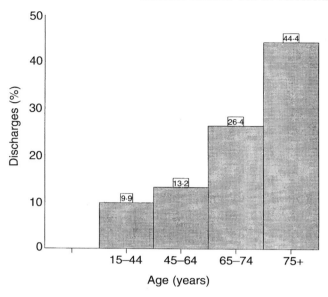

Fig 12.1   Annual hospital discharges per 100 people: United States 1991. (From US Department of Health and Human Services.[2])

Table 12.3   Mean length of stay (days)* in a general hospital in selected countries (1980s)

Country	Males					Females				
	65–69 years	70–74 years	75–79 years	80–84 years	85 + years	65–69 years	70–74 years	75–79 years	80–84 years	85 + years
Belgium (Brussels)	12	6	31	40	90	26	41	12	42	32
Finland (Tampere)	12	22	19	22	20	43	34	52	55	50
France (Midi-Pyrénées)	21	22	19	23	20	34	20	27	10	50
Germany (West Berlin)	29	62	30	32	52	43	34	52	55	50
Greece (rural)	55	79	80	46	10	39	50	50	28	73
Italy (Florence)	21	47	21	24	27	20	24	26	36	22
Kuwait	23	40	23	32	26	19	29	27	42	24
Poland (Bialystok)	23	30	35	28		37	46	42	21	
Rumania (Bucharest)	32	44	46	30	24	26	30	22	35	23
Former USSR (Kiev)	32	57	37	56	32	36	30	46	26	59

* Durations of stay have been rounded up.
From Heikkinen *et al*[3].

cerebrovascular disease, pneumonia, and fractures were the most common reasons for hospitalisation. Hospitalisation rates for all of these show age related increases except for neoplastic disease, which tend to decrease after age 75.[2]

Nursing home utilisation

Measures of nursing home (NH) utilisation parallel those for the hospital, but the label "nursing home" is often loosely used to describe different institutions catering to different clienteles and different needs, and it is crucial to be specific about what is being discussed. First are the custodial institutions (old age homes, senior centres, board and care homes, residential facilities, or retirement housing), where the services offered are essentially accommodation and food and which are intended for elderly people independent in most functional activities. At the other extreme are the hospices designed for the terminally ill, where the mandate is to help people make their final transition as smooth and dignified as possible. Between those two extremes are the NHs proper, which provide skilled nursing and personal care services for disabled or chronically ill persons who require constant care to cope with their disabilities but do not require hospitalisation. Such NHs are not homogeneous either—for example, some have substantial skilled nursing capacities and medical services, while others do not.

The NH clientele is similarly diverse. This diversity exists in several areas, including the degree of physical and/or mental impairment, the type of care required, and the duration of stay. The important distinction has been made between short stay patients (less than six months) and long stay patients (more than six months).[6] Short stay patients can be subdivided into two wholly different groups: firstly, patients needing rehabilitation (for instance, after a minor stroke or a fall) or convalescent care (for instance, after an acute illness), who are expected to be discharged home; and, secondly, the terminally ill patients (for example, end stage cancer or dementia), who could be considered hospice patients. Long stay patients can be divided into three groups: the cognitively impaired, the physically impaired (as a result of musculoskeletal, neurological, cardiac, or pulmonary disease), and those with combined impairment.

In the United States, the NH population grew by more than 24% between 1980 and 1990, with 5% of the over 65 year old population currently living in an NH. According to the two most recent and comprehensive surveys available,[7 8] the number of free standing American NHs reached 15 362 in 1992, with 1 625 383 functioning beds, whose occupancy rate averaged about 95%, thus accommodating an estimated 1 536 000 residents at any one time.

Relatively speaking, the United States ranks among the median group of industrialised countries in terms of the utilisation rate of NH facilities by the elderly population. Table 12.4 shows that the proportion of the elderly populations living in NHs differs widely among countries.[9] There is no obvious relationship between these rates and the relative size of the elderly population or the degree of industrialisation of the countries. Cultural differences, degree of family support, and availability of alternative care services are possible explanatory factors. Interpretation of these findings

Table 12.4 Percentages of the
elderly population over 65 in
nursing homes in selected
countries (circa 1984*)

Country	%
Lower group	
West Germany	4·1
Great Britain	4·0
Israel	4·0
Japan	3·9
Ireland	3·6
Median group	
Australia	6·4
Belgium	6·3
France	6·3
United States	5·7
Higher group	
Netherlands	10·9
Sweden	9·6
Switzerland	8·9
Canada	8·7
Denmark	7·0

* Figures refer to the early 1980s.
They are not strictly comparable
owing to differences in definitions
and coverage.
From Suzman et al.[9]

is further complicated by differences in definition of NH and financial coverage between countries.

Research efforts to identify determinants of NH use cover a wide spectrum, ranging from limited community samples to broadly based nationally representative surveys, and from simple enumeration of the characteristics of NH users to sophisticated multivariate modelling that quantifies the role played by various factors. The most common factors that correlate with NH use include age, diagnostic condition, living alone, activities of daily living (ADL) problem, marital status, mental status, white race, social support, poverty, outpatient admission, hospital admission, bed disability, female gender, type of residence, instrumental ADL assistance, and use of an ambulation aid.[10]

Age is the most obvious and probably the most important single determinant of NH use. Table 12.5 provides data from 15 countries on NH use and indicates the steadily increasing prevalence of use by age group.[9] This pattern is largely explained by the many other factors associated with advancing age, particularly the higher prevalence of chronic diseases, deterioration in physical and mental capacities, and increasing social isolation. After controlling for such variables, age itself becomes a much weaker predictor of NH use.[11] This emphasises the importance of

111

Table 12.5   Ageing and the rate of institutional use in selected countries (circa 1981)

Country	Age group			% increase with age	
	A 65–69 years	B 70–74 years	C 75 + years	A − B	B − C
Austria	1·6	2·4	7·3	150	304
Belgium	2·0	3·1	9·0	155	290
Canada	2·7	4·6	17·5	170	380
Denmark	1·6	2·8	13·4	175	478
France	2·2	2·9	9·1	132	314
East Germany	1·2	2·1	7·4	175	352
Italy	1·6	2·0	4·4	125	220
Japan	1·7	3·0	5·8	176	193
Luxembourg	2·7	4·4	11·6	163	263
Norway	0·9	2·1	11·0	233	552
Spain	1·2	1·8	3·7	150	205
Sweden	0·4	1·0	7·8	250	780
Switzerland	2·7	4·1	13·6	152	332
United Kingdom	1·2	1·9	7·8	158	410
United States	1·4	2·5	10·8	178	432

The last two columns are calculated. Institutional use includes both nursing homes and non-medical old age homes.
From Suzman et al.[9]

considering the interaction between the various independent explanatory variables.

Most studies have found that women have a significantly higher probability of NH use[12 13]; for instance, the lifetime probability of NH use for persons aged 65 and older in the United States is about 45% for women against 28% for men.[14] This sex differential exists for every elderly age subgroup but increases with advancing old age. This "gender gap" can be partially explained by the greater longevity of women, with decreased likelihood of spousal support, their higher prevalence of disabilities, their lower ADL scores, and their lower incomes.[3] It has been argued that when the effects of such variables are controlled for, older women may actually have a lower risk of NH use than older men.[15] Be that as it may, the current prototype of the NH dweller is still that of an older woman with multiple pathologies, taking several drugs,[16] most likely widowed, and incontinent.

Race is a determinant of special importance in the United States, unlike many other countries. Considerable data indicate that Americans identified as white use NHs more than those identified as black or Hispanic. A recent three year longitudinal study on NH admission in a biracial community found that, after adjustment for confounding factors, black residents were half as likely as white residents to be institutionalised.[17] The overall likelihood of NH use after age 65 was 23% for the former against 38% for the latter.[18] This situation can possibly be explained by various factors, including cultural and economic differences[19] and uneven access to long term care facilities.[20] Clarification of this issue is needed and requires further investigation.

Illness and health related factors are obviously major determinants of NH use. Behind each NH admission is some kind of disabling medical or functional condition. In Germany, illness was found to be the most important precipitating cause for institutionalisation, accounting for 39–61% of the reasons mentioned for entering an NH.[20] In the United States, Cohen *et al* used "perceived health status" as a subjective proxy for medical status and found it to be "the most powerful discriminant" between NH entrants and non-entrants after age and its interactions were taken into account.[12] Understanding of illness as a predictive variable is, however, complicated by the large number of diagnostic categories and severity levels for each.

Functional status is another important predictor. Persons independent in their ADL—whatever their age group—are clearly less at risk of entering an NH than dependent elderly persons in need of personal care. The burden that dependency throws on the care giver is often the direct cause of seeking institutionalisation. The risk for a person "in bed most of the time" was found to be 83% higher than the average risk of NH admission, regardless of age. The risk was only 56% higher if the disability required "help to get around", while simply being "housebound" or "having trouble getting around" were not associated with an increased risk.[12] The Barthel ADL index was found to be a simple and effective screening test for discriminating between patients really requiring NH placement and those who should be more appropriately kept at home or oriented towards a purely residential facility.[21] Of note in this context is that functional status depends on both physical and mental limitations. The degree of mental deterioration, especially among patients with dementia, was found to be the most significant factor of NH use in some studies.[22]

Social support includes assistance from family members (spouse and children), other relatives, friends, neighbours, and the local community in general. The kind of help or resources provided ranges from daily hands-on care, to mere contacts (visits or phone calls), to participation in communal activities, religious or otherwise. All are deemed to play a role in avoiding or at least delaying institutionalisation.[23] Although grouped under one category, these elements of social support and the different social structures from which they stem call for a multivariate approach in weighing their importance as NH determinants; for instance, the presence of a spouse, particularly for men, is usually much more important than phone contacts with relatives.[24] The role played by social networks is strongly conditioned by the prevailing socioeconomic system and the extent of its modernisation. The increasing female participation in the work force, the weakening of family ties, and the waning of communal solidarity common to many developed societies are such examples.

The Andersen behavioural model of health services utilisation (see p 116) is a conceptual model that defines three major determinants: predisposing

113

factors, need factors, and enabling factors. When applied to the use of NHs,[25] predisposing factors were being older, white, living alone, having a telephone, having fewer non-kin support, and not believing to have any control of personal health. Need factors were having difficulties with household ADL, such as meal preparation or shopping, and lower body limitations, such as impairment of gait, stooping, kneeling, or standing. Previous hospitalisation and NH use were also contributing factors.

Multivariate analysis is able to identify not only individual risk factors and their relative importance but also the effect of a combination of such factors. In one analysis, for example, a person over 85 had a 16% probability of institutional placement within 2·5 years. This probability decreased to 7% if a spouse existed, but was 19% if there was no spouse. In the latter case the risk increased to 62% if the person had other characteristics, such as a recent hospitalisation, lived in retirement housing, had one or more ADL problems, or had a mental problem. The risk decreased to 10% if those traits were absent.[26]

The picture that emerges from efforts devoted to study of NH utilisation seems fairly consistent despite differences in population samples and variables considered. As more data accumulate and better statistical tools are developed, our understanding and insight into the interrelationships involved will improve.

Community health care services

This category covers auxiliary and support health services and is usually subdivided into two: home care services (which include visiting nurses, hot meals, home health aid, or other special care delivered at home) and ambulatory care services (which include rehabilitation, counselling, speech therapy). Services offered by community centres, such as day hospitals and senior citizens centres, are also sometimes included.

Utilisation of these services has traditionally been low. In the National Health Interview Survey only 4% of respondents had reported using these services[27]; however, in recent years use of these services has markedly increased, especially in Europe and North America. Table 12.6 shows the great variation that exists between the different countries.[28]

The most important predictor of community services utilisation is a recent discharge from an acute hospital.[10 29] The increased use for patients over 65 years old after an acute hospitalisation is about 2–3 fold that of any other age group. Not all older patients discharged from an acute hospital need increased levels of community services. In a study of elderly patients followed after discharge, 65% returned to their baseline level of care, with only 10% needing a persistently higher level.[30]

Age is often considered a determinant of community services use but its exact role is unclear and in some studies the variance seen between different age groups was not significant after adjusting for need factors.[31 32] Other predictors of use have been poorly studied. In one study four risk factors

Table 12.6   Percentage of elderly people receiving home help in selected countries (1980s to early 1990s)

Country	Percentages
Denmark	20
Norway	14
Sweden	12
Finland	10
United Kingdom	9
Netherlands	8
United States	8
Australia	7
Belgium	6
Ireland	3
Canada	2
Austria	1
Italy	1
Portugal	1
Spain	1
Japan	0·5

From Organisation for Economic Cooperation and Development.[28]

for home health care utilisation were identified upon initial hospitalisation.[33] These included educational level below 12 years, less accessible social support, impairment in at least one activity of daily living, and previous home health care use. A risk stratification was created by adding one point for each risk factor present. With 0–1 risk factors present, 8% used home health care, with two 28%, with three 45%, and with four 76%.

Community care services have been often advocated as "alternatives" to more costly institutional services. While clearly useful in themselves, community care services have not been proven to prevent readmissions to hospitals or institutionalisation.[34-36] In fact several studies tend to suggest that readmitted patients are more likely to have recently seen a community nurse. Nor have these services been associated with decreased demands on the care givers.[29] Thus issues of cost effectiveness have often been cited as reasons why community care services are not more widely available.

Interrelationships

Utilisation of each service in the health care system discussed above is inexorably linked to use of other services. These linkages are difficult to analyse because of the complexity of the relationships as well as shortage of accurate information. In a 1991 study for the US Agency for Health Policy Research, Denson attempted to construct a diagrammatic movement pathway through the health care system for the American population.[37] This is shown in simplified fashion in fig 12.2. One can see that in a given year about 87% of the American population aged 75 and over will see a

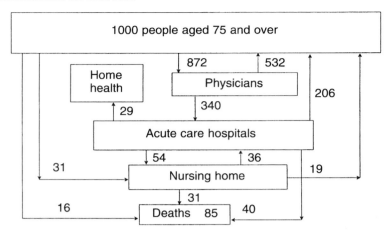

Fig 12.2 Movement of the elderly population through the health care system in the United States. (Adapted from Denson.[37])

physician, 34% will be hospitalised, 8·5% will enter a nursing home, 2·9% will receive home health care, and 8·5% will die. Also shown is the complexity of movement between many of the services.

Analytic aspects

Predictors of use

Clearly health services utilisation is determined both by medical need factors and by factors connecting these needs to services. This is of interest to the policy maker who designs the public measures for meeting long term care needs, to the state budget commissioner who must finance these measures, to the insurance industry fixing premiums for the different health plans, and to the health care industry itself, which must adjust its investments and price policies. A number of studies have explored predictors of use and a number of models have been put forth attempting to explain it. Among the most prominent has been the health behaviour model.

Health behaviour model

Even the most detailed and most comprehensive database does not speak by itself: the researcher needs a frame of reference in trying to understand and explain the findings. Such a framework in the present context is provided by the well known health behaviour model of Andersen.[38][39] Figure 12.3 depicts this model in a variant that tries to underline the issues raised in this chapter.[38]

116

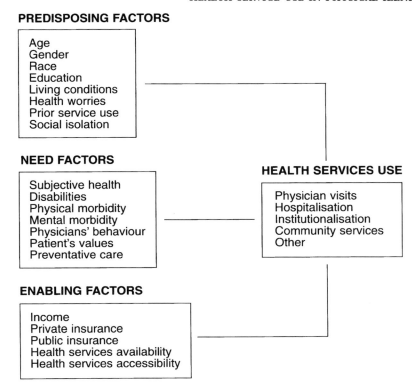

PREDISPOSING FACTORS

Age
Gender
Race
Education
Living conditions
Health worries
Prior service use
Social isolation

NEED FACTORS

Subjective health
Disabilities
Physical morbidity
Mental morbidity
Physicians' behaviour
Patient's values
Preventative care

HEALTH SERVICES USE

Physician visits
Hospitalisation
Institutionalisation
Community services
Other

ENABLING FACTORS

Income
Private insurance
Public insurance
Health services availability
Health services accessibility

Fig 12.3   Variant on the health behaviour or Anderson model. (Adapted from Andersen and Newman.[38])

This model describes the relationships between the various types of health service utilisation (the dependent variables) and the three groups of factors to which this utilisation can be attributed (the independent or predictor variables). In the model, health services use is explained by the bundle of factors in each of the three groups: the predisposing factors, the need factors, and the enabling factors. The predisposing and enabling factors will not be commented upon because the need factors are those that "drive the system"[38] and are the most relevant to the present discussion on physical illness.

As fig 12.3 shows, the set of need factors may be interpreted as a complex construct that includes distinct, though sometimes interrelated elements. Two of these elements are traditionally highlighted: *subjective health status* (so called "perceived" or "self rated" health status) and *disabilities*. The first is usually measured by scoring the answers to one question: "How do you rate your overall health status: excellent, very good, good, fair, or poor?" The second generally includes two or more components related to physical functioning—for example, basic ADL, more advanced or instrumental ADL, specific limitations, or other subdivisions of these limitations. Physical

117

disability is primarily a function of physical diseases. Arthritis and musculoskeletal diseases, in particular, but also cardiovascular, respiratory diseases, and stroke account for more than two thirds of the cases of physical disability.[40] These disabilities and their severity greatly influence subjective health status.

The third element, *physical morbidity*, is probably the most important. The primary clientele of health services are the sick. This has direct effects (for example, consulting a physician for an illness) and indirect effects through the impact of illness on subjective health status and on disability. The impact of specific diseases on health services utilisation by elderly persons has received relatively little attention. It is useful to distinguish between chronic diseases associated with ageing (for example, arthritis, hypertension, and cardiovascular diseases) and acute conditions (for example, myocardial infarction, stroke, or gastrointestinal haemorrhage). The first group has the greatest effect on service use as a consequence of their long duration. The severity of symptoms is also relevant: asymptomatic stages of a disease lead to a more passive attitude, while severe pain triggers an immediate visit to the physician and often a cascade of consultations.

Mental morbidity impact on health services are addressed elsewhere in this volume (see chapter 11). For the system as a whole, they have a relatively small effect on physical functioning. Among the diseases reported to cause difficulty with physical tasks, mental disorders come at the bottom of the list: 0·1 and 0·6% among men and women respectively, compared with 38·6 and 55·1% for arthritis and musculoskeletal diseases, and even below cancer (0·5 and 0·9%) or hypertension (0·4 and 1·7%).[40]

Physician behaviour has been added to the need set to recognise that some types of health services use (especially further visits, hospitalisations, and drug consumption) are made as a result of the treating doctor's recommendation, the patient awareness of a need being frequently a function of the physician's decision. This brings forth the whole issue of physician's practice styles, which disturbs the seeming simplicity of the link between morbidity, need, and health services use.

Older persons' health condition is often complex, largely due to prevalent comorbidity—in one French survey[1] many patients were documented to have 30 distinct diseases; there was marked vulnerability to adverse drug reactions and difficulty in devising clear cut treatment protocols. These considerations explain why diagnoses and prescriptions are far from homogeneous.[41] Many factors over and above old age conditions seem to contribute to such a diversity. A South African study[42] showed that medical schemes operating in a fee for service system were associated with higher rates of hospital utilisation and longer lengths of stay than those in which physicians worked for a salary from prospectively paid managed health care systems, such as health maintenance organisations. The difference was even larger in the number of physician visits, radiological procedures, and laboratory tests. Another study[43] showed that physicians differed in their propensity to make hospital referrals, depending on practice style.

Patients' values and attitudes toward their illness are also important factors. An older patient who is aware of a need for medical help may not be motivated enough to actually seek such help. This is especially common in less developed countries where older people—even when relatively young by Western standards—are still considered "survivors" and perhaps not deserving the health care resources required for their care, given the needs of younger generations and the belief that both illness and health are God sent. This fatalism may also partly explain the disinclination observed among many elderly persons in Western societies to make use of welfare services, towards which they may even feel hostility.[44]

Preventive care need is of utmost importance in the elderly population. Periodic immunisation, cancer screening, health education, and regular check ups are not generally conditioned by health status but rather by the socioeconomic status of the patients and their awareness of the need to prevent illness and to distinguish between ageing and disease. There has been no attempt to date to quantify the effect of this factor on health services utilisation.

Various relationships described by the Andersen model have been the object of statistical exercises aimed at testing their significance by analysing and processing data drawn from different samples. A heavily used sample stems from the 1976–84 Health Interview Survey (HIS), one of the principal sources of official statistics on health services utilisation in the United States.[45] A recent study done on 1984 HIS data evaluated the impact of specific diseases on utilisation of physician and hospital services by subjects over 65 years old.[46] Five chronic diseases were chosen as predictor variables: atherosclerotic heart disease, arthritis, cancer, diabetes mellitus, and hypertension, plus a sixth item grouping "other diseases". Outcome or dependent variables were physician visits and hospital stays. Disabilities and self rated overall health status were also included in the analysis.

Using sophisticated multivariate regression procedures, the study showed the strongest predictors of physician contact to be, in order of importance, hypertension, diabetes mellitus, cancer, and atherosclerotic heart disease, the rest having each less than a 4% marginal effect. In terms of number of visits the variables were the same but ranking changed. Effects on hospital contact and number of admissions were not well predicted by these variables.

Despite these interesting results one might ask whether they fully justify the impressive array of statistical procedures mobilised to achieve them. Of note is that the coefficients of determination (R^2) calculated were not more than 0·175 for the number of physician visits (as a function of the diseases plus disability and self rated overall health status) and 0·093 for the number of hospital stays. This means that 82·5 and 90% of the two utilisation variables respectively remained "unexplained".

Another perspective

Doubts have been expressed about the usefulness of such exercises. At best, multivariate regression models based on the health behaviour framework explain 25–30% of the variance in health services utilisation.[4 26 47 48] Wolinsky and Johnson, in their 1991 study, included 23 predictor variables in their model but the results obtained were again very modest, leaving most of the health services utilisation variables unexplained. The authors reached two sobering conclusions, namely, that "we do not really know what accounts for most health services use" and that "substantial improvements in R^2 will not likely result from further refinement or proliferation of the traditional measures of the predisposing, enabling, and need characteristics."[45]

Perhaps research is better oriented toward determinants on the supply side of health services: availability of hospital beds, supply of specialist physicians and surgeons, and variations in clinical practice and professional decision making.[47 49] While one can readily understand the basis of such supply side effects, it seems a sorry conclusion if administrative and bureaucratic concerns about financing health facilities, physician omnipotence, and individual practice tastes were the decisive factors determining health service use, not the patients' illnesses and their needs. Perhaps we must not lose sight of the fact that health services have basic similarities to other kinds of services, namely, commodities with markets where both supply and demand meet to determine how and to what extent these services are being used.

Adding new variables that encompass supply side factors to the behaviour model may improve its robustness. Substitution between physician and hospital use, between outpatient and inpatient services, between acute hospitals and nursing homes, and between formal and informal services, hopefully with some clarification of the role of different disease, may be helpful in this regard. Similarly, one can readily accept the need to explore the relationships—whether reciprocal or not—between the "explanatory" variables within the same group as well as between groups. Physical illness itself is a function of several variables, some of which already appear in the behaviour model (for example, age and socioeconomic status).

Finally, a possibility that should also be envisaged and openly discussed is that no systematic model can ever satisfactorily account for health services use by older persons because there are few discernible patterns or regularities in such use, given the basic heterogeneity of the older population.[48] Reality is always more complex than any necessarily simplifying model but there is no reason to capitulate or underestimate the potential achievements of further research efforts.

Predictors of outcome

A large number of studies have examined factors predictive of hospital outcomes for elderly people in a variety of settings and health care systems.[10 12 50–62] The majority of these are summarised in table 12.7. Outcomes most often examined in these studies were mortality, length

Table 12.7 Summary of studies examining factors associated with outcomes of hospitalised elderly persons

Reference, location	Facility type	Study design	Pt age (years)	Outcomes measured	Factors associated with adverse outcomes
Isaacs, 1965 England[50]	Geriatric hospital	Historical cohort (n=522)	≥65	Mort, LOS	Incr age, male, low funct and ment status
Farrow et al, 1976 England[51]	Geriatric service	10 year desc. analysis	≥60	Mort, LOS, disch loc, 2 year living loc, rehosp	Incr age (for mort and 2 year living loc)
Glass et al, 1977 New York[52]	Medical service	Adm cohort (n=256)	x̄=60	LOS	Age >80, low funct and ment status
Hodkinson and Hodkinson, 1980 England[53]	Geriatric service	Adm cohort (n=2022)	≥70	Mort, disch home	Incr age, low ment status, "constitutional upset", dehyd, emerg adm
Kane, 1983 California[10]	11 acute hospitals	1 year historical cohort (n=23 557)	≥65	NH adm	Living loc, age, sex, dx
Lamont et al, 1983 California[54]	Med/surg services	Historical adm cohort (n=205)	≥75	LOS, NH adm	Incr age, low funct and ment status
Donaldson and Jagger, 1984 England[55]	Geriatric hospitals	Cohort (n=3916)	≥65	Mort, disch loc, 6 month living loc	Incr age, "incapacity", prior LOS
Maguire et al, 1986 N Ireland[56]	Medical service	Adm cohort (n=419)	≥70	LOS	Incr age, low funct, stroke, confusion, falls
Rubenstein et al, 1986 California[57]	Acute hospital	Adm cohort (n=1427)	≥65	Mort, LOS, NH adm, 1 year rehosp	Clinical subgroup
Wachtel et al, 1987 Rhode Island[58]	Medical service	Adm cohort (n=367)	≥65	NH adm	Prior NH residence, age, low funct and ment status
Narain et al, 1988 California[59]	Acute hospital	Adm cohort (n=396)	≥70	Mort, LOS, NH adm, 6 month rehosp, living loc	Low funct and ment status, incr age, dx, living loc
Pompei et al, 1991 New York[60]	Acute hospital	Adm cohort (n=607)	x̄=63	Mort, LOS, cost, 1 year mort	Illness severity, low funct status
Cohen et al, 1986 N Carolina[12]	Acute hospital	Adm cohort (n=167)	≥75	2 year mort	Low funct status, incr age, NH adm
Incalzi et al, 1993 Italy[61]	Acute hospital	Disch cohort (n=178)	≥70	1 year mort, rehosp, funct worsening	Low funct status, cancer, heart dis
Dunlop et al, 1993 Br Columbia[62]	Acute hospital	Surg pt adm cohort (n=8899)	≥65	Mort, LOS	Illness severity, incr age

adm, admission; desc, descriptive; dehyd, dehydration; dis, disease; disch, discharge; dx, diagnosis; emerg, emergency; funct, functional; incr, increasing; loc, location; LOS, length of stay; med/surg, medical and surgical; ment, mental; mort, mortality; NH, nursing home; pt, patient; rehosp, rehospitalisation; x̄, mean.

121

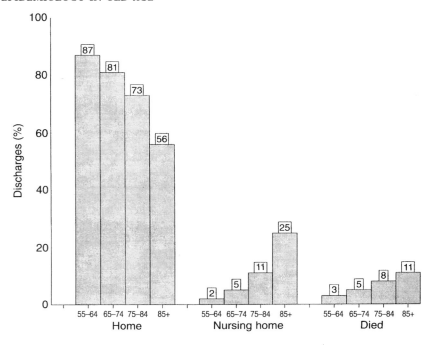

Fig 12.4   Hospital discharge locations by age for males United States 1987. (From US Department of Health and Human Services.[2])

of hospital stay, discharge location (including NH placement), re-hospitalization, and long term living location. Figure 12.4 shows us the distribution of discharges from hospital in 1987 in the United States, indicating major age effects on survival and nursing home placement.[2]

Factors most often associated with adverse hospital outcome were decreased functional status and mental status at hospital admission, advancing age, living location, illness severity, and a number of specific diagnoses (for example, stroke, heart disease, and cancer). Not surprisingly, factors most predictive of death were certain diagnoses (for example, cancer), their severity, being admitted from an NH, having impaired ADL, and mental status. Predictors of NH placement were certain diagnosis (for example, neurological problems), admission from NH, advancing age and having impaired ADL and mental status. The strongest predictor of adverse outcomes in most studies was impaired functional status, measured in a number of ways but usually including a measure of ADL.

Conclusion: the need for further international comparisons

An important though underresearched aspect of health services utilisation is the comparison of data from different countries and areas of the world.

Table 12.8   Health services utilisation among the elderly in five industrialised countries (1991)

	USA	Canada	UK	West Germany	Japan
Physician use in past six months					
None	40	31	33	14	1
Six or more	13	17	14	38	53
Mean contact	3·6	2·9	2·3	6·7	17·3
Average visit length (minutes)	30	20	14	18	12
Hospital use in past year					
Hospitalised (%)	18	18	14	16	10
Mean length of stay (days)	7	11	10	20	43

From Rowland D. A five-nation perspective on the elderly. *Health Affairs* 1992:205–16 (exhibit 4, p 211).

These comparisons can be very useful in trying to predict future trends in utilisation or possible impacts of health care reforms.

Table 12.8 compares utilisation among five industrialised countries. There are clearly major differences, and explanations are also very complex. Variations in coverage and definition in health system provision, in the standard of living, and in the cost and availability of services are among the variables to be taken into consideration. Even among societies that belong to the same culture and have similar per capita incomes, utilisation can differ widely. A wealth of information is available worldwide on service utilisation, but variability in health spectrums, socioeconomic conditions, and environmental factors makes it very difficult if not impossible to compare data and be definitive about trends and recommendations. Rather we have discrete pieces of information that may be useful for general guidelines. In coming years, with improved data sources and analytical techniques, more comprehensive conclusions should be feasible. Appropriately selected samples and international comparisons must be made to establish an international database from which researchers can start developing new theories and eventually new applications.

1 Velimirovic B. Balance between community-based and hospital-institutional care of the elderly. *Cah Sociol Demogr* 1990;**30**:509–42.
2 US Department of Health and Human Services. *Health United States, 1992.* Hyattsville, MD: USDHHS, 1993.
3 Heikkinen E, Waters WE, Brzeziriski ZJ. *The elderly in eleven countries: a sociomedical survey.* Copenhagen: WHO, 1983. (Public health in Europe No 21.)
4 Branch L, Jette A, Polansky M, Rose G, Diehr P. Toward understanding elders' health services utilization. *J Community Health* 1981;7(**2**):80–92.
5 Ouslander JG, Osterweil D. Physician evaluation and management of nursing home residents. *Ann Intern Med* 1994;**121**:584–92.
6 Boult C, Dowd B, McCaffrey D, *et al.* Screening elders for risk of hospital admission. *J Am Geriatr Soc* 1993;**41**:811–7.

7 Sirrocco A. Nursing Homes and Board and Care Homes. Data from the 1991 National Health Provider Inventory. *Advance Data from Vital and Health Statistics,* 1994;**244**.

8 *Managed care digest, long term care edition.* Kansas City: Marion Merrell Dow, 1993.

9 Suzman R, Kinsella KG, Myers GC. Demography of older populations in developed countries. In: Evans J, Williams T, editors. *Oxford textbook of geriatric medicine.* Oxford: Oxford Medical Publications, 1992: chapter 11.

10 Kane RL. The risk of placement in a nursing home after acute hospitalization. *Med Care* 1983;**21**:1055-61.

11 Greenberg J, Guin A. A multivariate analysis of the predictors of long-term care placement. *Home Health Care Serv Q* 1979;**1**:75-99.

12 Cohen MA, Tell EJ, Wallack SS. Client-related risk factors of nursing home entry among elderly adults. *J Gerontol* 1986;**41**:785-92.

13 Shapiro E, Tate RB, Roos NP. Do nursing homes reduce hospital use? *Med Care* 1987;**25**:1-8.

14 Kemper P, Murtaugh CM. Lifetime use of nursing home care. *N Engl J Med* 1991;**324**:595-60.

15 Doty P. Health status and health services use among older women—an international perspective. *World Health Stat Q* 1987;**40**:279-90.

16 Libow S, Starer P. Care of the nursing home patient. *N Engl J Med* 1989;**321**:93-6.

17 Salive ME, Collins KS, Foley DJ, George LK. Predictors of nursing home admission in a biracial population. *Am J Public Health* 1993;**83**:1765-7.

18 Murtaugh CM, Kemper P, Spillman BC. The risk of nursing home use in later life. *Med Care* 1990;**28**:952-62.

19 Wallace SP. The political economy of health care for elderly blacks. *Int J Health Serv* 1990;**20**:665-80.

20 Headen AE. Time costs and informal social support as determinants of differences between black and white families in the provision of long-term care. *Inquiry* 1992;**29**:440-50.

21 Miskelly FG, Subhani JM. Who needs a nursing home? A simple and effective screening test. *Br J Clin Pract* 1993;**47**:289-91.

22 Nygaard HA, Albrektsen G. Risk factors for admission to a nursing home. A study of elderly people receiving home nursing. *Scand J Prim Health Care* 1992;**10**:128-33.

23 Steinback U. Social networks, institutionalization and mortality among elderly people in the US. *J Gerontol Soc Sci* 1992;**49**:s183-90.

24 Freedman VA, Berkman LF, Rapp SR, Ostfeld AM. Family networks: predictors of nursing home entry. *Am J Public Health* 1994;**84**:843-5.

25 Wolinsky FD, Callahan CM, Fitzgerald JF, Johnson RJ. The risk of nursing home placement and subsequent death among older adults. *J Gerontol Soc Sci* 1992;**47**:s173-182.

26 Shapiro E, Kate R. Who is really at risk of institutionalization? *Gerontologist* 1988;**28**:237-45.

27 Evashwick C, Rowe G, Diehr P, Branch L. Factors explaining the use of health care services by the elderly. *Health Serv Res* 1984;**19(3)**:357-82.

28 Organisation for Economic Cooperation and Development. *New direction in care.* Paris: OECD, 1994. (Social policy studies, No 14.)

29 Hawe P, Gebski V, Andrews G. Elderly patients after they leave hospital. *Med J Aust* 1986;**145(6)**:251-4.

30 Davis JW, Shapiro MF, Kane RL. Level of care and complications among geriatric patients discharged from the medical services of a teaching hospital. *J Am Geriatr Soc* 1984;**32**:427-30.

31 Daatland SO. Use of public services for the aged and the role of the family. *Gerontologist* 1983;**23**:650-6.

32 Herman JM, Culpepper L, Franks P. Patterns of utilization, disposition and length of stay among stroke patients in a community hospital setting. *J Am Geriatr Soc* 1984;**32**:421-6.

33 Solomon DH, Wagner DR, Marenberg ME, *et al.* Predictors of formal home health care use in elderly patients after hospitalization. *J Am Geriatr Soc* 1993;**41**:961-6.

34 Bloom BS, Soper KA. Health and medical care for the elderly and aged population: the state of the evidence. *J Am Geriatr Soc* 1980;**28**:451-5.

35 Victor CR, Vetter NJ. The early readmission of the elderly to hospital. *Age Ageing* 1985;**14**:37-42.

36 Weissert WG. The national channeling demonstration: what we knew, know now, and still need to know. *Health Serv Res* 1986;**23**:175-87.

37 Denson P. *Tracing the elderly through the health care system*. Washington: Agency for Health Care Policy Research, 1991.

38 Andersen RM, Newman J. Societal and individual determinants of medical care utilization in the United States. *Milbank Mem Fund Q* 1973;51:95–124.

39 Aday LA, Andersen RM. A framework for the study of access to medical care. *Health Serv Res* 1974;9:208–20.

40 Ettinger WH, Fried LP, Harris T, *et al.* Self-reported causes of physical disability in older people: the cardiovascular health study. *J Am Geriatr Soc* 1994;42:1035–44.

41 Eisenberg JM. Physician utilization. The state of research about physician's practice patterns. *Med Care* 1985;23:461–83.

42 Broomberg J, Price MA. The impact of the fee-for-service reimbursement system on the utilization of health services. *S Afr Med J* 1990;78(3):130–2, 133–6.

43 Roos NP. Predicting hospital utilization by the elderly. The importance of patient, physician and hospital characteristics. *Med Care* 1989;27:905–19.

44 Ozaura MN, Marrow-Howell N. Service utilization by well-organized frail elderly individuals. *Int J Aging Hum Dev* 1992;35(3):179–91.

45 Wolinsky FD, Johnson RJ. The use of health services by older adults. *J Gerontol* 1991;46: S345–57.

46 Blaum CS, Liang J, Liu X. The relationship of chronic diseases and health status to the health services utilization of older Americans. *J Am Geriatr Soc* 1994;42:1087–93.

47 Nelson MA. Race, gender and the effect of social supports on the use of health services by elderly individuals. *Int J Aging Hum Dev* 1993;37(3):227–46.

48 Wolinsky FD, Arnold CL. A different perspective on health and health services utilization. *Annu Rev Gerontol Geriatr* 1988;8:71–101.

49 Morgan M, Mays N, Holland WN. Can hospital use be a measure of need for health care? *J Epidemiol Community Health* 1987;41:269–74.

50 Isaacs B. Prognostic factors in elderly patients in a geriatric institution. *Gerontol Clin* 1965; 7:202–15.

51 Farrow SC, Rablen MR, Silver CP. Geriatric admissions in east London 1962–72. *Age Ageing* 1976;5:49.

52 Glass RI, Mulvihill MN, Smith H, *et al.* The 4 score: an index for predicting a patient's non-medical hospital days. *Am J Public Health* 1977;67:751.

53 Hodkinson HM, Hodkinson I. Death and discharge from a geriatric department. *Age Ageing* 1980;9:220–8.

54 Lamont CT, Sampson S, Matthias R, *et al.* The outcome of hospitalization for acute illness in the elderly. *J Am Geriatr Soc* 1983;31:284.

55 Donaldson LJ, Jagger C. Outcomes of admissions of elderly people to hospitals and homes. *Public Health* 1984;98:270–6.

56 Maguire PA, Taylor IC, Stout RW. Elderly patients in acute medical wards: factors predicting length of stay. *BMJ* 1986;292:1251–3.

57 Rubenstein LZ, Josephson KR, Wieland GD, *et al.* Differential prognosis and utilization patterns among clinical subgroups of hospitalized geriatric patients. *Health Serv Res* 1986; 20:881–95.

58 Wachtel TJ, Fulton JP, Goldfarb J. Early prediction of discharge disposition after hospitalization. *Gerontologist* 1987;27:98–103.

59 Narain P, Rubenstein LZ, Wieland GD, *et al.* Predictors of immediate and 6-month outcomes in hospitalized elderly patients: the importance of functional status. *J Am Geriatr Soc* 1988;36:775–83.

60 Pompei P, Charlson ME, Ales K, *et al.* Relating patient characteristics at the time of admission to outcomes of hospitalization. *J Clin Epidemiol* 1991;44:1063–9.

61 Incalzi A, Gemma A, Capparella O, *et al.* Post-operative electrolyte imbalance: incidence and prognostic implications. *Age Ageing* 1993;22:325–31.

62 Dunlop WE, Rosenblood L, Lawrason L, *et al.* Effects of age and severity of illness on outcome and length of stay in geriatric surgical patients. *Am J Surg* 1993;165:577–80.

13 Community care

DAVID CHALLIS

Burden of care in the community

Similar pressures are evident upon the pattern of care of elderly people in many different countries, arising from the demographic pressures of an ageing population. Associated with this are the demands from age related conditions such as dementia. In the face of such "demand" pressures there is a common perception that previous patterns of care, particularly those for the very frail, based upon institutional solutions, are inappropriate and unsustainable. In countries as diverse as Australia, Sweden, Japan, the United States, and the United Kingdom the trend is to reduce reliance upon institutional care, placing a greater emphasis upon home based care, with improved coordination and care management to ensure that home care is deployed to best effect. The extent of the reliance on institutional forms of care varies markedly in different countries. To provide a comparison of the populations in institutional care in different countries gives an indication of the difference in the balance of care. The provision of such data is, however, by no means easy. This is due to variations in three factors. Firstly, there are differences in the definitions of institutional long term care used in the compilation of figures, including whether or not psychiatric beds are included; secondly, there are differences as to whether the rates are for age 60, 65, or 70; and, thirdly, there are differences as to which year the figures are available for. Table 13.1 none the less provides some comparative data.

The new policy in many countries has stressed the support of carers, reflecting a perception that to do so represents an investment if home care is to be effective. In the United Kingdom, estimates indicate that there are 6 million carers, of whom about three quarters look after a person aged 65 years and over. Two thirds of those providing intensive support are women, the remainder are generally men caring for their wives.[1] One major area of concern has been the effects of a shift in the balance of care towards the community in terms of stress and burdens upon carers of frail elderly people.

Structure, process, and outcome of community services

The pattern of provision in the United Kingdom reflects the 1971 and 1974 reforms of the social services and NHS respectively. The services of

126

Table 13.1   Populations in institutional care in different countries

Country	Institutional care (%)	Age (years)	Year
Australia[a]	9·7	70+	1988
Japan[b]	3·5*	65+	1986
Netherlands[c]	11·4	65+	1985
Sweden[c]	7·6	65+	1985
United Kingdom[d]	5·9	65+	1991
USA[e]	4·9†	65+	1989

* Including long stay patients in acute hospitals adds about another 2·4%.
† Resident in nursing homes.
[a] Department of Health, Housing, and Community Services. *Aged care reform strategy: mid term review 1990–91. Report.* Canberra: Australian Government Publishing Service, 1991.
[b] Tsuji T. An overview of health and welfare policies. In: Okazi Y, Tsuji T, Otomo E, Hayakawa K, Ibe H, Furuse T, editors. *Responding to the needs of an ageing society.* Tokyo: Foreign Press Centre, 1990.
[c] Kraan RJ, Baldock J, Davies B, *et al. Care for the elderly in three European countries.* Boulder, CO: Campus, 1991.
[d] Laing, Buisson. *Laing's review of private healthcare 1994.* London: Laing and Buisson, 1994.
[e] Rowland D, Lyons B. The elderly population in need of home care. In: Rowland D, Lyons B. *Financing home care: improving protection for disabled elderly people.* Baltimore: Johns Hopkins University Press, 1991.

local authority health departments—social workers, home helps, meals services, and day centres—became the responsibility of the then newly established social services departments; health care provision, such as community nursing, was transferred to the district health authorities. A clear separation of health and social care in organisational terms was created. There was not so great a separation in Northern Ireland where social services and health were part of integrated health and social services boards. Two main criticisms of this pre-1993 service system in the United Kingdom were that it was unable to provide sufficiently intensive and coordinated care to offer an alternative to institutional care, and that support to carers was lacking.

The current framework for community care was established in the 1990 NHS and Community Care Act and fully introduced in April 1993. The background for this lay in the rapid growth of residential and nursing home care in the 1980s. Entry to these homes was not determined by professional assessment of need but by the eligibility of the potential resident for financial support. Income support payments to people in these homes rose, at 1990 prices, from £33 million in 1980 to £1390 million in 1990.[2] In the face of growing needs arising from an ageing population the only substantial source of funds available for care was through the social security system, which enabled elderly people to enter private residential and nursing homes. Conversely, resources to develop home based care were restrained as part of an overall policy to reduce public spending. The Audit Commission

127

identified the perverse incentives created by this system of funding and criticised the organisational fragmentation and failure to match resources to need in community care.[3] The government appointed Sir Roy Griffiths to report upon possible solutions for community care. His report recommended a more coordinated approach to the funding and management of care, placing the responsibility for allocation of funds, assessment of need, and coordination of care with the local authority social services department. Care management was proposed to ensure a more effective use of resources.[4]

The majority of these recommendations were endorsed in the white paper *Caring for People* in 1989. This document identified six key objectives for community care as shown in box 13.1. The proposals meant a radical change in the nature of community care in the United Kingdom. The changes in responsibilities and funding are shown in box 13.2. The social services department was to act as a "lead agency" to coordinate assessment and act as the single source of public funding for the social care of elderly people. This was designed to provide an incentive for the development of alternative and less costly community care options. Social services departments were expected to appoint staff to act as care managers, to decide, on the basis of assessment, what combination of services best suits the needs and circumstances of an elderly person, and to monitor and review the quality of care provided. Greater coherence and specificity is given to the policy, compared with previous developments, as a result of the detailed guidance on different aspects of implementation issued to social service and health authorities. A greater diversity of provision, a

---

Box 13.1—Objectives of United Kingdom community care policy

- To promote the development of domiciliary, day, and respite services to enable people to live in their own homes wherever feasible and sensible
- To ensure that service providers make practical support for carers a high priority
- To make proper assessment of need and good case management the cornerstone of high quality care
- To promote the development of a flourishing independent sector alongside good quality public services
- To clarify the responsibilities of agencies and so to make it easier to hold them to account for their performance
- To secure better value for taxpayers' money by introducing a new funding structure for social care

Caring for People. London: HMSO, 1989. (Cmnd 849, para. 1.11)

Box 13.2—Main changes in service organisation in United Kingdom community care policy

- Local authority social service departments to be responsible, in collaboration with medical, nursing, and other interests, for assessing individual need, designing care arrangements, and securing their delivery within available resources. Assessment would be undertaken both for people seeking day and domiciliary care services and for those seeking admission to publicly funded residential and nursing home care. These activities would include the appointment of care managers for individuals such as the vulnerable elderly when it was appropriate
- A new funding structure placing responsibility for the financial support for those who enter residential care with the local authority, through its social services department, who would have to assess their need for such a placement. The social security funds spent upon residential care were to be transferred to the local authorities
- Local authorities will be expected to make maximum use of the independent sector in providing care services
- Local authorities will produce and publish clear plans for the development of community care services in their areas

---

mixed economy of welfare, is expected to develop and the public social services are expected to move from the role of monopoly provider into that of the "enabling authority" who, through purchasing, contracting, and planning, will not only be providers in a market but will also be those who create a market of care services that takes account of local needs and demands.

In this context of change, consideration of services and their efficacy must look back to provide a baseline, and forward to desired goals and shifts in the pattern of provision.

Border disputes

Arising from the community care reforms, border disputes revolve over which agency (health or social care) is responsible for providing long term care. The reduction in traditional long stay hospital beds is particularly contentious. Patterns of provision often reflect a balance between hospital care and residential care that owes more to historical accident and less to the rational allocation of roles between agencies. In the community there has been difficulty in discriminating between health and social care interventions in the provision of personal care. Implicit in the new reforms is a distinction between acute and chronic care, although it is never made fully explicit. In the Swedish reforms for care of the elderly this is explicit, with a mix of health and social care staff in each sector to undertake the different responsibilities of acute and long term care. Although boundary problems remain, the Swedish distinction is probably more comprehensible to all parties.

Patterns of service use

Numerous studies of community based services have been undertaken, often on a local basis, and substantial reviews exist; these will be cited here.[5 6]

Home help

Home help is the most frequently used service, provided to about 3% of people aged 65–74 and 18% of those aged 75 and over.[6] The most likely recipients of home help are those living alone, the very old and disabled, those in receipt of benefits, those in social classes IV and V, those not owning their own homes, and those with poorer quality housing. Other things being equal, men are more likely to receive help than women. Variations in levels of provision across England are substantial. Throughout the 1980s, policies have been designed to focus home help services more upon the most dependent elderly people and concomitantly to shift the balance from household activities towards more personal care. A study of the targeting of home care indicated that underprovision of care was a larger problem than inappropriate allocation. Between 1980 and 1985, increases in home care provision did not lead to an increase in provision for the most needy but rather spread the service more widely.[7]

There is little evidence about the growing range of private home care services. One estimate is that about 16% of retired households purchased private domestic help.[6] The growth of this sector and the use of it by local authorities after 1993 would suggest that the number receiving some or all of their home assistance from this source is considerably higher.

Community nursing

Community nurses have been estimated to spend about 90% of their time with patients over the age of 65. The level of provision in different areas varied from just over two to six per thousand over 65.[8] The balance of activities appeared to be that 40% of time was spent in technical nursing activities, such as injections, other nursing tasks took up 38% of the time, and advice, reassurance, and education 17% of time. The overlap with the work of home helps was greater for nursing auxiliaries, particularly as the former have moved towards undertaking personal care.[9] Patterns of contact with the social services appear to be markedly less effective with social services staff than with general practitioners, which is indicative of problems for integrated community care.

Meals on wheels

Home delivered meals are received by about 5% of those over the age of 75 and 1% of those aged 65–74. In common with home help, meals appear more likely to be received by those living alone, those who are housebound, and by men. The range of other meal provision beyond the traditional meals service has increased in recent years.

Day care

Day care has been notoriously difficult to define and there is enormous variety in the type, scale, and form of provision in different areas. About 4% of those aged 65–74 and 7% of those over 75 appear to use day care.[6] As with most services, receipt of day care appears to be associated with living alone and being over the age of 75.

Major trends in the provision of services have occurred during the 1980s, shifting the balance away from community care (fig 13.1).

Efficacy of community services

Evidence suggests that community services, particularly the most frequently used ones of home help and community nursing, are valued by those who receive them. Major issues include intensity and whether or not the services as organised and provided offer sufficient support to act as an alternative to institutional care. Critiques of community services have identified the problems as a mismatch between needs and resources, the inadequacy of appropriate initial assessment, and the lack of monitoring and review procedures. Domiciliary services appear to lack sufficient resources, provide low levels of help to individual cases, offer inflexible forms of provision, which do not reflect client's needs, and lack integration.[56] The lack of services oriented to carers has also been the cause of longstanding criticism of community services and is expected to be one of the areas for reorientation. The shift to community based care has required a focus upon intensity, avoidance of misplacement, coordinated care, and improved support for carers in the United Kingdom and in other countries.

Achieving better value for money

An underlying concern of the policy shifts in many countries has been to substitute at the margin more costly modes of care by less costly approaches—a strategy described in the Netherlands as "downward substitution". Three elements are important in this: alternative homes, enhanced home care, and care management and coordination.

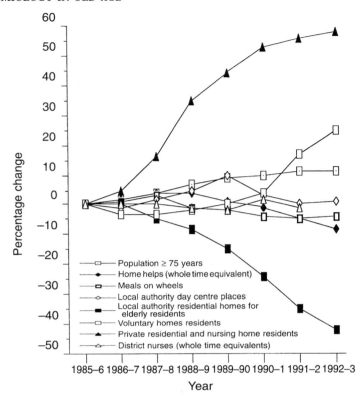

*Fig 13.1 Changes in community services, residential care, and population aged over 75 years: England 1985–1993. (Reproduced with permission from Impallomini M, Starr J. The UK Community Care Act (1990) and the elderly. Lancet 1994:**334**:1230. Copyright by the Lancet Ltd, 1994).*

Alternative homes

Although community care policies may be seen as downward substitution from institutional to home based care, more differentiated forms of sheltered housing have emerged in which care is also part of this process. Specialised nursing homes appear to offer a higher quality of care than long stay hospital care, at no greater cost.[10][11]

Enhanced home care

Studies have cast doubt upon whether a greater level of provision of home care as currently organised is sufficient to offer a realistic alternative to institutional care.[6][12] Reflecting this doubt there has been considerable interest in attempts to develop innovations in home care, offering more extensive forms of home support, providing long term care for the purpose

132

of freeing acute hospital beds by earlier discharge, and reducing the number of hospital long term care beds.

One form of enhanced home care has focused upon the need to assist in the discharge from acute hospital beds of elderly patients who experience social problems, or to prevent early readmission. A number of studies have been undertaken and successful outcomes appear to be associated with more focused services targeted upon those identified as being at risk and providing both domestic and personal care.[13 14]

A second focus of enhanced home care has been provision of more intensive long term care at home. Examples include an intensive home nursing and augmented home care service, providing up to 21 hours per week of home help, as an alternative to hospital care. Despite cost variations due to accommodation, it appeared on average to be a less costly alternative to long stay care for mentally intact but physically disabled elderly people, particularly those living with others.[15] Other intensive home care and respite services appear to indicate that, where such provision is effective, a degree of substitution of hospital beds or community nursing is possible from increased social care expenditure.[6 16] Even if such services are cost effective overall, from an individual agency perspective this may, however, not be the case because higher costs are incurred by the social services to reduce the provision of health services.

Care management

One important strand of British community care policy is designed to reduce inappropriate placement of publicly funded clients in nursing homes and residential care homes. Coordination of care for the more vulnerable individuals by care managers is designed to offer home care as an alternative to institutional long term care. Some of the earliest studies of care management for elderly people in the United Kingdom were the Personal Social Services Research Unit studies of care management in social care, primary care, and geriatric care settings.[9 17–19] The last also involved the use of multipurpose care workers who spanned the role of home help, nursing aide, and therapy aide. These were intensive forms of care management designed to provide frail elderly people with an alternative to admission to institutional care. Control of resources was devolved, within an overall cost framework, to individual care managers to permit more flexible responses to needs and the integration of fragmented services into a more coherent package of care.

These studies[9 17–19] indicated that care managers with greater budgetary flexibility were able to respond more creatively so that difficult care problems could be more effectively managed at home. The need for admission to institutional care for vulnerable elderly people was reduced. Table 13.2 indicates the greater probability of remaining at home and lower probability of entering institutional care over one year for recipients of the intensive care management studies. There were marked improvements in the levels of satisfaction of elderly people and their carers, and these were achieved at no greater cost to the social services, health service, or society as a whole.

It would appear that enhanced home care, in combination with intensive care management, offers a strategy for the pursuit of a degree of downward substitution in care. The extent of the shift in the balance of care desired between institutional and community settings in different countries and the cost of achieving this will, however, be likely to vary according to the initial levels of institutional care, as indicated in table 13.1. The likely cost and resource commitment of a percentage point shift towards home based care in the Netherlands, dealing with lower dependency percentile groups, is likely to be less than a percentage point shift in the United Kingdom or the United States. Hence there is the potential of diminishing returns and higher costs of change in the balance of care at different levels. Further, if policy is designed to bring about shifts there will need to be some indication of when that appropriate balance has been reached, which is a policy question requiring the contribution of systematic and possibly cross national, cost effectiveness studies.

Table 13.2   Care management studies: one year outcomes—percentage difference between experimental (E) and comparison (C) groups (E − C)

	Kent social care	Gateshead social care	Gateshead primary care	Darlington geriatric care
Own home	35	27	43	47
Residential nursing home	− 15	− 38	− 42	− 12
Hospital	− 1	3	− 4	− 45
Died	− 19	8	3	9

From Challis and Davies[17] and Challis et al.[9 18 19]

Research priorities for community care

Community care poses a range of research priorities, by no means all of them new; however, whenever new structural and administrative changes emerge there is a great deal of descriptive research. None the less, the "who gets what, with what consequences?" questions, cited as priorities over 10 years ago, still remain important in the new environment. Three other themes are likely to be important.

Carers have been shown to be a crucial element of community care and, whereas many studies have described the stresses and difficulties, there is a need for studies of the impact of different service responses upon carers in different circumstances.

Care management and assessment have been identified as the cornerstones of community care and the delineation of the different forms of these and the relative efficiency and effectiveness of each in providing long term care will be important in the evaluation of alternative approaches.

Related to the above is the degree to which health and social care services may jointly contribute to care management. The role of secondary health care services is particularly important here because the community care reforms in the United Kingdom do not allot them a specific role. This can be compared with Australia where geriatric assessment teams have a crucial role to play, both in screening elderly people for publicly funded places in residential and nursing homes and in some areas for care management.[9]

Finally, beyond the immediate health and social care context, provision of community care raises questions of funding, the effect of potentially catastrophic costs of entry to long term care, and the role of insurance and other means of broadening funding to match the new "mixed economy of care".[20]

1 Green H. *Informal carers: a study carried out on behalf of the Department of Health and Social Security as part of the 1985 general household survey.* London: HMSO, 1988.
2 Darton R, Wright K. Changes in the provision of long-stay care, 1970–1990. *Health Soc Care* 1993;1:11–25.
3 Audit Commission. *Making a reality of community care.* London: HMSO, 1986.
4 Griffiths R. *Community care: agenda for action.* London: HMSO, 1988.
5 Goldberg EM, Connelly N. *The effectiveness of social care.* London: Heinemann, 1982.
6 Sinclair I, Parker R, Leat D, Williams J. *The kaleidoscope of care.* London: HMSO, 1990.
7 Bebbington AC, Davies BP. Efficient targeting of community care: the case of the home help service. *J Soc Policy* 1993;22:373–91.
8 Dunnell K, Dobbs J. *Nurses working in the community.* London: HMSO, 1982.
9 Challis D, Darton R, Johnson L, Stone M, Traske K. *Care management and health care of older people.* Aldershot: Arena, Ashgate, 1994.
10 Bond S, Bond J. Outcomes of care within a multiple case study in the evaluation of the experimental National Health Service nursing homes. *Age Ageing* 1990;19:11–8.
11 Donaldson C, Bond J. Cost of continuing care facilities in the evaluation of experimental National Health Service nursing homes. *Age Ageing* 1991;20:160–8.
12 Davies BP, Bebbington A, Charnley H, Ferlie E, Hughes M, Twigg J. *Resources, needs and outcomes in community care.* Aldershot: Gower, 1990.
13 Townsend J, Piper M, Frank A, Dyer S, North W, Meade T. Reduction in hospital readmission stay of elderly patients by a community-based hospital discharge scheme: a randomised controlled trial. *BMJ* 1988;297:544–7.
14 Martin F, Oyewole A, Moloney A. A randomised controlled trial of a high support hospital discharge team for elderly people. *Age Ageing* 1994;23:228–34.
15 Gibbins FJ, Lee M, Davison P, et al. Augmented home nursing as an alternative to hospital care for chronic elderly invalids. *BMJ* 1982;284:330–3.
16 Donaldson C, Gregson B. Prolonging life at home: what is the cost? *Community Med* 1989;11:200–9.
17 Challis D, Davies B. *Case management in community care.* Aldershot: Gower, 1986.
18 Challis D, Chessum R, Chesterman J, Luckett R, Traske K. *Case management in social and health care.* Canterbury: PSSRU, University of Kent, 1990.
19 Challis D, Darton R, Johnson L, Stone M, Traske K. An evaluation of an alternative to long stay hospital care for the frail elderly: part II costs and outcomes. *Age Ageing* 1991;20:245–54.
20 Laing W. *Financing long-term care: the crucial debate.* London: Age Concern, 1993.

14 Value of screening in old age

IAIN CARPENTER

Definitions of screening

The value of screening has frequently been a subject of debate, and its value in old age is no exception. Multiple pathology is common in older people, yet problems are often attributed to age rather than medical illness, and admissions to institutions are frequently precipitated for "social" reasons. Length of stay in hospital is longer than for younger people and discharge is often delayed—also for "social" reasons. It has been shown that many admissions to institutions for long term residential or nursing care could have been avoided if the problems had been addressed more effectively and/or sooner.

Screening has been presented as the solution to these problems, yet its efficacy remains controversial. A proper understanding of the issues is helpful and one must be clear about what screening is and what has been carried out in the name of screening. "Screening is the detection of asymptomatic disease, for example early breast cancer, or the precursor of disease, for example high blood pressure or carcinoma in situ. The screening test itself is usually not definitive, indicating only an increased probability of disease and requiring further investigations to confirm the diagnosis."[1] Distinguishing screening from other activities aimed at identifying problems with the elderly is also helpful.

- *Screening* is a form of secondary prevention, namely, the search for a precursor disease in those who do not have the symptoms of the disease and who believe themselves to be free of it
- *Case finding* is a form of tertiary prevention in which established disease and resultant disability are sought in order to achieve earlier diagnosis and thus create better prospects for care (or alleviation) and rehabilitation[2]
- *Opportunistic case finding* is the systematic searching, at an opportunity presented by a consultation, for established disease and resultant disability other than that for which the consultation was intended
- *Assessment* is the formal means of examining the health status of a person against expected norms.

136

Brief history

The first "consultative clinic" for older people was developed by Ferguson Anderson in 1955.[3] In 1964 Williamson *et al* demonstrated that old people frequently had many physical and medical problems that were not known to their doctor, which patients may have been attributing to the normal effect of ageing and at least some of which were remediable.[4] These findings were repeated on many occasions but the costs of the programmes were high and the benefits not demonstrated beyond reports that the old people appreciated and valued the interest in their problems.

Attempts to reduce costs included using health visitors or district nurses, but they remained high because of the time required to assess all people over 75 in a given practice. A variety of other methods for screening and case finding have been developed, some of which cover the entire elderly population, while others try to identify groups at higher risk.[5] The identification of old people at risk is, however, not as simple as it might seem. Taylor *et al* found that visiting the 37% of the over 75 population responding to four of 10 questions on a postal questionnaire identified 83% of all "cases", a much higher yield than that of visiting those on a more conventional risk factor list.[6]

The issue

There seemed to be a paradox: people were admitted to hospitals and other institutions with remediable problems but attempts at early identification and remedy of the problems to prevent admission did not bring any identifiable benefit. Many of the problems identified by screening were chronic, irremediable, or of minor importance, or simply not medical. Attention to the processes that have been employed in the name of screening has helped to understand what is going on.

Recently the word "assessment" has become more widely used in this context, and comprehensive geriatric assessment (CGA) is the term that best describes the procedures that are commonly understood as screening and case finding. Under the banner of CGA some screening procedures, some case finding, and some review of existing known problems is carried out. Applying criteria described by Wilson and Jungner[7] before embarking upon a screening programme will help avoid many of the pitfalls (box 14.1).

The United Kingdom Department of Health contract for general practitioners (family physicians) requires annual health checks (social assessment, mobility, mental status, hearing and vision, continence, general functional assessment, and review of medication) of people over 75 years old.[8] This has been interpreted by general practitioners as screening, and in the absence of any clear evidence to show that screening is worthwhile

---

Box 14.1—Criteria for screening[7]

- The condition sought should pose an important health problem
- The natural history of the disease should be understood
- There should be a recognisable early stage
- Treatment of the disease at an early stage should be of more benefit than treatment started at a later stage
- There should be a suitable test
- The test should be acceptable to the population
- There should be adequate facilities for the diagnosis and treatment of abnormalities detected
- For diseases of insidious onset screening should be repeated at intervals determined by the natural history of the disease
- The chance of physical or psychological harm to those screened should be less than the chance of benefit
- The cost of the screening programme should be balanced against the benefit that it provides

---

has cast doubt on the exercise. The contract does not, however, say "screening"; it refers to a home visit and assessment, although it does not say how this should be carried out.

Screening

There is a number of conditions for which screening—"the search for a precursor disease in those who don't have the symptoms of the disease and who believe themselves to be free of it"—is now accepted to be of potential benefit in older people. These conditions are hypertension, cervical cancer, and breast cancer. Screening for colorectal cancer may soon be added to this list but the benefits/effectiveness remain to be demonstrated.

Hypertension

There is a strong relationship between raised blood pressure and mortality from stroke and myocardial infarction, systolic hypertension being apparently more important. Despite original scepticism, recent studies have demonstrated clear benefits in reducing hypertension in the elderly. This subject is discussed in more detail in chapter 26.

Cervical cancer

Women aged over 65 who have had regular negative cervical smears do not appear to benefit from continuing screening, but women over 65 who have never had a cervical smear should have triennial smears for several years.[9]

138

Breast cancer

Screening for breast cancer has demonstrated efficacy, with growing evidence of a cumulative effect from monthly breast self examination, yearly examination by a physician, and biennial mammography[10] (see chapter 34).

Colorectal cancer

Colorectal cancer is more common in older age groups, but effective screening for the disease is not simple or cheap. Faecal occult blood screening may detect 17% of expected cancers at a cost of $35 000 per year of life saved, and periodic sigmoidoscopy may be undertaken at a cost of between $43 000 and $47 000 per year of life saved.[11] Where there is a history of two or more first degree relatives with a history of colorectal cancer the benefits of screening are much higher and regular colonoscopy is indicated.

Comprehensive assessment

If one considers the breakdown of living at home or the admission to institution for long term residential or nursing care as the "disease", then an "asymptomatic" phase is recognisable. Increasing dependency—"the effect that a set of disabilities has on making a person dependent on the care of others"—is a recognised precursor of admission. If increasing dependency (the precursor) is the focus of screening, one may be able to avert the admission (the disease). Comprehensive assessment of older people (the screening test) leading to optimised treatment of identified problems has been the major contribution of geriatrics to medicine. The question is how to apply the principle in different settings at reasonable cost and provide useful results. It is probable that this can be achieved by adjusting the intensity of effort according to the likelihood of identifying remediable problems.

There are a variety of ways of carrying out comprehensive assessment. History has shown that examination and blood tests are not cost effective at this stage, but that a structured interview or questionnaire may be. Methods include postal questionnaires, regular home visiting with a structured conversation, and opportunistic case finding at general practitioner consultation.

Postal and self completed questionnaires

First used in 1979,[12] questionnaires and self completed instruments have been used frequently and there is evidence that they are a reliable way of gaining information about the health of elderly people.[13] Barber and Wallis's questionnaire identified too many people—a high false positive rate—to be

139

cost effective on a large scale.[12] Pathy *et al* found that a questionnaire focusing on function, with follow up by a specially appointed nurse, favourably influenced outcome and use of health care resources.[14]

Regular home visiting

Regular home visiting by qualified health professionals can be expensive, especially when clinical examination is undertaken. Visits that have been focused on a structured interview (without examination) covering health and social factors have, however, shown benefits,[15] even when unqualified personnel have undertaken the interview as a simple screening exercise.[16]

Opportunistic case finding

Opportunistic case finding has been described as a potentially effective way of identifying unreported health problems. This argument is based on the fact that old people do not "underconsult": 80–90% of people aged over 75 see their general practitioner at least once a year,[17 18] and those that do not are generally well.[19 20] Older people report their medical conditions, chronic or common acute ailments, to their doctor at least as frequently as younger people.[21] By asking questions about a list of topics not directly related to the problem for which a person is seeing the doctor, other problems which may require attention can be identified and appropriately managed. There have been no controlled trials of opportunistic case finding.

Content of the assessment

While there is still no standard list or structure for the content of comprehensive assessment questionnaires, the areas that should be covered include social contacts, mobility, foot care, hearing, vision, nutrition, dentition, continence, personal hygiene, mood, cognitive function, review of medication, house safety, awareness of welfare services, awareness of benefits, and availability and health of carers. Assessment should be structured so that repeated assessments can be compared.

Evidence of efficacy

A meta-analysis by Stuck *et al* studied the effect on mortality, living at home, hospital (re)admissions, and physical and cognitive function in 28 controlled trials of CGA in a variety of settings.[22] The trials were divided into five groups, geriatric evaluation and management units (GEMU), inpatient geriatric consultation services (IGCS), home assessment service (HAS), hospital home assessment service (HHAS), and outpatient assessment service (OAS) (box 14.2). They found that GEMU and HAS programmes reduced mortality, and GEMU, HAS, and HHAS programmes had a favourable effect on living location. All CGA types reduced hospital (re)admission (although four of six HAS programmes showed no significant effect), and only GEMU had a beneficial effect on physical function. Only seven of the 28 studies included an evaluation of cognitive function; of these, GEMU and IGCS programmes showed a benefit, with HHAS and OAS having no effect (table 14.1).

Box 14.2—Five settings for comprehensive geriatric assessment (CGA)[22]

- Geriatric evaluation and management units (GEMU)
- Inpatient geriatric consultation services (IGCS)

- Home assessment service (HAS)

- Hospital home assessment service (HHAS)
- Outpatient assessment service (OAS)

Designated inpatient units for elderly care
CGA provided on a consultative basis to hospitalised patients in non-designated units
In home CGA for community dwelling elderly persons
In home CGA for patients recently discharged from hospital
CGA provided in an outpatient setting

Table 14.1   *Benefit of different types of comprehensive geriatric assessment programme[22]*

Programme type	Mortality	Hospital (re)admission	Living at home	Physical function
GEMU	√	√	√	√
IGCS	√	√	X	X
HAS*	√	√	√	X
HHAS	X	√	√	X
OAS	X	√	X	X

√ Benefit demonstrated.
X No benefit demonstrated.
* Four out of six studies showed no effect.

The analysis included an examination of the effect of a number of covariates:

- Medical control over CGA recommendations
- Ambulatory follow up
- Exclusion of too healthy subjects
- Exclusion of subjects with poor prognosis.

Of these, "medical control over CGA recommendations" was associated with improved mortality and living location, and "ambulatory follow up" with reduced mortality in GEMU and improved physical function in the

141

combined institution based programmes (GEMU and IGCS). "Exclusion of too healthy subjects" was correlated with improved outcome in only one case (living at home for institution based studies at six months). Exclusion of subjects with poor prognosis did not show an association with effects.

These findings suggest that case finding without follow up may be less effective than CGA with follow up.

Identifying but not treating

Identifying unreported disease is not in itself a useful end. There is little point in identifying problems that will not benefit from further intervention because they are irremediable or because there are insufficient resources for the remedy, and it would be unreasonable to raise expectations in such circumstances. Regular home visiting with a structured interview may, however, change perceptions of health in old age and prompt people to ask for aids or help when otherwise they may have accepted the changes as inevitable. Frequently the assistance required is small, non-medical, and may be as simple as arranging for a higher chair, making getting up to go to the toilet a much easier task which "cures" incontinence of urine.

Priorities for research

The Medical Research Council (UK) is currently conducting a large scale trial of screening of the elderly in the community, which will make a significant contribution, examining the cost effectiveness of a number of methods of screening and follow up. There remain large gaps, however, particularly in the study of the effectiveness of screening for and treatment of depression and the early diagnosis of dementia, both of which are more common with increasing age. Depression is associated with increased resources for support, and they both increase the burden on informal carers.

A sound analysis of the cost implications must be included in all future studies.

Summary

Preventive screening techniques are of benefit in older people when appropriately applied. Screening for breast and cervical cancer and hypertension have proven benefits; cost effectiveness of screening for colorectal cancer remains to be demonstrated.

Comprehensive assessment has demonstrated benefits. In the community it should be two tiered, with a preliminary simple screening exercise by structured interview or appropriate postal questionnaire. It is likely to be most effective where there is monitoring of the interventions recommended and when the surveillance continues. Future research should address the problems of depression and dementia and must include good economic information.

Postscript

The number of people in older age groups is increasing in almost every country in the world. By 2020 people aged 65 and over in the developing world are expected to number a minimum of 470 million, more than double the number in the developed world. In many countries this represents a threefold increase. The greatest increase in the developed world will be in the very old, who have the highest prevalence of disability. These changes are a reflection of social, economic, and medical developments, which will shift future emphasis of health and welfare programmes from cure and survival to improved functional status and wellbeing,[23] a shift that has considerable training and resource implications. In the developing world there is no existing institutional base for residential or nursing care for the elderly population, and no resources to develop one. Effective, affordable, and comprehensive assessment, addressing problems early and targeting support services where and when they are needed to maintain people in their own homes, is of ever increasing importance.

1 Muir-Gray JA. Preventing disease and promoting health in old age. In: Evans J, Williams T, editors. *Oxford textbook of geriatric medicine.* Oxford: Oxford Medical Publications, 1992:709–14.
2 Williamson J. Screening, surveillance and case-finding. In Arie T, editor. *Essays in old age.* London: Croom Helm, 1981:194–213.
3 Anderson WF, Cowan NR. A consultative health centre for older people. *Lancet* 1955;**ii**: 239–40.
4 Williamson J, Stokoe IH, Gray S, *et al.* Old people at home: their unreported needs. *Lancet* 1964;**i**:1117–20.
5 Taylor RC, Buckley EG, editors. *Preventive care of the elderly: a review of current developments.* London: Royal College of General Practitioners, 1987.
6 Taylor RC, Ford G, Barber H. *The elderly at risk: a critical review of problems and progress in screening and case finding.* London: Age Concern, 1983.
7 Wilson JMC, Jungner G. *Principles and practice of screening for disease.* Geneva: WHO, 1968. (Public health paper, No 28.)
8 Department of Health. *General practice in the national health service: a new contract.* London: DoH, 1989.
9 Fahs MC, Mandelblatt J, Schechter C, Muller C. Cost effectiveness of cervical cancer screening for the elderly. *Ann Intern Med* 1992;**117**:520–7.
10 Robie PW. Cancer screening in the elderly. *J Am Geriatr Soc* 1989;**37**:888–93.
11 Wagner JL, Herdman RC, Wadwa S. Cost effectiveness of colo-rectal cancer screening in the elderly. *Ann Intern Med* 1991;**115**:807–17.
12 Barber JH, Wallis JB. A postal screening questionnaire in preventive geriatric care. *J R Coll Gen Pract* 1978;**30**:49–51.
13 Pannil FC. A patient completed screening instrument for functional disability in the elderly. *Am J Med* 1991;**90**:320–7.
14 Pathy MS, Bayer A, Harding K, Dibble A. Randomised trial of case finding and surveillance of elderly people at home. *Lancet* 1992;**340**:890–3.
15 Hendriksen C, Lund E, Stromgard E. Consequences of assessment and intervention among elderly people: a three year randomised controlled trial. *BMJ* 1984;**289**:1522–4.

16 Carpenter GI, Demopoulos GR. Screening the elderly in the community: a controlled trial of dependency surveillance using a questionnaire administered by volunteers. *BMJ* 1990;**300**:1253–6.

17 Williams EI. Characteristics of patients over 75 not seen during one year in general practice. *BMJ* 1984;**288**:119–21.

18 Freer CB. Care of the elderly: old myths. *Lancet* 1985;**i**:268–69.

19 Ebrahim S, Hedley R, Sheldon M. Low levels of ill health among elderly non-consulters in general practice. *BMJ* 1984;**289**:1273–5.

20 Goldman L. Characteristics of patients not seen for one year in general practice. *J R Coll Gen Pract* 1984;**33**:645.

21 Ford G, Taylor RC. The elderly as underconsulters: a critical reappraisal. *J R Coll Gen Pract* 1985;**35**:244–7.

22 Stuck AE, Siu AL, Wieland GD, Adams J, Rubenstein LZ. Comprehensive geriatric assessment: a meta-analysis of controlled trials. *Lancet* 1993;**342**:1032–6.

23 Steel K, Maggi S. Ageing as a global issue. *Age Ageing* 1993;**22**:237–9.

15 Preventive medicine

J A MUIR GRAY

The aim of this chapter is to outline the preventability of many of the problems in old age, the means by which they can be prevented, and the obstacles to prevention.

Preventability

As yet the ageing process is not preventable, but there is enormous scope for preventing many of the problems that occur in old age because many of these problems result not from the ageing process itself but from other processes.

Rise and fall

Most functional abilities, whether strength or skill or suppleness or intellectual ability, show a pattern of rise and fall throughout life. Figure 15.1 shows a simple graph of age in relation to walking ability, illustrating how there is a rapid increase in walking ability in the early years of life, a long plateau, and a decline during which the ability to walk even one metre may be lost.

For each individual this pattern varies. Some people die suddenly in good health and show no decrease in walking ability before death, whereas others become housebound or even chair or bedbound. Similar graphs can be drawn for almost any activity and the shape of the graph varies from activity to activity and from individual to individual. For intellectual ability, for example, it is not possible to draw a single graph because some intellectual skills peak at different ages from others. Short term memory, for example, almost certainly starts to decline in everyone from the age of about 20, whereas the ability to get on with and relate to other people does not show this early peaking and may continue to increase throughout the whole life of the individual in exceptional people.

Thus human life may be divided into two main stages: development and a phase of deterioration. In general, deterioration of physical abilities starts in the early 20s, although most people lead a life that is so physically undemanding that this does not become evident unless they are asked to take vigorous physical exercise.

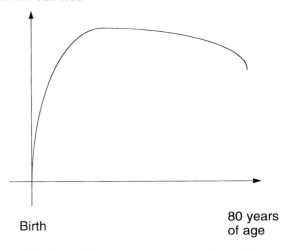

Birth

80 years
of age

Fig 15.1 Relationship of age to walking ability.

The preventable deterioration in performance results from the interaction of the ageing process with three interrelated processes: loss of fitness, disease, and social pressures (fig 15.2).

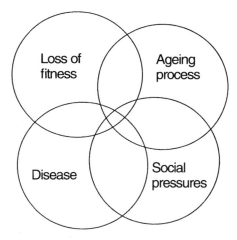

Fig 15.2 Interaction of the ageing process with loss of fitness, disease, and social pressures.

Loss of fitness

The fitness of an individual may be measured in two ways. One is the maximum work performance that the individual is able to attain. This is of importance for athletes but as we grow older a more important way of measuring fitness is by the response to an imposed challenge.

146

The best way to measure the fitness of a group of people is to subject them to some standard challenge—for example, running up a flight of stairs 10 times—and to measure the impact that this has on their resting cardiac and respiratory rates. The fitter one is, the less is the displacement and the quicker the return to the base rate.

Fitness gap

This principle is very important in old age. Older people cope very well when they are not challenged but it is when there is some challenge imposed on their cardiovascular system or balancing system that their loss of fitness becomes noticeable. Some aspects of cardiovascular performance decline as a result of the ageing process and are not preventable; for example, the maximum heart rate attainable by an individual declines with age. Even more important, however, is the fact that loss of cardiovascular fitness progressively occurs, with a gap between an individual's actual level of performance and the level of performance they could attain if fully fit, because there is a gap between how fit a person actually is and how fit a person could be. This gap, called the "fitness gap", widens progressively with age, as shown in fig 15.3.

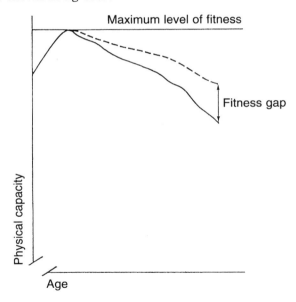

Fig 15.3   The fitness gap.

Consequences of loss of fitness

Because loss of fitness leads to a diminution in performance, loss of fitness alone may result in an individual's inability to respond to a

147

challenge—using the term "challenge" to include activities such as the ability to climb a flight of stairs. As can be seen from fig 15.3, loss of fitness may mean that an individual loses the ability as a result of loss of fitness, when it could have been maintained for five or 10 years longer had he or she remained fit and well.

Causes of fitness loss

At any age fitness is lost because of the lack of training—"training" being defined as work at a level that pushes the individual along at a level different from the natural daily work rate, with the result that the capacity for responding to increases in work in future is increased. Fitness training is by definition arduous and is felt by the individual as tiring and challenging, but it is very important because training can narrow the fitness gap at any age. There is good evidence to demonstrate that almost all aspects of performance, certainly strength, stamina, and suppleness, can be improved by training in old age.[1]

It is important to emphasise that the word "training" defines a level of work and not a particular style of work; training includes activities such as ballroom dancing, yoga exercises that increase suppleness, walking, and much of physiotherapy.

Training and ageing

There is an important relationship between training and biological ageing. One of the best ways of defining the effects of ageing is that it is a process, or set of processes, that reduces the body's ability to cope with challenges, whether those challenges are dehydration or infection or immobility. The important consequence of this for preventive medicine is that from the end of childhood it is important for us to continue to train and, because of the effects of the ageing process, from the age of about 20 onwards it is more important to train and to take challenging exercise more frequently each decade. The 20 year old can probably maintain reasonable levels of fitness with weekly exercise. By the 50s it is important and necessary to have exercise at a level sufficient to induce the training effect about three times a week.

Fitness, ageing, and social pressures

Biologically it is necessary to train more frequently as one ages; socially the pressure is to take less exercise as one ages. University students, for example, have an afternoon a week for training but when they enter another form of work physical exercise midweek is not allowed in the timetable, unless they happen to take a job in which exercise plays a central part. The more senior an individual becomes in an organisation, the less appropriate is it considered to take time off mid-week for exercise; the working day

148

may become longer and the added responsibilities of family life reduce the opportunities for exercise. In addition, there are also social pressures which mitigate against exercise; it would still be regarded as eccentric, although attitudes are changing, for the person in their 50s in a senior position to put on a tracksuit and exercise three times a week at lunchtime.

Disease and ageing

While it is true that older people have in general poorer health status than younger people, and this is due in part to the higher prevalence and incidence of disease in old age, it is essential to distinguish disease from ageing and to identify the part that the ageing process plays in the evolution of disease. The incidence of stroke increases with age, as does the incidence of cancer,[23] but this does not mean that ageing itself is a cause of these diseases and that they are therefore inevitable.

Ageing as a cause of disease

Ageing is a set of biological processes that are genetically determined; although it was thought in the past that ageing was the cause of a number of diseases due to a progressive "wearing out" of the body, it is now appreciated that much of the loss of functional ability that occurs in old age is due not so much to wearing out but to loss of fitness and to the onset of disease, with the ageing process playing only a part in the aetiology of disease.

It may well be that genes controlling division of cells or suppressing the production of certain types of proteins are involved in the causation of disease, and some genes suppress their effects as part of the general process of ageing, but in many diseases the cause is environmental and external to a greater degree than it is genetic and internal.

Prolonged exposure

One of the reasons why older people get disease more frequently than young people is that they have been alive, and exposed to the adverse environmental factors that cause disease, for a longer time. These factors may be external, as in the case of sunlight, which interacts with skin ageing to create lesions that become more common as individuals age.

The environmental factor, using the term "environmental" to mean external rather than internal, may be a chemical that becomes incorporated in the body; the effect of cigarette smoking is the most obvious example. Peripheral vascular disease is a disease that is principally caused by the effects of cigarette smoking. Similarly, the effects of diet influence the incidence of cancer of the gastrointestinal tract and the longer an individual has eaten a certain diet the more likely he or she is to develop cancer.

149

Thirdly, there are complex changes in the social environment that influence the physical environment and lifestyle of the individual and have an impact on the incidence and prevalence of disease. In a society that becomes wealthier, for example, meat eating and an increased ingestion of fat start to influence the pattern of disease in old age. Changes also occur in the age of first pregnancy and the number of children that women bear, and this change in the hormonal pattern of women influences the incidence of breast cancer in a population.

Cohort specific influences

Old people are not a homogeneous class and, within a group of people defined by a specific chronological age band, differences are greater than similarities. In addition, old people vary from one country to another, their health status is different in different parts of the same country, and the health status of older people is changing with time, principally due to the exposure of their particular cohort to adverse health influences in the past.

Those practising medicine with older people in the 1960s and 1970s, for example, dealt with many older men who had severe lung failure resulting not from ageing but from a single exposure to gas during the first world war. That cohort has now died and gas lung is no longer a cause of disability in old age. Chronic rheumatic heart disease is another condition, arising from an acute episode in childhood or early adult life, that was a common cause of disability but which, in the developed world at least, is now a much less common problem.

Patterns of disease change. The prevalence of smoking increased among men after the first world war and the increasing incidence of disease associated with this social trend became evident in the 1940s and 1950s. There is some evidence now that the incidence of smoking related disease in men is declining as the prevalence of cigarette smoking in some age and social groups is decreasing. In women, however, the pattern is different. Just as smoking became a widespread social phenomenon among men during the first world war, smoking became a much more widespread social phenomenon among women during the second world war as a consequence of the many changes in the status of women that occurred during that time. The smoking prevalence among women has increased since the second world war and we are now starting to see the health consequences of that as women now experience diseases (for example, lung cancer) that were at one time rare in that group.

Social environment and disease

There is no doubt that health and wealth are closely interrelated. In general the healthier a population or an individual is, the wealthier that population or person is, and within a country the subgroups who are wealthier are healthier than the subgroups who are poor. Older people are in general poorer than younger people, in part because they are not working, in part because of the inadequate pension arrangements that still exist in many countries, and in part because of decades of poverty that did not allow the older people to lay aside resources for their future. In considering the health problems of older people (hypothermia, for example) it is essential to remember that, although the ageing process reduces the individual's ability to adapt to changes in temperature, it is poverty that creates the environment that is the principal cause of hypothermia.

Preventive medicine

Health problems in old age are caused by four main forces: the ageing process (though relatively unimportant), loss of fitness, diseases caused by environmental stimuli, and social factors, including poverty. Thus medicine alone cannot prevent disease and action taken only in old age cannot prevent the problems of older people. There is the need for a combined approach that involves changes in the physical environment, changes in the social environment, and the provision of effective and acceptable health services. These three approaches are interrelated, as shown in fig 15.4.

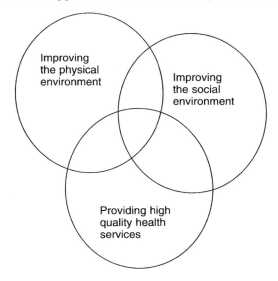

Fig 15.4   Combined approaches to preventive medicine.

Improving the physical and social environment

Elderly millionaires have health problems, but many health problems, and their consequences, seen by doctors are so complicated by inadequate income, poor housing, and poor social support that it is important never to underestimate the impact that changes in the physical and social environment might have on health in old age.[4] The professional working with an older person has, however, only limited opportunities to improve the physical and social environment, but these limited opportunities should be taken. Many older people, for example, do not receive all of the benefits for which they are eligible. There are two reasons for this. The first is that they are completely unaware of what is available; the second is that their attitude towards these benefits, and their fear of the consequences of applying, means that they are unwilling to apply for their rights. Every health professional who works with older people should know the basic facts about housing and income benefits and where more detailed information and help can be obtained.

Collectively the medical profession can press for better conditions for older people but it is only possible to do so if we are open and honest and accept that the profession is itself part of a system that ensures its members are wealthy while older people are poor. There is no law of nature that states that the salary of a doctor should be five, six, or more times that of the "salary" of a pensioner, for both, in the United Kingdom at least, are paid by the government.

Preventive health services

It is customary to divide preventive health services into three kinds: primary prevention or health promotion is the promotion of health and the prevention of disease; secondary prevention or screening is the identification and treatment of disease at an early stage; and tertiary prevention is the effective management of existing disease. All of these need to be developed but will only have their full impact if they are set in the context of the changes in the social and physical environment that are required to give old people health and wellbeing.

1 Gray JAM, Bassey J, Young A. The risks of inactivity. In: Gray JAM, editor. *Prevention of disease in the elderly.* Edinburgh: Churchill Livingstone, 1985:78–95.
2 World Health Organization. Tomatis L, editor. *Cancer: causes, occurrence and control.* Lyon: IARC Scientific Publications, 1990.
3 Hakulinen T, Kenward M, Luostarinen T, *et al. Cancer in Finland in 1954–2008. Incidence, mortality and prevalence by region.* Helsinki: Finnish Cancer Registry and Finnish Foundation for Cancer Research, 1989.
4 Murphy E. The social origins of depression in old age. *Br J Psychiatr* 1982;**141**:135–42.

16 Health promotion

ALEX KALACHE

There is at present a revived interest in health education and health promotion—sometimes wrongly interpreted as new. In fact the origins of such interest can be traced to a distant past. Health promotion in the 1990s has recognisable roots in earlier changes in the definition of public health. The nineteenth century saw the emergence of the "sanitation movement" comprising both environmental and individual health issues. This followed the industrialisation and urbanisation processes in western Europe; state intervention was required—often in order to "disinfect" the environment without challenging the social/political structures. Subsequently an emphasis on personal hygiene gradually emerged—an approach closely associated with the need to promote "natural efficiency". By the turn of the century it was regarded as imperative to control the "urban masses". Under the impact of the bacteriological revolution the focus was narrowed towards "isolation and purification", without much concern for personal lifestyles. An additional focus on "personal prevention" was only provided during the first decades of the twentieth century. The interwar years witnessed an increased interest in personal health and fitness; however, health services were still largely uninvolved with promotion of health.

After the second world war prevention and health promotion were redefined. In Britain this was influenced by the reorientation of public health following the establishment of the National Health Service and the development of epidemiology. At an international level the work of the World Health Organization and other agencies has shaped such redefinition. This chapter provides an outline of the developments that have culminated in the current conception of health promotion; it attempts to differentiate health promotion and ageing from health promotion in old age; it states why elderly people are a special group; it provides some specific examples of interventions and calls for the need for establishing criteria for priority action and for evaluation.

Context in which health promotion gained prominence in public health

With the establishment of WHO immediately after the second world war, health was for the first time defined as not merely absence of disease.

However utopian, the "state of complete physical, mental and social wellbeing" captured the imagination of a whole generation of health professionals but it took another 30 years for the Alma-Ata declaration to be proclaimed. The core message of the declaration was unequivocal: "the need for urgent action by all governments, all health and development workers, and the world community to protect and promote the health of all people of the world." The foundations of primary health care were firmly established: prevention and promotion as the central focus of health care. The declaration regarded health as an asset to be protected and a fundamental human right. The attainment of the highest possible level of health was seen by the signatories as a vitally important worldwide social goal whose realisation "requires the action of many other social and economic sectors in addition to the health sector." From the foundations provided in Alma-Ata emerged the WHO Health for All movement, which can be encapsulated by its six principles: (a) equity, (b) health promotion/ disease prevention, (c) community participation, (d) intersectoral collaboration, (e) the importance of the primary health care sector, and (f) international cooperation.

WHO approach to health promotion

Against this background a momentum was generated and by the early 1980s a clear "WHO approach" to health promotion could be identified. Its main tenets are (a) cultural specificity; (b) basic resources for health

---

Box 16.1—The Ottawa charter

Health promotion action means:
- Build healthy public policy—different sectors, different levels
- Create supportive environments—a socioecological approach required
- Strengthen community action—ownership, development and involvement of local people
- Develop personal skills—lifelong learning, choices conducive to health
- Reorientation of health services—towards a greater emphasis on health promotion

Ottawa commitment to health promotion
- Political commitment to health and equity in all sectors
- Counteract effects of harmful products, environments, and living conditions
- Respond to the health gap within and between societies
- Acknowledge people as the main health resource
- Reorientate health services towards health promotion, sharing power with people themselves
- Recognise health and its maintenance as a major social investment and challenge

---

are income, shelter, and food; (c) complementary requisites are information/ knowledge about health factors, appropriate skills for health, and supportive environments to enhance health and opportunities for healthier choices. It combines personal choice with social responsibility to create a healthier future.

The underlying idea is that people should be able to increase their control over their health. In order to facilitate control, "access to health" needs to become universal—that is, inequalities need to be reduced and "environments conducive to health" stimulated. Furthermore, the WHO approach emphasises the importance of strengthening social networks and social support as well as the need for observing societies' predominant ways of life.

Eventually, in 1986, WHO organised the first international conference on health promotion in Ottawa, Canada. Its main resolutions are encapsulated in the Ottawa charter for health promotion and are shown in box 16.1.

Definition of health promotion

Health promotion consists of a range of interventions that lead to improvement, maintenance, and prevention of decline in health status. It benefits from a range of disciplines and requires action from different sectors of society. Four main components are identifiable within its framework:

- *Health education*: the process of giving information where the aim is to promote health through conventional and innovative techniques (for example, peer education, multimedia use, social participation)
- *Disease prevention*: refers to interventions used in early diagnosis or prevention of specific diseases (for example, screening, immunisation)
- *Health maintenance*: treatment interventions used to prevent a decline in health status, particularly in vulnerable groups, and to promote wellbeing (physical, social, and mental) are emphasised
- *Healthy public policy*: policy interventions that contribute to health promotion directly or by creating a supportive climate; examples include legal and fiscal policy, public transport policies, international conventions, advertising regulations, and health system organisation.

Effective health promotion strategies include all four elements. As suggested in fig 16.1, the more they overlap the stronger the health promotion impact and the commitment to a healthier public policy.

Health promotion is an evolving concept. Much has, however, been written about it recently (some further reading is suggested among the references of this chapter); its very interdisciplinary nature indicates different philosophies, languages, and time frames, which require further classification and precision.

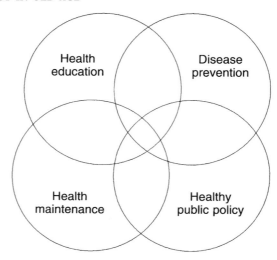

Fig 16.1   The four elements of health promotion: greater overlap indicates stronger health promotion impact.

Health promotion and ageing

Ageing is associated with health *unless* there is sickness or disability. The vast majority of healthy ageing individuals are a testimony to this. As people age, however, they increase their risk of acquiring diseases and disabilities; these could often be avoided altogether—but when they have occurred, preventive action might have mitigated or deferred them. Individuals age differently and there is more "diversity" in old age than at any other point in life. While hereditary factors may play a role, life habits, living conditions, and environmental factors are of paramount importance. Functions can be maintained at adequate levels for longer, depending on, for instance, lifestyles—which can also precipitate a decline into disability. Health promotion and ageing deals with stimulating habits and lifestyle conducive to a better old age in the future—that is, health promotion can play a crucial role in determining how different individuals reach old age. Maintaining health into old age requires investment during earlier stages of life, basically through healthier lifestyles and lifelong health promotion. This notion has been encapsulated by the term "healthy ageing", a concept actively promoted by agencies such as WHO,[1] Age Concern,[2] and the European Union.[3]

Health promotion in old age

Recognition that health can be promoted even for individuals already in the "old age" category has increased over the last few years. In 1986 WHO looked into possibilities for the promotion of health in old age and for the

156

postponement of diseases and disabilities. This initiative triggered action at country level, such as the outline of a national plan for health promotion in older age in Britain.[4] Elsewhere the academic community, national governments, and non-governmental organisations have conducted a series of meetings and published specific reports.

Effective health promotion interventions in old age require the perception of elderly people as a special group, as indicated in box 16.2.

Box 16.2—Features characteristic of the elderly as a special group

- Heterogeneity
- Increased risk of diseases/disabilities
- Multiple pathologies often present
- Iatrogenic problems common—and frequently unrecognised
- Social deficits frequent
- Low adaptability to changes (social, environmental, and biological)
- Premature intervention may trigger dependency
- Negative stereotypes created by society nurture negative attitudes to old age (by society, professionals, and elderly people themselves)

Promoting health in old age implies in the first place an acceptance of ageing as a process—not a disease to be prevented. With chronological ageing there is indeed a progressive decline in the ability to respond to the stresses of a dynamic environment that may result in functional impairment. The ageing process can, however, be accelerated/complicated by extrinsic factors such as those associated with lifestyles, environmental conditions, and diseases. The effects of ageing can be positively dealt with. These include social changes/deficits that tend to occur as individuals age, decline in functional capacity, increased risk of diseases and disabilities, and loss of adaptability to challenges (environmental, social, or biological). These factors frequently overlap, which makes disentangling their relative contributions particularly difficult.

Social and health services can considerably improve individuals' responses. Self help/self care approaches are particularly relevant, as are those that seek to strengthen the informal care sector. Most disabled elderly people remain in the community and are looked after by relatives and friends—mostly women, often old and frail themselves and in need of support if they are to perform their caring roles effectively. In all these respects health professionals have a fundamental role to play, provided that in addition to being providers of care they also act as promoters of health for elderly people, as mediators, facilitators, advocates, disseminators, and trainers. This changing role is a challenge; it is translated in practice into an interaction in which information and skills have to be shared; health promotion requires individuals to be well informed and to acquire new skills.

In practice this demands that health professionals share knowledge—that is, share power, which is not something easy to do unless there is a great awareness of the benefits to be gained.

Specific examples of health promotion in old age

The practical implementation of health promotion in old age is still in its infancy and the number of established programmes—most of them in North America and western Europe—is therefore relatively small at present. An overview of such programmes follows.

Most of the existing health promotion programmes for the elderly cover one of the following areas; physical exercise[5-10] and healthy living,[11-16] prevention of frailty and injury,[17] smoking cessation,[18] chronic disease management,[19 20] appropriate medication,[21] healthy nutrition,[22 23] social empowerment,[24] immunisation,[25 26] holistic wellbeing,[27] and combined self care and healthy lifestyle.[28-31]

The vast majority of programmes involve elderly people living in the community,[5-7 10-24 26-30] with only three being targeted towards elderly in institutions.[8 9 25] Typically the programmes are set in various community centres,[5 6 9-11 19 23 27 30] medical health centres,[8 15 17 20 28] primary care practices,[14 18] hospitals,[7 26] or a combination of hospital and community centre.[13]

Although most programmes use groups led by professionals or trained volunteers, sometimes together with peers,[5-10 17 19-21 24 28 30] some (including those focusing on smoking cessation, healthy nutrition, immunisation, and two of those concerning healthy lifestyles) employ an individual approach.[12 14 18 22 23 25 26] A combination of both peer and professional leadership is used by three of the healthy lifestyle programmes.[11 13 15]

Apart from two programmes which involve only postal and no personal contact,[12 23] all programmes involve a personal contact between the "health promoters" and the participant. Active participation of elderly people in development and implementation of the programme, in line with the concept of empowerment, is employed in a few of the programmes.[5 13-15 24 29 30]

Most projects (apart from those conducted exclusively by post) have a theoretical and a practical component, the latter involving, for example, physical exercise classes[5-8] or the teaching of practical self care skills.[19 20 28] Finally, some of the health promotion programmes are part of a comprehensive care "package" involving additionally traditional medical and pharmacological interventions.[13 15]

Criteria for selecting interventions

Screening and case finding are valuable approaches to secondary prevention of disease. Unfortunately they are sometimes taken as the only effective contributions in promoting health in old age. Thus in selecting interventions it is important to define precise objectives and to consider the general principles of health promotion previously outlined in this chapter. Criteria for establishing priorities should include (a) most prevalent factors associated with premature/avoidable death and disability; (b) prominent societal concerns; (c) neglected topics currently supported at inadequate levels; and (d) amenability to intervention—that is, the literature provides evidence of effective ways to deal with the problem. All these dimensions have their own difficulties. Reliance on existing sources of data—for example, mortality, morbidity, and disability data—may be misplaced when statistics related to older people are notoriously deficient. Societal concerns are often the subject of sensationalist media attention and the vested interests of industries and/or of politicians. Adequate levels of support require reliable indicators for proper definition. Effectiveness has to be demonstrated by good research, which in turn cannot be conducted unless appropriate levels of funding are made available.

Until relatively recently the research community largely neglected the common problems of old age. Results of investigations conducted in predominantly middle aged (male) individuals were (and still are) extrapolated as relevant to those in old age; for instance, clinical trials on problems common after the age of 65 used almost systematically to exclude elderly people from their samples. There is now an emerging awareness that these distortions must be corrected, but much remains to be done.

The difficulties are further compounded by the barriers to gaining approval:

- There is a long interval between the intervention and the outcome
- The benefits are often in terms of wellbeing/comfort, gains in healthy years, or quality of life; consistency in assessing quantitative and qualitative outcomes is always difficult to achieve
- Many innovations focus on responsibilities of different organisations and agencies, making them unusually difficult to cost and assess
- Current sources of information on the health of the elderly population are particularly patchy and poor; the database with which to monitor health improvements in older age rarely exists
- Methods of measuring the benefits to individuals or the cost effectiveness of specific proposals are still largely unsatisfactory
- Approaches such as quality of life measures remain controversial
- Opportunity costs of alternative interventions are rarely assessed
- Local initiatives are widespread but uncoordinated
- Regulatory discrimination against elderly people is still very common, reflecting a lack of organised political power.

Some of the challenges ahead

A policy for the aged is a policy for being healthy. In this context the concept of health should also include the ability to cope adequately with

159

stress, health problems, social losses, limitations, and handicaps.[32] Incorporation of this dimension into the thinking of policy makers is one of the challenges for gerontologists at the turn of the twenty first century. In addition, there is the problem of the choice of adequate indicators. The use of economic indicators—"valuation" of various states of health when elderly people are no longer "contributing" to the wealth of the community—is a negative bias (see chapter 9). Effort in generating indicators more sensitive to non-monetary outcomes is necessary.

Another challenge relates to resources: activities for health promotion in old age may often bring about a temporary increase in demand for health services. At times of zero or negative growth in health expenditure this may be a major impediment to progress.

Last but not least, there is an urgent need to evaluate appropriately and rigorously the impact of interventions. The ability to influence policies depends on the ability to demonstrate the effectiveness of various courses of action. Epidemiology will continue to be a core discipline—particularly when associated with qualitative evaluation techniques—because scientific evidence of efficacy is increasingly demanded by policy makers and health service purchasers.

1 Hermanova HM. *Health promotion for the elderly*. International workshop; 1992 Nov 16–17; Jerusalem. Geneva: ESHEL JDC Brookdale Institute, Ministry of Health, and World Health Organization, 1992.
2 Eurolink Age. Age well conference. Eurolink age bulletin. London: Age Concern, 1992.
3 Anderson R, Daunt P, Drury E, *et al. The Coming of Age in Europe*. London: Age Concern and Eurolink Age, 1992.
4 Kalache A, Warnes T, Hunter DJ. *Promoting health among elderly people: a statement from a working group*. London: King's Fund, 1988.
5 Attig GA, Chanawongse K. Elderly people as health promoters. *World Health Forum* 1989; **10**:186–9.
6 Ebrahim S, Williams J. Assessing the effects of a health promotion programme for elderly people. *J Public Health Med* 1992;**14**:199–205.
7 Morey MC, Crowley GM, Robbins MS, Cowper PA, Sullivan RJ. The gerofit program: a VA innovation. *South Med J* 1994;**87**:S83–7.
8 Morey MC, Cowper PA, Feussner JR, *et al.* Evaluation of a supervised exercise in a geriatric population. *J Am Geriatr Soc* 1989;**37**:348–54.
9 Kinion ES, Christie N, Villella AM. Promoting activity in the elderly through interdisciplinary linkages. *Nurs Connect* 1993;**6**:19–26.
10 Haber D. Health promotion to reduce blood pressure level among older blacks. *Gerontologist* 1986;**26**:119–21.
11 Clifford PA, Tan S-Y, Gorsuch RL. Efficacy of a self-directed behavioural change program: weight, body composition, cardiovascular fitness, blood pressure, health risk, and psychosocial mediating variables. *J Behav Med* 1991;**14**:303–23.
12 Fries JF, Bloch DA, Harrington H, Richardson N, Beck R. Two-year results of a randomized controlled trial of a health promotion program in a retiree population: the Bank of America study. *Am J Med* 1993;**94**:455–62.
13 Scharlach AE, Mor-Barak ME, Katz A, Birba L, Garcia G, Sokolov J. Generation: a corporate-sponsored retiree health care programme. *Gerontologist* 1992;**32**:265–9.
14 Schmidt RM. Health Watch: Health promotion and disease prevention in primary care. *Methods Inf Med* 1993;**32**:245–8.
15 Roger J, Grower R, Supino P. Participant evaluation and cost of a community-based health promotion program for elders. *Public Health Rep* 1992;**107**:417–26.
16 Sutherland M, Cowart M, Heack C. A rural senior citizens health promotion demonstration project. *Health Educ* 1989;**20**:40–3.

17 Ory MG, Schechtmann KB, Miller JP, *et al.* for the FICSIT group. Frailty and injuries in later life: the FICSIT trials. *J Am Geriatr Soc* 1993;**41**:283–96.

18 Vetter NJ, Ford D. Smoking prevention among people aged 60 and over: a randomized controlled trial. *Age Ageing* 1990;**19**:164–8.

19 Petrie DA. A community-based health promotion project for persons with chronic respiratory disease. *Can J Public Health* 1990;**81**:310–1.

20 Bremer-Schulte M, Kestner A, Pluym B, Sutherland C. Health promotion and self care in the case of cardiovascular disease. *J Clin Epidemiol* 1990;**43**:817–25.

21 Cormack MA, Sweeney KG, Hughes-Jones H, Foot GA. Evaluation of an easy, cost-effective strategy for cutting benzodiazepine use in general practice. *Br J Gen Pract* 1994;**44**:5–8.

22 Roseman JI. Massachusetts sponsors the first statewide farmers' market coupon program for elders. *J Nutr Elderly* 1989;**9**:41–50.

23 Mayeda C, Anderson J. Evaluating the effectiveness of the "Self CARE for a healthy heart" program with older adults. *J Nutr Elderly* 1993;**13**:11–22.

24 Minkler M. Community organizing among the elderly poor in the United States: a case study. *Int J Health Serv* 1992;**22**:303–16.

25 Patriarca PA, Weber JA, Parker RA, *et al.* Efficacy of influenza vaccine in nursing homes. *JAMA* 1985;**253**:1136–9.

26 Sims RV, Steinmann WC, McConville JH, King LR, Zwick WC, Schwartz S. The clinical effectiveness of pneumococcal vaccine in the elderly. *Ann Intern Med* 1988;**108**:653–7.

27 Ruffing-Rahal MA. Evaluation of group health promotion with community-dwelling older women. *Public Health Nurs* 1994;**11**:38–48.

28 Simmons JJ, Nelson EC, Roberts E, Travis Salisbury Z, Kane-Williams E, Benson L. A health promotion program: Staying Healthy After Fifty. *Health Educ Q* 1989;**16**:461–72.

29 Age Concern Institute of Gerontology. *Age well. The first five years.* London: Age Concern, 1991.

30 Echevarria KH, Ross V, Bezon JF, Flow J. A successful aging project: pooling university and community resources. *J Gerontol Nurs* 1991;**17**:27–30.

31 Benson L, Nelson EC, Napps SE, Roberts E, Kane-Williams E, Travis Salisbury Z. Evaluation of the Staying Healthy After Fifty program: impact on course participants. *Health Educ Q* 1989;**16**:485–508.

32 Lehr U. The challenge of ageing well. In: *Ageing well—a call for European action.* London: Age Concern and Eurolink Age, 1992.

17 Successful ageing

MARGRET M BALTES

Successful ageing seems an oxymoron. In the face of an increasingly negative balance between gains and losses, can one ever age successfully? Does successful ageing imply not ageing at all? Some interpret the interest of gerontologists in successful ageing as exactly that—namely, the desire to impose middle aged values of productivity and social involvement on late life.[1 2]

Successful ageing cannot mean denying ageing or perpetuating middle age. Attempting to extend the middle years will inevitably lead to despair and eventual defeat.[3 4] Any model of successful ageing needs to take into account both the losses and the gains of ageing. Successful ageing must thus describe and explain successful adaptation to age specific losses and challenges. At the same time, however, a model of successful ageing also needs to accommodate growth and development in old age.[5]

The intent of this chapter is first to hint at the empirical basis on which we can argue for positive or successful ageing. Then, in discussing success and successful ageing, a pluralistic view towards criteria, norms, and standards used to measure success will be developed. Finally, a meta-model of successful ageing, "selective optimization with compensation", that accommodates a multitude of criteria and norms and defines three processes, each harbouring a great diversity of psychological strategies and mechanisms by which successful ageing can be accomplished, will be described.

Three facts of ageing

There are a number of empirical data that can be considered facts about ageing; Paul Baltes has presented them as seven theses.[6] In this context, three seem to have particular weight: heterogeneity, plasticity, and limits in plasticity or reserves.

To date, empirical evidence for *heterogeneity* in the elderly population is abundant.[7 8] Its causal base can be summarised in the idea of lifelong development as a process of individuation and specialisation. The resulting large interindividual differences are an accumulation of differences in genetic factors and environmental conditions as well as an outcome of the active role each person plays in the design of his or her development. The

162

environment and niche the person is proactively or reactively searching for or creating and the environments that are offered or available to the person will have to "fit" if development and ageing are to be successful. The concept of fit is at the core of Lawton and Nahemow's[9] person–environment model in which fit means a balance between resources and demands leading to just manageable difficulty levels.[10]

Like heterogeneity, the use of the word *plasticity* (of the elderly organism) has become common—referring to unused and latent potentials. Evidence is primarily found in the domain of cognitive ageing[11-13] and the physical/biological domain,[14-16] but also in the social domain.[17 18] Unused potentials are activated when conditions are favourable, stimulating, and challenging.

This is not to say that ageing declines can be "intervened away". Evidence pointing to the *limits in plasticity* or reserves has accumulated.[19] Increasing biological vulnerability in ageing reduces the breadth and scope of existing reserves. Thus, in the face of demands of life an elderly person will exhaust his or her reserves more quickly, may have to overtax resources, rely on supportive resources, or search for less demanding environments to cope with the problem at hand.

Taken together these ageing facts suggest that successful ageing will have many faces, will have to flourish against the odds of diminishing reserves, but will also allow for growth. How can we then define success and successful ageing?

Success and successful ageing

Most adult developmental and gerontological theories specify an ideal end state towards which the person is to develop.[20-30] In all these theories successful ageing has come to imply specific end states in physical and mental health, satisfaction with life, and high morale. No one criterion, or even pattern of criteria, has been widely accepted as a cogent prescription for or explanation of successful ageing. A multicriteria approach is surely preferable to a monocriterion approach.[29] Unless we accept all criteria as equally important—which would render the numbers of successful ageing people extremely small—we are, however, left with the problem of heterogeneity. Success and successful ageing means different things to different people, cultures, or subgroups at different historical and individual times.[5]

Throughout history success has been defined in strikingly different ways.[31] In early times success was the result of fate or good fortune. Success was then construed as the ratio between gains and losses, and still later it was considered the result of effort and achievement. Successful attainment was related to both hedonistic and utilitarian goals. It is only today that we associate success and successful attainment almost exclusively with economic and material gain.[32] Association of success with productivity and materialism is at the root of our uneasiness in talking about successful ageing. It smacks of capitalist ideology.[5 33]

There is, however, no rule, hindering us from tying success to non-materialistic goals and to norms and standards that do not comply with a free market system and do not measure up to one universal standard. Elsewhere[34 35] we have proposed defining success and successful ageing as goal attainment, whereby the goal can be defined by different authorities (the person, a group of people, a culture, etc), different criteria of assessment (objective v subjective), and different norms (functional, statistical, ideal, etc). In this sense, denying successful ageing would mean denying the elderly to have goals and to strive towards reaching these goals.

Setting and reaching goals is a human affair. To have and strive towards goals despite losses endemic to ageing is the essence of successful ageing. I argue that the demonstration of adaptability in the light of obstacles on the way to one's goals and the manifestation of reserves in the face of losses are what characterises successful ageing. To this end the elderly person will have to make use of three processes: selection, optimisation, and compensation.

Meta-model of successful ageing: selective optimisation with compensation

This meta-model defines three processes that assist in the adaptation to challenges of old age; thus, the focus of the model is *how* people age successfully. It does not specify *what* is successful ageing, save for a general description of adaptivity. In line with a life span perspective, with its multidimensional and multidirectional conception of development, adaptability is regarded as the efficacious functioning of the individual in an identified system (biological, social, psychological), domain (family, work, sports, leisure, etc), or task (cognitive performance, social integration, self actualisation, etc). The domain or goal of successful adaptation is not prescribed, nor is it measured against a universal standard. Rather the interplay, the fit, between personal and environmental resources and situational demands is the yardstick, using a functional, ideal, or individual norm.

The processes of selection, compensation, and optimisation also comprise a multitude of different strategies and mechanisms and thus allow for interindividual differences. Strategies such as downward social comparison, socioemotional selectivity, self efficacy beliefs, accommodative coping, or secondary control can all serve selection. Similarly, compensation can refer to any kind of mental or physical prosthetics, to behavioural dependency, passive control, or proxy control. Strategies of optimisation may entail effort, deliberate practice, creative thinking, upward social comparison, assimilative coping, etc.[34] If implemented, the three processes, using these diverse strategies, can empower people in their pursuit of successful ageing despite or perhaps even because of losses and increasing vulnerabilities.

164

Definition of the three processes

Selection refers to an increasing restriction of one's life world to fewer domains of functioning as a consequence or in anticipation of losses in personal and environmental resources. Selection may mean avoidance of one domain altogether or it can mean a restriction in tasks and goals within one domain or a number of domains. The adaptive task of the person is to concentrate on and select those domains, tasks, goals, and expectations that are of high priority and involve a convergence of environmental demands, individual motivations, skills, and biological capacity.

Selection implies that an individual's expectations are readjusted and reassessed. It can be proactive or reactive. It encompasses environmental changes (for example, relocation), active behaviour changes (for example, reducing the number of commitments), or passive adjustment (for example, avoiding climbing stairs or allowing somebody to take responsibility). Proactively, people can monitor their functioning, predict future changes and losses (for example, death of the spouse), and make efforts to look and search for tasks and domains that will remain intact after losses. Selection is reactive when unpredictable or sudden changes force the person to make a selection.

Compensation, the second component facilitating mastery of loss in reserves, becomes operative when specific behavioural capacities or skills are lost or reduced below the level required for adequate functioning. The question here is: do I have other means of reaching the same goal, accomplishing the same outcome in a specific domain? Losses in specific behavioural capacities loom particularly large when situations and goals require a wide range of activity and a high level of performance (for example, competitive sports, rush hour traffic, accumulation of daily irritations, and situations that require quick thinking and memorisation).

Compensatory efforts can be automatic or planned. If a goal within a domain that includes a large number of activities and means is well elaborated, the person will not experience much trouble in counterbalancing or compensating for a specific behavioural deficiency. If the deficiency is large in scope or if the domains and goals are defined by one or very few activities, compensatory efforts will be more difficult. Compensation is not necessarily dependent on existing behaviours or means. It sometimes requires the acquisition of new skills or means not yet in one's repertoire.

The component of compensation thus differs from selection in that the target, the domain, the task, or the goal, is maintained, but new means are enlisted to compensate for a behavioural deficiency in order to maintain or optimise previous functioning. The element of compensation involves aspects of both the mind and technology.

Optimisation, the third component of the meta-model, involves the processes of enriching and augmenting reserves or resources and thus enhancing function in selected life domains. Optimisation and growth may relate to the development of existing goals and expectations (for example,

165

with regard to generativity). They may also reflect new goals and expectations in line with developmental tasks of the third phase of life, such as acceptance of one's own mortality.

How much selection and compensation must be invested in order to secure maintenance and stimulate optimisation is an empirical question. Intervention studies in gerontology suggest that, in principle, many elderly people have the necessary resources and reserves to optimise functions but face restrictive or overprotective environments that inhibit optimisation. There is no doubt that the process of optimisation will to a large extent be contingent on stimulating and enhancing environmental conditions. Thus society plays a central role in providing environments that facilitate optimisation. In fact the success of relatively simple interventions suggests that the elderly often live in a world of underdemand rather than overdemand. Optimisation is dependent upon available opportunities unless older people actively seek new terrain and frontiers.[36]

All three components can be activated more easily and readily when there is a rich and broad array of resources to draw from. When resources become depleted an increasingly fine tuned and subtle interplay among the three components is necessary. We contend, however, that even very frail people can select, compensate, and optimise to maximise goal attainment. B.F. Skinner,[37] for example, in an account of his own ageing gave eloquent advice on intellectual management to preserve and continue high productivity in light of failing reserves. It was clear from his writings that the intellectual domain was of high priority and that his life was arranged to maximise function in this selected domain as opposed to others.

Summary

Recent findings about ageing, as well as vital statistics about the population of the elderly, present us with the obvious fact that there are more elderly living relatively healthy and independent lives than there are elderly who need to be taken care of or live in institutions. In both gerontology and in our societies we have come to be more concerned about the security and safety of the elderly, their problems, and dependencies than about the enrichment, enhancement, and stimulation of the elderly, their growth and autonomy. Successful ageing has been described as putting elderly people to the task instead of letting them enjoy their late freedom.

The meta-model of selective optimisation with compensation proposes three processes that are needed for adaptation to the losses of ageing, at the same time having and striving for goals. Success is defined as goal attainment whereby the goals can be set by different actors and can be measured by different standards and norms. Successful ageing thus implies having goals and striving for goals against the odds of ever diminishing reserves and increasing vulnerabilities. Three processes, selection, compensation, and optimisation, are considered to empower the elderly to strive towards goal attainment in the face of losses.

1 Cole TR. The "enlightened" view of aging: Victorian morality in a new key. *Hastings Cent Rep* 1983;**13**:34–40.
2 Rosenmayr L. Wandlungen der gesellschaftlichen Sicht und Bewertung des Alters. [Changes in society's perspective toward and evaluation of ageing.] In: Baltes MM, Kohli M, Sames K, editors. *Erfolgreiches Altern: Bedingungen und Variationen*. [Successful aging: conditions and variations.] Bern: Huber, 1989:96–101.
3 Butler RN. Successful aging and the role of the life review. *J Am Geriatr Soc* 1974;**22**: 529–35.
4 Erikson EH. The problem of ego identity. *Psychol Issues* 1959;**1**:101–64.
5 Baltes PB, Baltes MM, editors. Psychological perspectives on successful aging: the model of selective optimization with compensation. In: *Successful aging: perspectives from the behavioral sciences*. New York: Cambridge University Press, 1990:1–34.
6 Baltes PB. The aging mind: potentials and limits. *Gerontologist* 1993;**33**:580–94.
7 Maddox GL. Aging differently. *Gerontologist* 1987;**27**:557–64.
8 Schaie KW. The optimization of cognitive functioning in old age: predictions based on cohort-sequential and longitudinal data. In: Baltes PB, Baltes MM, editors. *Successful aging: perspectives from the behavioral sciences*. New York: Cambridge University Press, 1990:94–117.
9 Lawton MP, Nahemow L. Ecology and the aging process. In: Eisdorfer C, Lawton MP, editors. *Psychology of adult development and aging*. Washington: American Psychological Association, 1973:619–74.
10 Brim OG. Losing and winning: the nature of ambition in everyday life. *Psychol Today* 1988;**9**:48–52.
11 Baltes PB, Lindenberger U. On the range of cognitive plasticity in old age as a function of experience: 15 years of intervention research. *Behav Ther* 1988;**19**:283–300.
12 Perlmutter M, editor. *Late-life potential*. Washington: Gerontological Society of America, 1989.
13 Baltes MM, Reichert M. Successful aging: the product of biological factors, environmental quality, and behavioral competence. In: Ebrahim S, editor. *Health care for older women*. Oxford: Oxford University Press, 1992:236–56.
14 Bortz WM. *We live too short and die too long*. New York: Bantam Books, 1991.
15 Stones MJ, Kozma A. Physical performance. In: Charness N, editor. *Aging and human performance*. New York: Wiley, 1985:261–91.
16 Whitbourne SK. *The aging body*. New York: Springer, 1985.
17 Baltes MM. The etiology and maintenance of dependency in the elderly: three phases of operant research. *Behav Ther* 1988;**19**:301–19.
18 Mosher-Ashley PM. Procedural and methodological parameters in behavioral–gerontological research: a review. *Int J Aging Hum Dev* 1986–7;**24**:189–229.
19 Baltes PB, Kliegl R. Further testing of limits in cognitive plasticity in old age: negative age differences in a mnemonic skill are robust. *Dev Psychol* 1992;**28**:121–5.
20 Atchley RC. A continuity theory of normal aging. *Gerontologist* 1989;**29**:183–90.
21 Bühler Ch. *Der menschliche Lebenslauf als psychologisches Problem*. [The human life course as psychological problem.] Leipzig: Hirzel, 1933.
22 Cumming E, Henry WE. *Growing old: the process of disengagement*. New York: Basic Books, 1961.
23 Erikson EH. *The life cycle completed. A review*. New York: Norton, 1982.
24 Havighurst RJ, Albrecht R. *Older people*. New York: Longman, 1953.
25 Jahoda M. *Current concepts of positive mental health*. New York: Basic Books, 1958.
26 Jung CG. Die Lebenswende [Life's turning point.] In: *Seelenprobleme der Gegenwart*. [Psychological problems of today.] Zürich: Rascher, 1931:248–74.
27 Maddox GL. Fact and artifact: evidence bearing on disengagement theory from the Duke geriatrics project. *Hum Dev* 1965;**8**:117–30.
28 Maslow A. *Toward a psychology of being*, 2nd ed. New York: Van Nostrand, 1968.
29 Ryff CD. Beyond Ponce de Leon and life satisfaction: new directions in quest of successful aging. *Int J Behav Dev* 1989;**12**:35–55.
30 Rogers CR. *On becoming a person*. Boston: Houghton Mifflin, 1961.

31 Simpson J, Weiner E, editors. *The Oxford English dictionary*, 2nd ed, vol XVII. Oxford: Clarendon Press, 1989:92–93.
32 Bellah RN, Madison R, Sullivan WK, *et al*, editors. *Habits of the heart. Individualism and commitment in American life*. Berkeley: University of California Press, 1986.
33 Cole TR. Aging, meaning, and well-being: musings of a cultural historian. *Int J Aging Hum Dev* 1984;**19**:329–36.
34 Baltes MM, Carstensen LL. The process of successful aging. *Ageing and Society* 1996;(in press).
35 Marsiske M, Lang FR, Baltes PB, Baltes MM. Selective optimization with compensation: life-span perspectives on successful human development. In: Dixon RA, Bäckman L, editors. *Psychological compensation: managing losses and promoting gains*. Hillsdale, NJ: Erlbaum, 1995.
36 Rosenmayr L. *Die späte Freiheit*. [The late freedom.] Berlin: Severin & Siedler, 1983.
37 Skinner BF. Intellectual self-management in old age. *Am Psychol* 1983;**38**:239–44.

Part II
Risk factors and health status

18 Nutritional status

KAY-TEE KHAW

Nutrition has a key role in health at all ages. The importance of adequate nutrition in pregnancy, childhood, and adolescence, and of nutritional deficiency diseases is well recognised. Malnutrition is still a major problem in many communities worldwide and numerous deficiency diseases are still endemic; these include protein calorie malnutrition, iodine deficiency leading to goitre and related conditions, iron deficiency and anaemias, and specific vitamin deficiency diseases such as scurvy, pellagra, and osteomalacia. For many of these conditions the causes and remedies are known: the issues are largely those of practical implementation of solutions. The health challenges facing industrialised nations appear somewhat different; high among them is disability in an ageing population due to chronic diseases such as cardiovascular disease, cancer, osteoporosis, arthritis, and the dementias. Nevertheless, it is increasingly appreciated that nutrition also has a large, though perhaps more subtle, impact on health and disability in ageing populations. This chapter focuses on this particular aspect of nutrition in older persons.

Measurement

Dietary intake and nutritional status are related, but distinct, aspects of nutrition.[1][2] Several factors influence the relationship between the two.

Dietary intake simply indicates food, including any nutritional supplements, eaten. Several direct methods of quantification of dietary intake are commonly used. Dietary histories are based on food records, either by recall or prospectively, with various degrees of accuracy, such as weighing meals over 24 hours or several days. Food frequency questionnaires documenting usual frequencies of specified foods are more summary measures.[1] The difficulties of measuring dietary intake in free living populations are obvious, owing to the large day to day variability in individuals as well as the numerous sources and varying composition of food. All methods suffer from difficulties with compliance, measurement error in estimation of quantities, variability of nutrients in different foods, and inadequacy of nutrient and food databases.

Indirect measurements include 24 hour urinary estimations, suitable for only a limited number of nutrients, such as sodium, potassium, and nitrogen, used, for example, to assess protein intake; these are based on sometimes questionable assumptions of steady state balance and negligible excretion from other sites.

A separate issue revolves around eating patterns, including meal frequency during the day, and weekly or seasonal variation.

Nutritional status is a more complex entity, reflecting not just dietary intake but metabolic processes and interactions. It is influenced by amount of nutrient absorbed in the gut (and thus, digestive enzyme, gut bacteria, and luminal activity) as well as factors influencing metabolic processes, including physical activity, concurrent illnesses, or other environmental exposures, such as sunshine (necessary for skin manufacture of vitamin D) or smoking (affecting free radical load and hence antioxidant availability).

Nutritional status can be measured in a number of ways[2]: the simplest are anthropometric measures, including height, weight, and weight for height measures such as body mass index (weight/height squared), and measures of fat distribution such as waist:hip ratio or skin fold thickness at different sites. Then there are specific biochemical measures that reflect

---

Box 18.1—Examples of measures of dietary intake or nutritional status and outcomes

Dietary assessment
- Food history/records   Average 24 hour intake of foods
    Average 24 hour intake of nutrients
    Meal patterns/frequency of food consumption in 24 hours
    Weekly or seasonal variability of foods and nutrients
- Urine collection   24 hour urinary excretion of nutrients

Nutritional status
- Anthropometric   Weight, height, and weight for height measures – for example, body mass index
    Fat distribution – for example, waist:hip ratio, skinfold thickness
- Biochemical   Blood levels of proteins, albumin, vitamins – for example, ascorbic acid (C), tocopherol (E), carotenes and retinol (A), fatty acids

Intermediate variables
- Physiological   Blood pressure, bone mass, muscle strength, respiratory function
- Biochemical   Lipids, haemoglobin, haemostatic factors, hormones

Health outcome
- Clinical   Stroke, heart attack, fracture, cancer, cataract
- Functional   Cognitive ability, psychological wellbeing, mobility

---

both intake and metabolism; these include serum levels of vitamins, proteins (albumin), minerals, haemoglobin, hormones, enzymes. Biochemical indices also have limitations: laboratory measurement methods are often not well validated or standardised, and how these measures relate either to intake or to functional outcome is unclear.

Examples of methods are listed in box 18.1. The choice of method used depends on the question being addressed and the precision required; most dietary surveys rely on either food frequency or daily diet records to obtain estimates of average 24 hour intake in different groups.

Age and sex patterns in nutritional status

Figures 18.1 and 18.2 and table 18.1 show mean body mass index and mean waist:hip ratio in men and women by age in a British population sample.[3] Mean body mass index increases with increasing age in both men and women until age 60 or so, after which it declines; mean levels do not differ greatly in men and women, particularly after the age of 60 years. In contrast, mean waist:hip ratios increase steadily with increasing age throughout life and women have significantly lower mean waist:hip ratios than men at all ages. Increasing age is associated with a reduction in muscle and bone mass and a relative increase in percentage of fat, particularly central abdominal fat, consistent with both the body mass index and waist: hip ratio patterns. How much this is due to physiological ageing and how much to changing lifestyle, such as physical activity and diet, is not clear. Data from other industrialised countries show similar patterns; nevertheless, secular changes in industrialised countries (in which mean body mass index levels have increased in the last few decades) and differences in some non-industrialised countries (which show no increase in body mass index with age) suggest that many of these changes are not concomitants of ageing but are susceptible to lifestyle influences.

There are few population based survey data that directly compare dietary intake or biochemical status in young and old adults; in Britain, the 1986 dietary and nutritional survey[2] only examined persons aged 16–64 years. Two surveys, in 1968 and 1972, on British men and women aged 65 years and over[4] reported both sex and age differences in energy and nutrient intake. Table 18.2 shows mean daily intakes of energy and nutrients in men and women in two age groups. Total energy intake fell with age and was also lower in women; since nutrient density of the diet tended to remain similar, absolute levels of nutrient intake also fell with age. Malnutrition was diagnosed in about 3% of the people over 65 seen. Assessment of the prevalence of poor nutrition was more problematic: the survey highlighted the lack of information on which a sound estimate of requirements for nutrients or nutritional norms can be based. In general, caloric needs are influenced by physical activity and thought to decline with age: table 18.3 shows estimated daily caloric requirements with age.[5] Whether this is

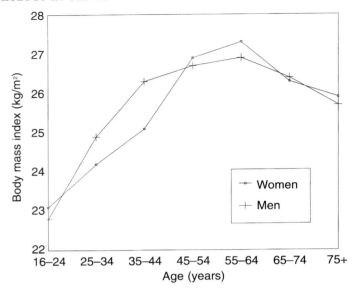

Fig 18.1   Mean body mass index by age and sex: health survey for England 1991.

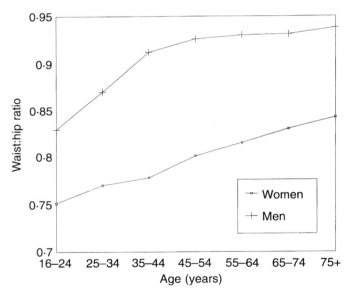

Fig 18.2   Mean waist:hip ratio by age and sex: health survey for England 1991.

desirable or not is debatable. Additionally, dietary habits are not static: profound secular and longitudinal changes in diet in older persons, such as declining caloric intake, correspond to secular changes in the population as a whole.

174

Table 18.1   Mean body mass index and waist:hip ratio by age and sex in British adults

	Age (years)						
	16–24	25–34	35–44	45–54	55–64	65–74	75+
Body mass index (kg/m²)							
Men	22·8	24·9	26·3	26·7	26·9	26·4	25·7
Women	23·1	24·2	25·1	26·9	27·3	26·3	25·9
Waist:hip ratio (cm:cm)							
Men	0·829	0·870	0·912	0·926	0·930	0·931	0·938
Women	0·751	0·770	0·778	0·801	0·815	0·830	0·842

Table 18.2   Mean daily intakes of energy and nutrients in British men and women aged 65 years and over (DHSS survey of the elderly 1972[4])

	Men		Women	
	65–79 years	80 + years	65–79 years	80 + years
Daily dietary intake				
Energy (kcal)	2217	2024	1679	1559
(MJ)	9·3	8·5	7·0	6·5
Animal protein (g)	47·5	47·8	39·3	36·4
Total protein (g)	71·2	68·9	57·5	52·6
Fat (g)	100	93	81	72
Carbohydrate (g)	255	235	189	182
Calcium (mg)	890	870	780	690
Iron (mg)	11·6	11·0	9·3	8·6
Vitamin A (μg)	1120	1050	1050	980
Thiamin (mg)	1·0	0·9	0·8	0·7
Riboflavin (mg)	1·5	1·4	1·3	1·1
Nicotinic acid (mg)	14·4	12·3	10·3	9·7
Pyridoxine (mg)	1·3	1·2	0·9	0·9
Vitamin C (mg)	46	38	40	37
Vitamin D (μg)	2·4	2·7	2·1	2·3
Added sugars (g)	71·6	66·0	48·8	48·5
Energy from protein (%)	13·1	13·7	13·9	13·7
Energy from fat (%)	40·6	41·0	43·2	41·8
Energy from added sugars (%)	12·7	13·2	11·5	12·2
Biochemistry				
Serum total proteins (g/l)	73·1	73·4	72·4	72·0
Serum albumin (g/l)	43·4	42·1	43·4	42·7
Alkaline phosphatase (KA units)	7·9	9·5	8·4	9·2
Serum calcium (mmol/l)	2·36	2·36	2·38	2·36
Serum phosphate (mmol/l)	0·93	0·93	1·10	1·07
Leucocyte ascorbic acid (μg/10⁸ cells)	22·8	21·8	27·0	23·3
Plasma ascorbic acid (μmol/l)	27·8	29·0	28·4	31·2
Red cell transketolase (activation count)	1·14	1·14	1·13	1·11
Red cell glutathione reductase (activation count)	1·27	1·26	1·25	1·25

175

Table 18.3   Estimated average daily requirements for energy[5]

Age (years)	Men		Women	
	MJ	kcal	MJ	kcal
19–50	10·60	2550	8·10	1940
51–59	10·60	2550	8·00	1900
60–64	99·93	2380	7·99	1900
65–74	9·71	2330	7·96	1900
75+	8·77	2100	7·61	1810

Associations and causal links with disease

Diet, nutritional status, and health

A central question must be what recommended dietary intakes should be for older persons and, related to this, whether there are optimal ranges for nutritional status.[6] This depends on what the objectives of such recommendations are. If the main aim is optimum health, then many methods used to make judgements in the past about recommendations are subject to criticism. Some recommendations are based on normative ranges, that is, statistical definitions such as percentiles derived from surveys, but these are not particularly helpful because they vary from population to population; what is statistically normal is not necessarily desirable. Others relate to findings from metabolic studies, such as absorption and balance experiments. Estimates of requirements may thus be based on intakes needed to maintain a given circulating level or degree of enzyme saturation or tissue concentration. How these may relate to health is not always clear. Some recommendations (for example, for vitamins) are based on the minimum required to prevent deficiency diseases; however, these minimal levels may not be optimal. Even when overt deficiency diseases are not present, low levels of nutrients may be associated with increased risk of many chronic conditions; for example, vitamin D deficiency is undoubtedly a cause of osteomalacia, but persons with low levels of vitamin D (though above those that lead to osteomalacia) may be at increased risk of osteoporosis and fracture as well as muscle weakness. Similarly, anaemia and peripheral neuropathy associated with severe folate or B_{12} deficiency is well recognised; but suboptimal intake of B vitamins is also associated with increased homocysteine levels and atherosclerosis risk, and impaired neurological and cognitive function.[7] For many diseases risk is related in a continuous manner to level of intake or biochemical status. Thus, while extreme values associated with toxicity or deficiency can be defined, within a large middle range, the functional significance is unknown.

Ultimately, the standard for recommendations should be the level associated with optimum health outcome, which is not the same as the

176

level to prevent clinical deficiency. There are several types of study that may contribute towards our understanding of the association between nutrition and health; apart from laboratory work demonstrating biologically plausible mechanisms, and metabolic ward studies, epidemiological data including ecological, case control, and prospective studies, and, strongest evidence of all, intervention studies, are required. Unfortunately, studies on nutrition and health outcome in human populations are particularly hard to carry out. Assessment of dietary intake in free living human populations is laborious and difficult, confounding is a particular problem, and the long time scale and size of the population required to measure health end points are problematic. Intervention studies are even more difficult because it is hard to change one nutrient without changing many others in a diet, quite apart from the problems of compliance.

Why might the elderly differ from the young?

The generalisability of studies carried out in younger age groups to the elderly is debatable because older persons may differ in many respects as a result of physiological changes with age, and cohort and selective survival effects. Many metabolic processes, gut, endocrine, hepatic, and renal function change with age, so requirements in older people may differ. Digestive and luminal changes with age may affect the ability to absorb nutrients ingested, such as calcium; for a given dose of ultraviolet light older persons manufacture less vitamin D in their skin compared with younger persons; older persons appear less able to excrete a sodium load and may be more susceptible to the blood pressure raising effect of high dietary sodium. The impact of illness, so common in older persons, is even less well understood.

Evidence for optimal levels of nutritional status or dietary intake in older persons

Anthropometry

While obesity has been associated with many chronic age related conditions, such as diabetes, cardiovascular disease, and arthritis, the relationship between body mass index and health in older persons is controversial. There appears to be a U shaped relationship between body mass index and mortality, and optimum body mass index in terms of health outcome appears to increase with increasing age[8]; this may be due to selective survival or mortality or to changing metabolic processes. Table 18.4 shows the body mass index level associated with lowest mortality from the US build study 1979.[8] The US national health and nutrition examination study, which measured functional status outcome for men and women in the community aged 65–86 years, also indicated a U shaped relationship with body mass index: very high or very low values were associated with worse functional status.[9] The optimum range was wide: for women it was 18·9–31·0 and for men 21·9–29·3.

Table 18.4   Body mass index (kg/m²) level at different ages associated with lowest mortality (US body build and blood pressure study 1979[8])

Age (years)	Men	Women
20–29	21·4	19·5
30–39	21·6	23·4
40–49	22·9	23·2
50–59	25·8	25·2
60–69	26·6	27·3

In contrast, numerous studies have shown that waist:hip ratio, a measure of central abdominal obesity, is a strong predictor of subsequent health; indeed, some population studies have shown that persons in the lowest waist:hip ratio decile show much less rise in cardiovascular mortality with age.[10] Body mass index (a weight for height measure) may be a poorer surrogate measure of the metabolic consequences of inappropriate nutrition in adults than waist:hip ratio, which reflects fat distribution; low waist:hip ratio is a better predictor of health in older persons.

Both body mass ratio and waist:hip ratio reflect not just dietary intake but also physical activity, and increased levels of physical activity are associated with better health in older persons.[11]

Dietary intake

Early experiments reporting that severe food restriction (though resulting in many early deaths) increased longevity in surviving rats led to the widespread belief that caloric restriction would delay ageing in humans[12]; however, this is largely unsupported by evidence in humans. Findings from rats in strictly controlled experimental conditions are not easily applicable to free living humans.[13] In fact prospective population studies have shown an inverse relationship between mortality and caloric intake.[14 15] It is likely that the higher caloric intake associated with better health outcome in humans may reflect both higher levels of physical activity patterns that are beneficial and higher intake of protective nutrients.

Many different types of study have reported the relationship between nutrients and health outcomes; some of these are listed in box 18.2 and reviewed fully elsewhere.[16–20] Many chronic diseases associated with ageing are related less to overnutrition, as rat experiments would lead us to believe, than to inappropriate or undernutrition—in particular, low levels of apparently protective nutrients such as vitamins and minerals. It is also notable that the foods and nutrients that appear beneficial are very similar for many chronic diseases, such as cardiovascular disease and cancer.

178

Box 18.2—Examples of dietary factors associated with disease

Condition	Dietary factor
● Stroke	Adverse: sodium, alcohol (high dose)
	Protective: potassium, vitamin C, magnesium, fruit and vegetables
● Coronary heart disease	Adverse: saturated fat, *trans*-fatty acids, dietary cholesterol
	Protective: ω-3 fatty acids, α linolenic acid, oleic acid, non-starch polysaccharides, starch, potassium, magnesium, calcium, phyto-oestrogens, antioxidants – for example, vitamins E, C, flavonoids, carotenoids, selenium, folate/riboflavin
● Osteoporosis/fractures	Adverse: caffeine, animal protein, sodium, alcohol (high dose)
	Protective: calcium, vitamin D, ω-3 fatty acids, alcohol (low dose), phyto-oestrogens
● Macular degeneration	Protective: carotenoids, vitamin C, ω-3 fatty acids
● Cataracts	Protective: antioxidants, riboflavin, vitamin B_{12}
● Rheumatoid arthritis	Protective: ω-3 fatty acids
● Osteoarthritis	Adverse: saturated fat, meat
● Dementia	Adverse: aluminium
	Protective: antioxidants—for example, vitamin E, B vitamins
● Large bowel disease	Adverse: sulphite, meat, fat
	Protective: non-starch polysaccharides, starch
● Diabetes	Adverse: non-milk extrinsic sugars
	Protective: ω-3 fatty acids, antioxidants, soluble non-starch polysaccharides

---

Interventions and evaluations of efficacy

While abundant clinical, observational, and laboratory data support the importance of nutritional factors and health, there is a paucity of evidence from randomised controlled intervention trials, and trials including older subjects are even more scarce. Nevertheless, several trials lend support to the notion not only that nutritional interventions influence health in the elderly but also that the absolute impact may in fact be as great or greater in older persons. A French trial of vitamin D and calcium supplementation in women aged 75 years and over showed 30% reduction in fractures after 18 months[21]; two secondary prevention trials following myocardial

179

infarction (which may be relevant in the elderly, who may have already established disease) showed, in one case, advice to eat fatty fish twice weekly was associated with a 30% reduction in mortality[22]; in the second, a Mediterranean diet (substituting monounsaturated fat for other fats, increasing fruit intake) resulted in a 70% reduction in four year mortality.[23] A multinutrient (vitamins and minerals) supplement improved immunological function and decreased infections by half in healthy men and women aged 65 years and over.[24] While the generalisability of such findings to the whole elderly population is debatable, and more quantitative data relating intakes to health outcomes are required, the profound secular changes and international variations in disease and dietary patterns are consistent with trial findings.

Nutritional status in institutionalised elderly people

Numerous surveys have been published indicating that undernutrition is a particular issue in institutionalised elderly people. A major difficulty in interpretation of such data is that institutionalised elderly people are heterogenous and highly selected in different ways depending on the reasons for institutionalisation, which may vary between different institutions and countries and indeed over time.[25] Groups that have been studied include hospitalised elderly, residents of old age homes, residents of nursing homes, and those institutionalised with chronic mental illness. Some institutions may only admit healthy elderly; others may admit those who are already severely debilitated. Thus the nutritional status of those in institutions reflects a complex mixture not just of dietary intake but also of existing health status, which depends on the selection criteria for institutionalisation. Many studies indicate that for whatever reasons, including existing physical illness or disability, poor dentition and loss of appetite, low palatability and nutritional content of mass catered food, as well as social factors, institutionalised elderly are at increased risk of protein calorie malnutrition and biochemical evidence of micronutrient deficiencies.[26-28]

While overt specific clinical deficiency diseases, such as scurvy or pellagra, are relatively unusual, the clinical impact may be profound: non-specific consequences including general weakness and debility, susceptibility to infection, loss of muscle strength, and depression have been attributed to undernutrition, and poor nutritional status is associated with increased mortality.[29 30] Some intervention studies have reported that nutritional supplements may be beneficial in the convalescence period after hospitalisation for acute events, such as fracture of femur or chest infections, although the relevance of these findings to long term institutionalised elderly groups is less clear.[31 32]

Poor nutritional status is not, however, an invariable feature of institutionalisation: other surveys have reported that institutionalised elderly compared favourably in nutritional status with those elderly living in the community.[33] Inconsistency in findings probably reflects selection differences for different institutions and illustrates how generalisation of findings from various studies of elderly living in institutions is problematic.

Dietary recommendations and health policy

Factors apart from diet, not discussed here, clearly have a major influence on health; these are illustrated in box 18.3. Nevertheless, nutrition has a critical role in the health of the elderly.

Box 18.3—Factors influencing nutrition and health

Element	Factors influencing
• Food intake	Socioeconomic—for example, knowledge preference, accessibility, income
	Physiological—for example, dentition, swallowing
• Nutritional status	Environmental—for example, sunlight exposure
	Behavioural—for example, physical activity, smoking
	Metabolic—for example, digestion, absorption
• Health outcome	Host factors—for example, genetic susceptibility, concurrent illness
	Environmental—for example, other exposures (for example, toxins, smoking, infection)

While precise recommendations for daily allowances for specific nutrients are controversial because of paucity of data, the overall evidence to date does support strongly particular eating and nutritional patterns concomitant with good health. The 1994 recommendations of the Committee on Medical Aspects of Food Policy[20] stress the importance of adequate intake of nutrients such as vitamins and minerals, and of ω-3 fatty acids, achieved by diets high in fresh fruit, vegetables, and complex carbohydrates such as bread and potatoes, and by fatty fish intake (at least once a week). Conversely, reduction in dietary sodium and saturated or *trans*-fatty acid intake can be achieved by reduction in certain processed foods or substitution with oils and fats rich in monounsaturated fatty acids. There is insufficient evidence on benefits to recommend widespread use of vitamin or other nutritional supplements in healthy persons if dietary guidelines are followed and there is concern about possible toxicity.

Extremes of weight, as indicated by either very high or very low body mass indices, are adversely associated with health; to maintain adequate nutrition while keeping body mass index within a desirable (albeit wide) range implies regular physical activity.

181

While better data are always needed, the evidence to date supports the recommendations of the Working Party on the Nutrition of Elderly People[5]:

the majority of people aged 65 years or more should adopt, where possible, similar patterns of eating and lifestyle to those advised for maintaining health in younger adults. Physical activity improves muscle tone and power, and leads to higher energy expenditure. A diet which provides an adequate intake of all nutrients can more easily be obtained if the energy intake remains at a level close to that recommended for younger adults. There needs to be greater awareness of the importance of good nutrition for maintaining the health of elderly people and of its contribution to recovery from illness. Nutrition and health promotion programmes should include this population group.

Dietary recommendations are of course only one aspect of clinical or health policy. Dietary intake is influenced by a host of social and cultural factors, including choice, access, availability, and income. Older persons who are at high risk of poor nutrition and health include those who may already have poor health, with poor dentition or inability to swallow, those with physical disability, mental illness, malabsorption, those who are taking medications that interfere with nutrition, and those who are poor or isolated or in ignorance of basic nutritional facts. The social framework and policies necessary for improvement of nutrition include consideration of issues such as labelling, advertising, foods for subsidy, education, and incomes.

1 Bingham S. The dietary assessment of individuals: methods, accuracy, new techniques and recommendations. *Nutr Abs Rev* 1987;**57**:705–42.
2 Office of Population Censuses and Surveys Social Survey Division. *The dietary and nutritional survey of British adults.* London: HMSO, 1990.
3 Office of Population Censuses and Surveys Social Survey Division. *Health survey for England 1991.* London: HMSO, 1993.
4 Department of Health and Social Services. *Nutrition and health in old age.* London: HMSO, 1979. (Report on health and social subjects, No 16.)
5 Department of Health. *The nutrition of elderly people.* London: HMSO, 1992. (Report on health and social subjects, No 43.)
6 Department of Health. *Dietary reference values for food energy and nutrients for the United Kingdom.* London: HMSO, 1991. (Report on health and social subjects, No 41.)
7 Rosenberg IH, Miller JW. Nutritional factors in physical and cognitive functions of elderly people. *Am J Clin Nutr* 1992;**55**:1237–43S.
8 Andres R, Elahi D, Tobin JD, Muller DC, Brant L. Impact of age on weight goals. *Ann Intern Med* 1985;**103**:1030–3.
9 Galanos AN, Pieper CF, Cornoni-Huntley JC, Bales CW, Fillenbaum GG. Nutrition and function: is there a relationship between body mass index and the functional capabilities of community dwelling elderly? *J Am Geriatr Soc* 1994;**42**:368–73.
10 Larsson B. Regional obesity as a health hazard in men—prospective studies. *Acta Med Scand* 1988;**723**(suppl):45–51.
11 Donahue RP, Abbott RD, Reed MD, Yano K. Physical activity and coronary heart disease in middle aged and elderly men. *Am J Public Health* 1989;**78**:683–5.
12 McCay CM, Sperling G, Barnes LL. Growth, aging, chronic diseases and lifespan in rats. *Arch Biochem* 1943;**2**:469–79.
13 Widdowson EM. Physiological processes of aging: are there special nutritional requirements for elderly people? Do McCay's findings apply to humans? *Am J Clin Nutr* 1992;**55**: 1246–9S.
14 Kromhout D, De Lezenne Coulander C. Diet, prevalence and 10 year mortality from coronary heart disease in 871 middle aged men. *Am J Epidemiol* 1984;**119**:733–41.

15 Lapidus L, Andersson H, Bengtsson C, Bosaeus I. Dietary habits in relation to cardiovascular disease and death in women. *Am J Clin Nutr* 1986;**44**:444–8.
16 World Health Organization study group. Diet, nutrition and the prevention of chronic diseases. *WHO Tech Rep Ser* 1990;797.
17 US Department of Health and Human Services. *The Surgeon General's report on nutrition and health.* Washington: USDHHS(PHS), 1988. (Publication No 88-50210.)
18 Munro HM, Danford DE, editors. *Nutrition, ageing and the elderly.* New York: Plenum Press, 1989.
19 Horwitz A, MacFadyen DM, Munro H, Scrimshaw NS, Steen B, Williams TF, editors. *Nutrition in the elderly.* Oxford: Oxford University Press, 1989.
20 Department of Health. *Nutritional aspects of cardiovascular disease. Report of the Cardiovascular Review Group committee on medical aspects of food policy.* London: HMSO, 1994.
21 Chapuy MC, Arlot ME, Duboeuf F, *et al.* Vitamin D3 and calcium to prevent hip fractures in elderly women. *N Engl J Med* 1992;**32**:1637–42.
22 de Lorgeril M, Renaud S, Mamelle S, *et al.* Mediterranean alpha linolenic rich diet in secondary prevention of coronary heart disease. *Lancet* 1994;**343**:1454–9.
23 Burr ML, Fehily AM, Gilbert JF, *et al.* Effects of changes in fat, fish and fibre intakes on death and myocardial infarction. *Lancet* 1989;**ii**:757–61.
24 Chandra RK. Effect of vitamin and trace-element supplementation on immune responses and infection in elderly subjects. *Lancet* 1992;**340**:1124–7.
25 Goodwin JS. Social, psychological and physical factors affecting the nutritional status of elderly subjects: separating cause and effect. *Am J Clin Nutr* 1989;**50**:1201–9.
26 Rudman D, Feller AG. Protein-calorie undernutrition in the nursing home. *J Am Geriatr Soc* 1989;**37**:173–83.
27 Infante-Rivard C, Krieger M, Gascon-Barre M, Rivard GE. Folate deficiency among the institutionalised elderly. Public health impact. *J Am Geriatr Soc* 1986;**34**:211–4.
28 Morgan DB, Newton HM, Schorah CJ, Jewitt MA, Hancock MR, Hullin RP. Abnormal indices of nutrition in the elderly: a study of different clinical groups. *Age Ageing* 1986;**15**:65-76.
29 Rudman D, Mattson DE, Nagraj HS, Caindec N, Rudman IW, Jackson DL. Antecedents of death in the men of a Veterans Administration nursing home. *J Am Geriatr Soc* 1987;**35**:496–502.
30 Woo J, Chan SM, Mak YT, Swaminathan R. Biochemical predictors of short term mortality in elderly residents of chronic care institutions. *J Clin Pathol* 1989;**42**:1241–5.
31 Delmi M, Rapin CH, Bengoa JM, Delmas PD, Vasey H, Bonjour JP. Dietary supplementation in elderly patients with fractured neck of femur. *Lancet* 1990;**335**:1013–6.
32 Woo J, Ho SC, Mak YT, Law LK, Cheung A. Nutritional status of elderly patients during recovery from chest infection and the role of nutritional supplementation assessed by prospective randomised single blind trial. *Age Ageing* 1994;**23**:40–8.
33 Sahyoun NR, Otradovec CL, Hartz SC, *et al.* Dietary intakes and biochemical indicators of nutritional status in an elderly, institutionalised population. *Am J Clin Nutr* 1988;**47**:524–33.

19 Classical cardiovascular risk factors

RUTH BONITA

The standard or "classical" cardiovascular risk factors refer to those that are major, well established, and modifiable. These are smoking, raised blood pressure, and, at least for coronary heart disease, raised cholesterol. There are many other potentially modifiable risk factors, including obesity and physical inactivity, as well as psychosocial factors—for example, poor social networks, and lack of social support—that are associated with cardiovascular disease; social class is a major determinant of cardiovascular disease risk. Non-modifiable risk factors for cardiovascular disease include a previous vascular event (myocardial infarction, stroke, angina, or peripheral vascular disease), family history of coronary heart disease, male gender, and, above all, increasing age.

Of what relevance are these risk factors in older people, who, by their very age, are at an increased risk of cardiovascular disease? Despite the fact that over 80% of cardiovascular disease deaths occur in people over the age of 65, the significance of the classical risk factors for cardiovascular disease in older people has only been confirmed recently. This chapter examines the evidence concerning cigarette smoking, raised blood pressure, and raised cholesterol levels and their association with cardiovascular disease, coronary heart disease, and stroke in particular.

Smoking

Cigarette smoking is the most important modifiable risk factor for cardiovascular disease for young and old alike. Fortunately, smoking is usually less prevalent in older people than in younger people. Although there have been reductions in the prevalence of cigarette smoking in some countries, this is not shared by all age and gender groups. For example, in the United States smoking declined in men aged 65 years and over from 28% in the mid-1960s to 15% in 1990; meanwhile smoking increased from 10 to 12% in women in the same age group.[1]

The increased relative risk of coronary heart disease associated with cigarette smoking tends to decrease in older age groups, although this could be the result of a selective loss of smokers due to premature death.

184

Reductions in stroke and coronary heart disease from cessation of smoking have been well established.[2] Rates decline as time since quitting increases, but some benefits are realised immediately. For example, stroke risk decreases after two years' abstinence from cigarette smoking and becomes the same as that of never smokers after five years.[3]

The public health significance of the association between smoking and cardiovascular disease in elderly people is shown in table 19.1, which compares current smokers with never smokers and shows both the relative risks and deaths attributed to smoking for younger (35–64 years) and older (65 years and over) adults. The number of deaths attributable to smoking are greater in the older ages, despite lower relative risks, because death rates increase steeply with age. Although relative risks for coronary heart disease and stroke are about the same in men and women, the excess number of deaths attributable to smoking is much higher for men because of higher rates of cardiovascular disease in men.

Table 19.1   Relative risk (RR) and population attributable risk (PAR)* in current smokers compared with never smokers, by age group, United States 1985[1]

Age (years)	Coronary heart disease				Stroke			
	Men		Women		Men		Women	
	RR	PAR	RR	PAR	RR	PAR	RR	PAR
35–64	2·8	34 000	3·0	11 000	3·7	5 500	4·8	5 200
65+	1·6	44 000	1·6	26 000	1·9	12 000	1·5	4 800

* Deaths attributable to smoking.

In summary, the relationship between smoking and cardiovascular disease in older people, while not as strong or as consistent in relative terms as in younger people, is of great importance in terms of absolute risk. The benefits of quitting smoking, even at older ages, are wide ranging and include reduction of risk for cardiovascular disease and improvements in total mortality.

Blood pressure

Elevated blood pressure is common in elderly people. Systolic blood pressure increases with age, at least until the eighth decade. In contrast, diastolic blood pressure rises only until about 50 years of age and levels off or decreases thereafter. These divergent trends in systolic blood pressure and diastolic blood pressure lead to the increase with age of pulse pressure and the increasing prevalence of isolated systolic hypertension. The prevalence of isolated systolic hypertension (defined as systolic) blood pressure ≥ 160 mm Hg and diastolic blood pressure ≥ 90 mm Hg) rises from around 5% at age 60, to 12% at age 70, and 23% at age 80.

Most estimates of the prevalence of hypertension have been based on casual measurements; the proportion of people who have sustained hypertension is considerably lower and likely to be between a quarter and a third of those with casual hypertension. In the United States about one half of the population aged 65–74 years are on treatment for hypertension or have a systolic blood pressure ≥ 160 mm Hg and/or a diastolic blood pressure ≥ 95 mm Hg. Cardiovascular complications in older people are more closely related to systolic blood pressure than to diastolic blood pressure. High blood pressure is the most important risk factor for both ischaemic and haemorrhagic stroke.

A number of clinical trials focusing on older people have now demonstrated that reducing blood pressure reduces the risk of both stroke and coronary heart disease, although the relative benefits are greater for stroke.[4] A noteworthy feature of these clinical trials in older people is the tiny proportion of the population who were eligible for the studies, casting doubt on the applicability of these findings to the general population.

In summary, blood pressure is a major risk factor for cardiovascular disease and reducing blood pressure by treatment has been shown to be beneficial in patients up to the age of 80 years; the relative benefits of reduction are less for coronary heart disease than for stroke, but the absolute benefits are greater for coronary heart disease (see chapter 26).

Cholesterol

Elevated serum cholesterol is common in older people. Men and women tend to run a parallel course in mean blood cholesterol levels until the sixth decade, when mean levels for women become higher. In the Framingham cohort free of coronary heart disease at age 65 years, 37% of men and 61% of women had cholesterol levels greater than 6·0 mmol/l.[5]

Total serum cholesterol predicts coronary heart disease death in older men and women, with the absolute excess risk greater at older ages.[6] Other studies have reported either a J shaped relationship or an inverse relationship between total cholesterol and coronary heart disease and total mortality; the latter finding may be partly explained by pre-existing disease, heavy smoking, and lipid lowering drugs.

There are only limited data on the effect of lipid fractions and coronary heart disease in older people. High low density lipoproteins and low levels of high density lipoprotein cholesterol are associated with an increased risk of coronary heart disease, particularly in older people with high triglyceride levels[7]; high density lipoprotein cholesterol is inversely related to coronary heart disease in older women but not older men.[6] The association of serum cholesterol and stroke appears to be in oppositive directions for non-haemorrhagic (direct association) and haemorrhagic stroke (inverse association).[8]

In summary, total serum cholesterol is a risk factor for coronary heart disease in both men and women and this relationship persists into very old age. With regard to stroke, total serum cholesterol is positively associated with cerebral infarction but inversely associated with haemorrhagic stroke.

Intervention

Prevention of cardiovascular disease at older ages presents challenges and opportunities that are different from those experienced at younger ages. There is less information about the efficacy of specific interventions at older ages, especially in women. Until this information is available, extrapolation from mid-aged adults to older people must be cautious.

Cardiovascular risk reduction requires attention to all modifiable classical risk factors. The dramatic decline in cigarette smoking in many wealthy countries shows that smokers can be persuaded to give up smoking. In many countries the cohorts of women who started smoking during and after the second world war are now entering old age, indicating the importance of including elderly women in smoking cessation programmes.

Management of mild elevations of blood pressure in elderly people can be achieved by non-pharmacological measures, including reduction of salt and excess alcohol consumption, weight control, and physical activity.[9] For patients with moderate to severe hypertension, randomised controlled trials of elderly hypertensives have demonstrated a significant reduction in cardiovascular disease mortality using diuretics and β blockers. Newer drugs, such as angiotensin converting enzyme inhibitors, α blockers, and calcium antagonists, probably should not be considered for first line treatment until trials show that they are at least as effective as diuretics and β blockers in reducing cardiovascular disease events.

Whether cholesterol lowering will have similar effects on the risk of coronary heart disease in older people is uncertain, although current trials are assessing this issue. As with younger people, drug therapy should be initiated only after serious dietary therapy has been attempted. At present there are no data showing that treatment decreases cardiovascular disease events above age 80; diagnosis and treatment after this age is not generally indicated.

Cost effectiveness

Inexpensive interventions directed at the whole population offer the best value for money, especially where there is a high prevalence of risk factors.[10] The gains in cost effectiveness of any intervention are greatest where absolute risk is increased, at older ages, and when other risk factors are present. In addition, the benefits of treatment accumulate sooner in older compared with younger patients. Most cost effectiveness studies have underestimated the potential benefit from treatment of the elderly by exclusion of elderly people and their ability to benefit in the models.

A large percentage of older women have cholesterol levels above the cut off points recommended for either vigorous dietary or drug therapy; however, the evidence is insufficient to justify population screening for high cholesterol in older people, particularly when the economic costs are considered, unlike opportunistic screening for raised blood pressure, which adds little extra cost.[11]

Health policy

The increasing number of elderly people in all societies and the high burden from cardiovascular disease in elderly people make it urgent that appropriate health policy recommendations are made for this important and growing group. In particular, the special features of old age—the presence of comorbidity, the influence of social and economic factors, and the importance of drug interactions—require tailoring of programmes to suit the needs of older people.

Health and social policy needs to be guided by scientific evidence, which is likely to become increasingly available. Until recently, research on the importance of risk factors in older people has lagged behind that in younger people. Relative risk of an association of a risk factor with cardiovascular disease has received more attention than the absolute risk, yet it is the latter which is of more relevance in determining treatment strategies in older people. The high prevalence of cardiovascular disease risk factors in older people, particularly raised blood pressure and raised serum cholesterol, has the potential to lead to widespread treatment of older people. Greater emphasis needs to be directed at primary prevention beginning earlier in life.

Conclusions

Worldwide, cardiovascular disease is the leading cause of disability and death in the population aged 65 years and above. The variation in cardiovascular disease mortality rates in people over 65 years of age between and among countries indicates the potential for prevention. Declines in cardiovascular disease mortality rates, including people in the oldest age groups, are occurring in many countries, but not all; rates are increasing in some eastern and central European countries. Older people share the same risk factors as younger populations. Furthermore, while risk measured in mid-age predicts the development of cardiovascular disease in old age, risk factors measured in older age also predict the development of cardiovascular disease. Since elevated risk factor levels are common in older people, even small increases in relative risk are of great public health importance because of the higher absolute rates of disease in this population.

188

There is great potential for the prevention of cardiovascular disease in older populations and individual treatment strategies should be guided by the scientific evidence. At present the evidence is best for the treatment of elevated blood pressure in older people and for smoking cessation.

1 US Department of Health and Human Services. *Reducing the health consequences of smoking: 25 years of progress. A report of the Surgeon General.* Washington: USDHHS, 1989. (Publication (CDC) 89–8411.)
2 Jajich CL, Ostfeld AM, Freeman DH. Smoking and coronary heart disease mortality in the elderly. *JAMA* 1984;**252**:2831–4.
3 Wolf PA, D'Agostino RB, Kannel WB, Bonita R, Belanger AJ. Cigarette smoking as a risk factor for stroke: the Framingham study. *JAMA* 1988;**259**:1025–9.
4 SHEP Cooperative Research Group. Prevention of stroke by antihypertensive drug treatment in older persons with isolated systolic hypertension. Final results of the Systolic Hypertension in the Elderly Program (SHEP). *JAMA* 1991;**265**:3255–64.
5 Harris T, Cook EF, Kannel WB, *et al.* Proportional hazards analysis of risk factors for coronary heart disease in individuals aged 65 or older. *J Am Geriatr Soc* 1988;**36**:1023–8.
6 Manolio TA, Pearson TA, Wenger NK, *et al.* Cholesterol and heart disease in older persons and women. Review of an NHLBI Workshop. *Ann Epidemiol* 1992;**2**:161–76.
7 Castelli WP, Wilson PWF, Levy D, *et al.* Cardiovascular risk factors in the elderly. *Am J Cardiol* 1989;**63**:12–9H.
8 Iso H, Jacobs DR Jr, Wentworth D, *et al.* Serum cholesterol levels in 6-year mortality from stroke in 350 977 men screened for the Multiple Risk Factor Intervention Trial. *New Engl J Med* 1989;**14**:904–10.
9 Geleijnse JM, Witteman JCM, Bak AAA, den Breeijen JH, Grobbee DE. Reduction in blood pressure with a low sodium, high potassium, high magnesium salt in older subjects with mild to moderate hypertension. *BMJ* 1994;**309**:436–40.
10 Goldman L, Gordon DJ, Rifkind BM, *et al.* Cost and health implications of cholesterol lowering. *Circulation* 1992;**85**:1960–8.
11 Fletcher AE. Cost effectiveness analyses in the treatment of high blood pressure. *J Hum Hypertens* 1992;**6**:437–45.

20 Exercise

ARCHIE YOUNG

Exercise of some kind or other is almost essential to the preservation of health in persons of all ages—but in none more so than in the old.

Daniel MacLachlan

Physician and Surgeon to the Royal Hospital, Chelsea (1840–1863). *From a practical treatise on the disease and infirmities of advanced life,* 1863.

The health benefits of exercise are of particular importance in old age. Their evaluation, however, is complicated by the need to define the frequency, intensity, duration, and type of exercise, and by the need to demonstrate the physiological effects conceptually necessary for a causal link between the exercise and the health benefits.

Measurement

Habitual physical activity

There are several questionnaires for the measurement of the habitual physical activity of older people but the absolute levels of habitual physical activity encountered amongst elderly people vary widely, from elite veteran athletes running perhaps 50 km every week to people housebound by the disabling effects of stroke and arthritis. As a result, no single questionnaire can be assumed to be appropriate for measuring the habitual physical activity of all elderly people. The purpose of the measurement will dictate the relative importance of ceiling effects, floor effects, and sensitivity to change and so dictate the choice of questionnaire.

All questionnaires depend on accurate recall. There is little reason to suppose that recall of habitual physical activity will be any more reliable in elderly people than in other study populations. Hence the interest in attempts to make direct measurements of habitual activity by means of unobtrusive monitors that provide either a cumulative or, in some cases, a continuous record of activity over periods of at least 24 hours. These instruments may record movement, footfall, heart rate, or energy expenditure. They too have important limitations: for example, the instrumentation itself necessarily limits these studies to small numbers of subjects. Also, if the exercise stimulus is of sufficient intensity some of its beneficial effects may be achieved with only rather infrequent performance (perhaps only three times a week) of rather brief exercise (perhaps only 10 minutes at a time). Even the most accurate cumulative record of physical activity cannot provide this crucial degree of discrimination. The conventional analysis of 24 hour recordings must be modified to yield estimates of the frequency of episodes of activity whose duration and intensity exceed predetermined critical values.

Strength

An isometric contraction is one in which the muscle's action is pitted against an immovable object, so that the length of the active muscle remains unchanged. In an isokinetic contraction the length of the active muscle does change, but specialised instrumentation ensures that this is at a constant velocity. Provided muscle strength is measured in an action that involves only a single joint, and the adjacent limb segments are firmly secured, a practised operator can readily obtain reliable measurements of muscle strength (table 20.1) as the force (or torque) exerted in maximal voluntary isometric or isokinetic contractions.

Table 20.1 Coefficients of variation for measurements of physical performance in healthy older subjects[3]

	70–79 years	80–89 years
Isometric strength		
Handgrip	3%	
Knee extension	8%* or 6%	4%
Elbow flexion	6%	
Lower limb extensor power	9%	
Cardiac frequency during progressive exercise tests (by interpolation):		
Treadmill walking		
at $\dot{V}o_2 = 10\,ml\,kg^{-1}\,min^{-1}$	4%	
at $\dot{V}o_2 = 15\,ml\,kg^{-1}\,min^{-1}$	7%	
Cycle ergometry		
at $\dot{V}o_2 = 10\,ml\,kg^{-1}\,min^{-1}$		6%†
at $\dot{V}o_2 = 15\,ml\,kg^{-1}\,min^{-1}$		4%†

* From Young and Stokes.[1]
† Unpublished data.

Eccentric contractions (in which the muscle is stretched, increasing the length, while it is active) are of considerable physiological interest but probably need not concern the epidemiologist.

In some studies, strength has been measured as the "1-repetition maximum" (or "1-RM"), the heaviest weight that can be lifted once. Interpretation, especially in training studies, is complicated by the scope for increased skill (rather than increased strength of individual muscles) considerably to enhance the performance of this manoeuvre.

Power

Contrary to widespread clinical practice, the words "strength" and "power" are not interchangeable. Whereas strength is a measure of force or torque (expressed in newtons or newton.metres), power (expressed in watts) is the *rate* of performing work—that is, *power = force × speed*. For some functional activities, measurements of power may be more relevant than measurements of strength. Moreover, as explained below, there are circumstances in which the age related decline in power may be even more dramatic than the decline in strength. Nevertheless, maximal short term power output is rarely measured. This is partly because of neglect of the conceptual distinction between strength and power. It is also because the usual measurement techniques have been unsuitable for use with frail subjects, involving, for example, measuring the speed of a sprint up a flight of stairs or the height of a standing jump. Fortunately an instrument (the Nottingham power rig) is now available for the safe and reliable measurement, in seated subjects, of the explosive power of a single contraction of the lower limb extensors.[2]

Aerobic exercise

If exercise is to be sustained for more than a few minutes its oxygen cost must be met while it is being performed. This is termed aerobic exercise. Maximal aerobic power (or maximal oxygen uptake, $\dot{V}O_2max$) is the greatest rate at which oxygen can be taken up from the atmosphere, transported from the lungs, and utilised by the working muscles. It is usually measured during exercise of progressively increasing intensity on a treadmill or a cycle ergometer. Direct measurements of $\dot{V}O_2max$ require that the rate of oxygen uptake during a progressive test can be shown to have plateaued and that it is therefore a true measure of the subject's physical limit. Criteria used for this purpose with young adults are less suitable with older adults. With older subjects, for example, the progressive increments in work rate must be smaller (to ensure an adequate length of test and an adequate number of increments), making it technically harder to demonstrate a plateau (a statistically meaningful similarity between consecutive values) of oxygen consumption. With younger adults the peak values achieved for heart rate and for plasma lactate concentration are used as criteria to define a "maximal" test. Both fall with inceasing age, however, and the literature contains few data from which to judge whether an older individual's peak heart rate or peak plasma lactate concentration are likely to be true maxima.

More usually, the ability to perform aerobic exercise is judged by predicting $\dot{V}O_2max$ from measurements of oxygen consumption and heart rate at submaximal work rates. This too is fraught with problems. Firstly, the prediction of $\dot{V}O_2max$ from submaximal data depends on an age based estimate of the individual's maximal heart rate; not only is this subject to error due to considerable interindividual variation, there are even several different formulas for the relationship between age and maximal heart rate in older adults. In addition, the prediction of $\dot{V}o_2$max depends upon extrapolation of a regression line calculated from a set of data points less widely dispersed than those provided by a younger subject's exercise test. If seeking to demonstrate a change in aerobic fitness it is probably preferable to seek evidence of a reduction in the heart rate at an arbitrary submaximal interpolated value of oxygen consumption (table 20.1), rather than to attempt to demonstrate an increase in an extrapolated prediction of $\dot{V}o_2$max.

Flexibility and balance

These attributes are also important determinants of exercise performance and functional ability. Flexibility and balance have been measured in large scale surveys but there is even less experience in the use of such measures (and of their limitations) than is the case for either strength or aerobic power.

Variation

Subject selection

This is an important issue in all human gerontological studies, and crucial in exercise studies. The unfortunate stereotyping effect of the expression "the elderly" encourages the assumption that all those aged over 65 are similar. On the contrary, substantial age related effects are seen within the elderly age range. Subject selection must also recognise the effects of the rising prevalence of a variety of chronic diseases with increasing age.

The aim of one study might be best served by subjects who are representative of their contemporaries, with all the chronic disorders and medication that this implies. The aim of another study might require subjects who, although atypical, are "normal" (free of disease and of medication). For such a study how far should the investigator go in attempting to exclude the presence of disease? It would usually be impractical to require a complete clinical, radiological, and laboratory screen. Moreover, detection would still be far from complete; there is high prevalence of undiagnosed disease at postmortem examination. Just as the SENIEUR protocol[3] was developed to identify healthy subjects for immunogerontological studies, we have suggested exclusion criteria that might influence safety or alter exercise performance.[4] To study age related changes in cardiac output, Lakatta's group went further, specifically excluding subjects with abnormalities on myocardial imaging.[5]

Finally, no exclusion criteria can alter the fact that it is highly likely that a study of exercise performance will preferentially attract volunteers with a personal interest in physical activity and with a corresponding lifestyle.

Seasonal effects

Ambient temperature varies with the time of year. Cooling a muscle greatly reduces the explosive power that it can generate. This may be especially important in those elderly people who are immobile, thin, and living in poorly heated accommodation, perhaps contributing to the increased incidence of falls and fractures in cold weather.

In addition, there may be seasonal differences in habitual activity, and as a result in measures of physical fitness. In a study conducted in Wisconsin, 10 women (aged 65–86 years) were 34% less active in winter than in summer and showed a corresponding seasonal variation in thigh muscle strength of some 10%[6].

Social effects

Habitual participation in vigorous exercise varies inversely with employment grade.[7] Social class differences in physical activity persist (and may even increase) after retirement and contribute to differences in muscular performance. There may be other associations between social class and physical abilities in addition to those explicable on the basis of differences in habitual activity.[8]

There may be important ethnic differences in participation in physical recreation. In addition, ethnic differences in body build may complicate the interpretation of observed differences in physical ability.[9 10]

Age trends

Habitual physical activity

The absolute level of habitual activity declines with increasing age, but maximal oxygen uptake declines with age; therefore, rather than comparing absolute levels of activity, a more appropriate comparison might be in terms of the duration and frequency of episodes of activity above, say, 60% of $\dot{V}o_2max$. Judged on this basis it seems quite likely that elderly people may be more "active" than young people. Indeed, the Olympic athlete and the elderly patient may have a lot in common! Both must perform frequently and consistently at the limit of their physical ability.

Strength and power

The loss of muscle strength begins in middle age.[11] Across the age range 65–89 even highly selected healthy men and women have differences in strength that imply annual "losses" of some 1–2% (of the value for a 77 year old), and in lower limb extensor power implying an annual "loss" of some 3–4%.[12] Extreme weakness is common amongst elderly patients; for example, in women who have had surgery to repair a hip fracture, even

194

when they are ready for discharge the extensors of the uninjured leg are some 40% weaker and 70% less powerful than in their healthy contemporaries.

The most important factor causing muscle weakness in old age is the greatly reduced muscle mass (fig 20.1). Much of this so called "sarcopenia" is the consequence of loss of muscle fibres, probably the result of incompletely compensated, slowly progressive denervation.[13 14] Elderly muscle may also regenerate less effectively after damage.[14]

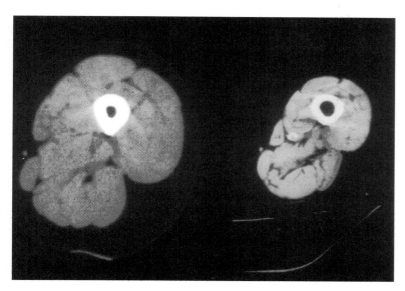

Fig 20.1 Computed tomographic cross-sectional images at mid-thigh from a healthy woman in her 20s (left) and a healthy woman in her 80s (right), to the same magnification.

The loss of strength and power with increasing age cannot be explained merely on the basis of a declining level of habitual physical activity. The inexorable decline is also seen in the performances of highly trained, highly competitive, elite veteran sportsmen.[15 16] It seems likely that the loss of muscle fibres is obligatory. In addition, atrophy of remaining muscle fibres may also be found in biopsies from some elderly subjects,[17] becoming more common after 70 years of age.[14] This may perhaps reflect individual variation in habitual activity and may therefore be susceptible to improvement.[18 19]

In addition, older muscle may be weak for its size.[14] Data from women of different ages suggest that a reduction in the ratio of the strength of the adductor pollicis muscle to its cross-sectional area may occur suddenly at the menopause.[20]

The force–velocity relationship describes the fact that a muscle can develop greater force in a slow contraction than in a fast contraction (fig 20.2). The power–velocity relationship (derived from the force–velocity relationship) shows that there is an optimal speed of contraction for the generation of power (fig 20.2). A reduction in strength means that a slower contraction is required in order to achieve the same absolute force. Working against the same absolute external resistance, the weaker muscle may have to use a contraction speed slower than that which is optimal for the generation of power. The power that a weakened muscle can generate against an unchanged external resistance is thus reduced in two ways: by the same proportion as the reduction in strength; and by an additional amount due to the slower contraction's suboptimal position on the power–velocity curve. Elderly patients therefore face a double jeopardy; not only are they weak but when moving an unchanged body weight their weakness is such that they must use a contraction velocity below the peak of their power–velocity curve. As a result, deficits in power in such tasks are even greater than deficits in strength. This functionally important phenomenon is reflected in measurements (such as those at the beginning of this section) made with the Nottingham power rig because the weight of its flywheel is constant irrespective of the severity of weakness of the subject.

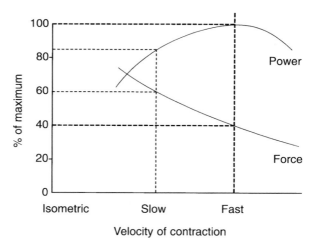

Fig 20.2   Force–velocity and power–velocity relationships of muscle.

Aerobic exercise

The decline in maximal oxygen uptake ($\dot{V}o_2$max) with age (some 10% per decade) may in part be due to the diminishing total muscle mass.[4] Once again, it is possible to use the age related decline in the performances of elite veteran athletes (this time in endurance events) to demonstrate that the age related decline in $\dot{V}o_2$max cannot be explained as merely the result of habitual inactivity.[21 22]

Associations and causal links with health

Ageing and functional ability

Elderly women have lower power:weight ratios than elderly men of the same age.[12] A young person's strength includes a generous safety margin but large numbers of healthy elderly women have strength (and power) below or near to functionally important thresholds and so have lost or are in danger of losing the ability to perform some important everyday tasks.[23] This helps explain the lower step heights achievable by healthy elderly women.[12] It may also contribute to the greater prevalence of disability and of falls amongst elderly women than amongst elderly men and to the age related decline in the percentage of elderly women using public transport on their own.

The age related decline in $\dot{V}o_2max$, especially when combined with the effects of disease, means that many elderly people need only a small further decline to render some everyday activities either impossible or so dependent on anaerobic metabolism as to be unpleasant to perform.[23]

Box 20.1—Health benefits of exercise in old age[28]

Exercise prevents . . .

Disease, such as:
- Osteoporosis
- Non-insulin dependent diabetes
- Hypertension
- Ischaemic heart disease
- Stroke

Disability caused by:
- Intermittent claudication
- Angina pectoris
- Heart failure
- Asthma
- Chronic bronchitis
- Age related weakness

Immobility, which can cause:
- Faecal impaction
- Incontinence
- Deep vein thrombosis
- Pulmonary embolism
- Gravitational oedema
- Skin ulceration

Isolation, which can cause:
- Loneliness
- Depression

Ageing, exercise, and ill health

The health benefits of exercise in old age[24] include the prevention of disease and the prevention of disability in the presence of established disease (box 20.1). For those who are severely disabled, movement itself (even in the absence of a training effect) is crucial in preventing some of the serious complications of immobility. Recreational exercise also offers psychological benefits, including important opportunities for socialisation and socially acceptable non-clinical physical contact.

Intervention

Effects of training

Randomized controlled trials (including one with healthy women aged 76–93[26] and one with frail institutionalized subjects aged 72–98[27] confirm that elderly muscle retains its responsiveness to strength training and that training-induced improvements in strength may improve selected functional abilities. Nevertheless, maximal functional benefit from improved strength may also require practice of the necessary skills.[26]

Up to 70 years of age it seems that a 10–20% improvement in $\dot{V}o_2$max can be expected from endurance training.[23] This cannot be assumed to be true for older people. Nor can functional benefit be assumed. This is an important area for further research.

Evaluations of efficacy

As always, the most important problem is to identify implementation strategies that will ensure that beneficial effects identified in tightly supervised research studies can also be induced through sustainable low cost, high compliance changes in lifestyle. There are a few promising early indications.[28 29]

Health policy

Elderly people must not be excluded from a general drive to get the population moving more vigorously and more frequently. The widespread adoption of a combination of recreational brisk walking and swimming could be expected to produce important improvements in the health of older people. There is considerable scope for improving their use of recreational sports facilities. Many will welcome the opportunity to participate in a supervised exercise group, for guidance, for encouragement, and for socialisation. The supervision of a seniors' exercise group is a specialised skill (boxes 20.2 and 20.3).[25] Efforts to increase the number of such groups and to ensure their success and safety should include insistence that group leaders hold an appropriate specialist qualification.[25]

Box 20.2—Fitness sessions for older people: recommendations I[28]

For teachers
- Emphasise posture and technique
- Give more teaching points and repeat more often
- Give more warning of directional and step changes
- Improve own body language and demonstration skills
- Improve own observation, monitoring, and correction skills
- Offer more choices
- Be polished and punctual

Box 20.3—Fitness sessions for older people: recommendations II[28]

For programming
- Include older people in planning and staffing
- Include older people in promotional material
- Progressive and multilevel programme
- Mixture of activities
- Ensure essential facilities
- Appropriate scheduling and costing
- Include socialisation time

I am indebted to the following collaborators: David Levy and Ai-Lyn Yeo for unpublished data on strength and power after hip fracture; Katie Malbut, Susie Dinan, and Harald Verhaar for unpublished data on cycle ergometry in the ninth decade; Katie Malbut for discussions of criteria for $\dot{V}o_2$max; and Susie Dinan for boxes 20.2 and 20.3.

1 Young A, Stokes M. Non-invasive measurement of muscle in the rehabilitation of masters athletes. In: Sutton JR, Brock RM, editors. *Sports medicine for the mature athlete.* Indianapolis: Benchmark Press, 1986:45–55.

2 Bassey EJ, Short AH. A new method for measuring power output in a single leg extension: feasibility, reliability and validity. *Eur J Appl Physiol* 1990;**60**:385–90.

3 Ligthart GJ, Corberand JX, Geertzen HGM, Meinders AE, Knook DL, Hijmans W. Necessity of the assessment of health status in human immunogerontological studies: evaluation of the SENIEUR protocol. *Mech Ageing Dev* 1990;**55**:89–105.

4 Greig CA, Young A, Skelton DA, Pippet E, Butler FMM, Mahmud SM. Exercise studies with elderly volunteers. *Age Ageing* 1994;**23**:185–9.

5 Lakatta EG. Hemodynamic adaptations to stress with advancing age. *Acta Physiol Scand* 1986;**711**(suppl):39–52.

6 Cress ME, Thomas DP, Johnson J, *et al.* Effect of training on $\dot{V}o_2$max, thigh strength, and muscle morphology in septuagenarian women. *Med Sci Sports Exerc* 1991;**23**:752–8.

7 Marmot MG, Davey Smith G, Stansfeld S, *et al.* Health inequalities among British civil servants: the Whitehall II study. *Lancet* 1991;**337**:1387–93.

8 Rantanen T, Parkatti T, Heikkinen E. Muscle strength according to level of physical exercise and educational background in middle-aged women. *Eur J Appl Physiol* 1992;**65**: 507–12.

9 Ebrahim SBJ, Patel N, Coats M, *et al.* Prevalence and severity of morbidity amongst Gujarati Asian elders: a controlled comparison. *Fam Pract* 1991;**8**:57–62.

10 Era P, Rantanen T, Avlund K, *et al.* Maximal isometric muscle strength and anthropometry in 75-year-old men and women in three Nordic localities. *Scand J Med Sci Sports* 1994; **4**:26–31.

11 Young A. Strength and power. In: Evans JG, Williams TF, editors. *Oxford textbook of geriatric medicine.* Oxford: Oxford University Press, 1992:597–601.

12 Skelton DA, Greig CA, Davies JM, Young A. Strength, power and related functional ability of healthy people aged 65–89 years. *Age Ageing* 1994;**23**:371–7.

13 Young A. Muscle function in old age: In: Peripheral Nerve Change In The Elderly. *New Issues Neurosci* 1988;**1**:141–56.

14 Faulkner JA, Brooks SV, Zerba E. Skeletal muscle weakness and fatigue in old age: underlying mechanisms. *Ann Rev Gerontol Geriatr* 1990;**10**:147–66.

15 Meltzer DE. Age dependence of Olympic weightlifting ability. *Med Sci Sports Exerc* 1994; **26**:1053–67.

16 Moore DH. A study of age group track and field records to relate age and running speed. *Nature* 1975;**253**:264–5.

17 Lexell J, Taylor CC. Variability in muscle fibre areas in whole human quadriceps muscle: effects of increasing age. *J Anat* 1991;**174**:239–49.

18 Aniansson A, Grimby G, Hedberg M. Compensatory muscle fiber hypertrophy in elderly men. *J Appl Physiol* 1992;**73**:812–6.

19 Klitgaard H, Mantoni M, Schiafino S, *et al.* Function, morphology and protein expression of ageing skeletal muscle: a cross-sectional study of elderly men with different training backgrounds. *Acta Physiol Scand* 1990;**140**:41–54.

20 Phillips SK, Rook KM, Siddle NC, Bruce SA, Woledge RC. Muscle weakness in women occurs at an earlier age than in men, but strength is preserved by hormone replacement therapy. *Clin Sci* 1993;**84**:95–8.

21 Saltin B. The ageing endurance athlete. In: Sutton JR, Brock RM, editors. *Sports medicine for the mature athlete.* Indianapolis: Benchmark Press, 1986:59–80.

22 Greig C, Young A. Aerobic exercise. In: Evans JG, Williams TF, editors. *Oxford textbook of geriatric medicine.* Oxford: Oxford University Press, 1992:601–4.

23 Young A. Exercise physiology in geriatric practice. *Acta Med Scand* 1986;**suppl 711**: 227–32.

24 Young A. Exercise. In: Fowler G, Gray M, Anderson P, editors. *Prevention in general practice.* Oxford: Oxford University Press, 1993:170–90.

25 Young A, Dinan S. Fitness for older people. In: McClatchie G, Harries M, King J, and Williams, C, eds. *ABC of sports medicine.* London: BMJ Publishing Group, 1995:69–72.

26 Skelton DA, Young A, Greig CA, Malbut KE. Effects of resistance training on strength, power, and selected functional abilities of women aged 75 and over. *J Am Geriatr Soc* 1995;**43**:1–7.

27 Fiatarone MA, O'Neill EF, Ryan ND, *et al.* Exercise training and nutritional supplementation for physical frailty in very elderly people. *N Engl J Med* 1994;**330**: 1769–75.

28 Frändin K, Johannesson K, Grimby G. Physical activity as part of an intervention program for elderly persons in Göteborg. *Scand J Med Sci Sports* 1992;**2**:218–24.

29 Browne D. Encourage active community life. *BMJ* 1994;**309**:872.

21 Migration and ethnicity

SHAH EBRAHIM

Nature of migration

Migration as a variable of interest in the study of aetiology of diseases and outcomes of health and social care is not a single factor.[1,2] The act of migration is confounded by the ethnicity of migrants, their social and economic circumstances, their health status at the point of migration, and the place in which they settle.[3,4] Thus study of health and social problems of migrants is linked with the study of social and economic disadvantages associated with racism and prejudice.[5-7]

It is tempting to assume that migration of so called "visible" immigrants (particularly from the new Commonwealth countries of south Asia) will have to cope with more adversity, and study of such populations has tended to be the chief priority. The health and social circumstances of much larger migrant populations, such as the Irish in the United Kingdom or the United States, have received much less interest.

This chapter will focus on the problems of black and Asian migrants, illustrating features of migration and ethnicity from a British perspective. By doing so it is not the intention to negate the very real problems experienced by Irish, Mediterranean, and European migrants. Where possible the precise country of birth will be used to describe migrant groups but much of the literature has grouped people together without regard for culture, migrant history, or religion.

Migration to the United Kingdom: natural history

Migration has occurred in several waves, with West Indians and Indians being the earliest groups to arrive in substantial numbers shortly after the second world war, until the early 1960s. With the need to rebuild post-war Britain a large and healthy labour force was required and was obtained from the colonies.[4,8,9] This desire to recruit young fit men led inevitably to two phenomena: firstly, the more youthful passport age; and, secondly, the migration of men before wives and families. Before that time migrants tended to be concentrated around ports and to be drawn from the traditional migrant occupation of merchant seamen.

Successive migrant groups arrived from east Africa, particularly from Uganda and Bangladesh, as a consequence of civil unrest and political and economic pressure during the 1970s. In response to a perceived threat to jobs and housing for the white population of Britain, ever more complicated immigration legislation was enacted and resulted in a dramatic reduction in the numbers of migrants. During the late 1980s the only groups that arrived in any numbers were people fleeing wars and severe oppression from places such as Somalia, Turkey, and South East Asia.

The background and circumstances of migration must have a profound effect on health and social circumstances and it is likely that the more recent arrivals, not selected for health and vigour in the workplace, will have health and social status more representative of the countries from which they have come.

Ethnicity

Ethnicity is a complex concept. It comprises skin colour, culture, language, religion, birth place, food, beliefs, and behaviour. It is impossible to define clearly and in most contexts refers to the "otherness" of people who do not belong to the predominant population. The Office of Population Censuses and Surveys classification[10] emphasises the "visible" criterion of skin colour, reflecting British views of ethnicity (box 21.1). Not surprisingly, people who share a skin colour do not necessarily have much else in common.

Box 21.1—Classification of ethnicity used in the British census (1991)

- White
- Black—Caribbean
- Black—African
- Black—other
- Indian
- Pakistani
- Bangladeshi
- Chinese
- Asian—other
- Other

The aim of obtaining better information about ethnicity has prompted investigators to ask more complicated questions than simply place of birth. The accuracy of even simple questions about ethnicity has proved low,[11 12] particularly when the reasons for asking such questions may be understood as being part of immigration monitoring or attempts to repatriate.

Ethnicity has supplanted race as a classifier in descriptive studies because the poor value of race as a "genetic" or biological marker of any importance is now realised.[13] As the meaning of ethnicity is by no means clear, however, and is likely to vary over time and between places, its value is suspect. Of fundamental importance in any consideration of the relationship between ethnicity and health is the role of poverty, deprivation, and discrimination.[14] The tendency for the observation of ethnic differences to be viewed as causal rather than as an effect of underlying social, economic, or environmental factors has been noted.[15] The term "Asian" is a major barrier to sensible communication because of the major heterogeneity of ethnic groups covered by such a term.[16]

Demographic trends

The numbers of people belonging to different ethnic groups are relatively small—about 5% overall.[17] Most ethnic minorities in the United Kingdom are young compared with the white British population; with only 5–10% of the population aged over 65 years. All these populations are ageing rapidly as people who arrived in the United Kingdom in the 1950s and 1960s in their 20s and 30s reach retirement. The numbers of older people from ethnic minorities will increase dramatically over the next two decades. The distribution of ethnic minorities in Britain is strongly biased towards inner city areas of major industrial towns.

The subpensioner age group shown in table 21.1 outnumbers the pensioner group by ratios of 2–6 fold. Since it is unlikely that much of this subpensioner population will die before reaching their 60s, it is likely that the next decade will see massive increases in the numbers of older migrants.

Table 21.1   Numbers of migrants by country of birth at ages 40–60/65 and 60/65* in thousands

	40–60/65		60/65	
	1981	1991	1981	1991
India	104	187	44	44
Caribbean	101	132	16	40
Pakistan	34	76	5	12
Bangladesh	9	26	4	2·5

* The category 60/65 refers to women aged 60 + and men aged 65 + (the pensionable ages in the United Kingdom). From Office of Population Censuses and Surveys. *Census for Great Britain 1981* and *1991*. London: HMSO.

Cultural aspects

Extended family

The extended family is a major strategy for the social support of elderly people in all cultures but, because of the nature of migration and the extended family living arrangements in many countries, multigenerational households are relatively more common than among the white British population (table 21.2). This leads to one of the more serious myths associated with migrants: "they will look after their own."

203

Table 21.2   Living arrangements of elderly migrants resident in Birmingham, UK

	Asian	Afro-Caribbean
Alone	5	36
With one other	13	32
With 2–5	11	30
With 6+	71	2

Values are percentages.
From Blakemore.[18]

Surveys[18 19] have examined the extent of family support in inner cities and have documented that the problems of a high proportion of elderly migrants cannot be met by means of family because they live alone or as husband and wife couples. It is clear from such data that reliance on the extended family, particularly living in the same house, is an unrealistic sole option for social support.

Language

Many elderly migrants, particularly women, are unable to speak adequate English and those from poorer countries, such as Bangladesh, are frequently illiterate in their own language. This has major implications for the provision of information about services. The use of simple translated—or in Britain transliterated—material is unlikely to achieve successful communication. Even video and tape material (often made at great cost) can be unproductive because it is made within the migrant culture accessible to those who have money to spend on health education and social welfare. These contacts are invariably the able educated minority within the migrant population.

Use of health and social services

Levels of use of statutory social services by elderly migrants is low (table 21.3) and this is the result of several forces: the services may be inappropriate; they may be complicated to access; language may be a major barrier; they may be too expensive; they may be viewed as belonging to and for the white British population; their use may be stigmatising. It is frequently assumed by managers that if the service is not used then it is clearly not needed because if problems were bad enough people would be happy to use any available service.

204

Table 21.3   Use of Social and Health Services in Birmingham. Figures are percentages having contact in the three months before interview

	Indigenous	Asian	Afro-Caribbean
Meals on wheels	6	0	2
Home Help	19	0	9
Health Visitor	0	1	3
Community Nurse	6	1	8
Family Doctor	53	70	68

From Blakemore.[18]

The use of health services, unlike social services, is not a problem of access. Indeed researchers and policy makers have been guilty of phrasing their questions in terms of "overconsultation" and "high admission rates" and effort has been made to discover ways of "normalising" the rates. While access to services is not difficult, it is not clear whether the quality of care offered is adequate; for example, while hospital admission rates are higher the proportions followed up in outpatient clinics are lower.[20] The frequent attendance in primary care reported in all studies[21 22] may be a cause of frustration to doctors if no solution is found. This demonstrates the western preoccupation with cause and effect: the notion that all problems have solutions.

Health problems

The common health problems of migrants tend to differ in degree, rather than in kind, from the indigenous population[23] and it has been suggested that understanding of migrants' health needs, the attitudes of health care providers, and the orientation of research must change if burdens of illness are to be reduced.[24]

Healthy migrant effect

If all causes mortality is used as an index of health, migrants tend to be healthier than those who remain in their own country because the process of migration requires fitness.[25 26] In the United States, however, mortality patterns among the black and white populations show interesting differences (table 21.4). Life expectancy starts off worse in black people, reflecting high infant mortality rates, which may be due to worse health services.[27] By the age of 70, life expectancy is similar in both black and white people. The explanation of this crossover in life expectancy is not understood but a "survival of the fittest" hypothesis—black people die sooner as a consequence of increased illness and poorer services, leaving behind a relatively indestructible group of elders—has been suggested.[28] Whether British ethnic migrants will share this American advantage in longevity remains to be seen.

Table 21.4   Life expectancy at various ages by race and sex, United States 1978

Age (years)	White		Non-white	
	Male	Female	Male	Female
0	70·2	77·8	65·0	73·6
20	52·0	59·1	47·4	55·6
40	33·6	39·9	30·4	37·0
60	17·2	22·3	16·5	21·2
70	11·1	14·8	11·6	14·8
80	6·7	8·8	8·8	11·5

From National Center for Health Statistics. *Life Tables: Vital Statistics of the United States 1978*. Washington DC: Government Printing Office, 1980.

The health problems experienced by migrants fall into four main categories: influences of the old country; influences of the new country; selection of who migrates; and the process of migration and adaptation.[25 26] This model helps in understanding the patterns of migrant mortality and morbidity experienced in Britain.

A general review of disease in ethnic groups has been published[29] and some specific problems will be discussed briefly here. Tuberculosis is a problem in the old country and migrants in effect bring this problem with them, although the conditions for spread of tuberculosis are rife in Britain (overcrowding, poverty, poor nutrition) and the disease is enjoying something of a vogue again. Ischaemic heart disease, stroke, diabetes, and asthma appear to be diseases that are associated with changes in way of life, in particular the move from rural to urban settings. They reflect the pattern of disease in the new country and may be associated with specific predispositions to disease in the face of changes in diet, stress, or activity.[30 31]

The process of migration and adaptation is often viewed as the reason for an excess of psychotic illness amongst Afro-Caribbean migrants, although the issue is clouded by criteria used for making the diagnosis in ethnic minorities, and increased psychiatric illness is not found in Asian migrants.[32] The multitude of non-specific symptoms that many migrants present to their doctors is almost certainly a reflection of the process of adaptation to the uncertainties and pressures of a new life that is complicated by prejudice and racism.

The precise burden of disease experienced by migrants is not easy to quantify except by relating deaths for particular conditions to the population at risk. Standardised mortality ratios have been calculated but are now rather out of date.[25 26] These mortality ratios demonstrate that some migrant groups are healthier than might be expected (the so-called "healthy migrant" effect), reflecting the selection pressures on who migrates. When specific diseases are considered, however, it is clear that Indian and Caribbean migrants have higher mortality from tuberculosis, cancer of cervix, stroke, and accidents and violence. Caribbean migrants have lower levels of heart disease, whereas Indians have higher levels than expected.[25]

Further data on morbidity have been reported from hospital admission statistics[33] and ad hoc surveys in primary care.[20-22] Among older people a better indicator of the burden of illness can be obtained from examining levels of disability. Surprisingly little work has been done in this area but the figures that are available suggest that, age for age, migrants have worse levels of disability than members of the white British population. The data shown in table 21.5 demonstrate disability levels among very old Pakistani people living in Leicester.[34] Unfortunately no age–sex matched reference population was studied but a similar questionnaire was used in a nearby market town.

Table 21.5 Levels of independence in activities of daily living among Asians aged ≥ 75 years in Leicester compared with white British in Melton Mowbray

	Asians	Indigenous
Mobility outdoors	41	63
Climb stairs	41	91
Mobility indoors	61	81
Dressing	76	94
Bathing	82	64
Urinary continence	82	90

Values are percentages.
From Donaldson.[34]

It is possible that these increased levels of disability among ethnic elders are a result of ethnic differences in age associated declines in physical capacity, which are well recognised (see chapter 20). Evidence of lower levels of muscle strength among Gujarati elders compared with age and sex matched white British people has been reported,[31] which would support this hypothesis. The underlying mechanism for this difference in muscle strength remains to be explored.

Meaning of illness

Little work has been done on the meaning of illness among migrants, who will have experienced a very different pattern of disease in their home countries and yet will have to cope with a new disease profile in Britain[35]; for example, in countries where serious acute infectious disease (such as dysentery, meningitis, malaria) is common, it makes good sense to lie down, sweat it out, and either survive or die after a few days. When faced with a stroke or heart failure such practice will only be rewarded with non-fatal but terrible consequences of incontinence, pressure sores, contracture of joints, and loss of ability.

Much more work with local communities is required to uncover and use cross cultural understanding of the meaning of illness and our responses.

207

Most cultures have a multilayered understanding of aetiology ranging from evil forces, witchcraft, and religious interpretations to infection, risk factors, and so on. It is quite easy for people to move between different belief systems and to hold apparently inconsistent beliefs simultaneously.

Conclusion

Much work has been carried out involving people from ethnic minority groups in vain hopes and expectations of improving their access to services and in reducing their health problems. Researchers need to be more critical in their use of ethnicity as a construct and more willing to confront society's (and their own) views of the meaning of ethnicity in the context of health, illness, and use of services.

1 Fennell G, Phillipson C, Evers H. Race, ethnicity and old age. In: *The sociology of old age.* Milton Keynes: Open University Press, 1988:114–34.
2 Ebrahim S, Hillier S. Ethnic minority needs. *Rev Clin Gerontol* 1991;**1**:195–9.
3 Moore JW. Situational factors affecting minority aging. *Gerontologist* 1971;**11**:88–92.
4 Watson JL. *Between two cultures: migrants and minorities in Britain.* Oxford: Blackwell, 1977.
5 Bulmer M. Race and ethnicity. In: Burgess RC, editor. *Key variables in social investigation.* London: Routledge and Kegan Paul, 1988.
6 Dowd JJ, Bengtson VL. Ageing in minority populations: an examination of the double jeopardy hypothesis. *J Gerontol* 1978;**33**:427–36.
7 Norman A. *Triple jeopardy: growing old in a second homeland.* London: Centre for Policy on Ageing, 1985.
8 Barker J. *Black and Asian old people in Britain.* Mitcham: Age Concern Research Unit, 1984.
9 Rose EJB. *Colour and citizenship.* Oxford: Oxford University Press/Institute of Race Relations, 1969.
10 Office of Population Censuses and Surveys. *Census for Great Britain, 1991.* London: HMSO, 1993.
11 Office of Population Censuses and Surveys Monitor 1981 Census. *Developing a question on ethnic origin.* London: HMSO, 1978. (CEN 78/4.)
12 Office of Population Censuses and Surveys Monitor 1981 Census. *Tests of an ethnic question.* London: HMSO, 1980. (CEN 80/3.)
13 Hill A. Molecular markers of ethnic groups. In: Cruickshank J, Beevers D, editors. *Ethnic factors in health and disease.* Bristol: Wright, 1989:25–31.
14 Ahmad W, Kernohan E, Baker M. Health of British Asians: a research review. *Community Med* 1989;**11**:49–56.
15 Sheldon T, Parker H. Race and ethnicity in health research. *J Public Health Med* 1992; **14**:104–10.
16 Bhopal RS, Phillimore P, Kholi HS. Inappropriate use of the term "Asian": an obstacle to ethnicity and health research. *J Public Health Med* 1991;**13**:244–6.
17 Anonymous. Estimates of the ethnic minority population of Great Britain. *Population Trends* 1992;**67**:1.
18 Blakemore K. Health and illness among the elderly of minority ethnic groups living in Birmingham: some new findings. *Health Trends* 1982;**14**:69–72.
19 Blakemore K. Ethnicity, self-reported illness and use of medical services by the elderly. *Postgrad Med J* 1983;**59**:668–70.
20 Ebrahim S, Patel N, Coats M, *et al.* Physical capacity, ill-health and use of health services by Gujarati elders: a comparative study. *Fam Pract* 1991;**8**:57–62.
21 Gillam SJ, Jarman B, White P, Law R. Ethnic differences in consultation rates in urban general practice. *BMJ* 1989;**299**:953–7.
22 Balarajan R, Yuen P, Raleigh VS. Ethnic differences in general practitioner consultations. *BMJ* 1989;**299**:958–60.

23 Black N. Migration and health. *BMJ* 1987;**295**:566.

24 Colledge M, vanGuens HA, Svensson P-G, editors. *Migration and health: towards an understanding of the health care needs of ethnic minorities.* Copenhagen: WHO Regional Office for Europe; London: HMSO, 1986.

25 Marmot M, Adelstein AM, Bulusu L. Lessons from the study of immigrant mortality. *Lancet* 1984;**i**:1455–7.

26 Marmot M, Adlestein AM, Bulusu L. *Immigrant mortality in England and Wales (1970–78): causes of death by country.* London: HMSO, 1984. (OPCS studies of medical and population subjects, No 47.)

27 Clarke M, Clayton DG. Quality of obstetric care provided for Asian immigrants in Leicestershire. *BMJ* 1983;**286**:621–3.

28 Manton KG. Sex and race specific mortality differentials in multiple cause of death data. *Gerontologist* 1980;**20**:480–93.

29 Cruickshank JK, Beevers DG, editors. *Ethnic factors in health and disease.* London: Butterworth, 1989.

30 McKeigue PM, Miller GJ, Marmot MG. Coronary heart disease in south Asians overseas—a review. *J Clin Epidemiol* 1989;**42**:597–609.

31 Polednak AP. *Racial and ethnic differences in disease.* Oxford: Oxford University Press, 1989.

32 Cochrane R. Psychological and behavioural disturbance in West Indians, Indians and Pakistanis in Britain: a comparison of rates among children and adults. *Br J Psychol* 1979; **134**:201–10.

33 Ebrahim S, Smith C, Giggs J. Elderly immigrants—a disadvantaged group? *Age Ageing* 1987;**16**:249–55.

34 Donaldson L. Health and social status of elderly Asians: a community survey. *BMJ* 1986; **293**:1079–82.

35 Donovan J. Ethnicity and health—a research review. *Soc Sci Med* 1984;**19**:663–70.

22 Gender

KASTURI SEN

Gender penetrates and fashions sex. Becoming a child, a youth and then an adult is a social process, woven through biological age

LM Verbrugge

This chapter will provide an overview of literature on gender in later life. It is rare to find data from developing countries on sex differentials in mortality, and the evidence for patterns of morbidity is restricted to a handful of country case studies, often supplemented by inferences from the overresearched realm of reproductive health.

For developed countries, on the other hand, the past two decades have witnessed a growing body of literature that focuses almost exclusively on sex differentials in mortality and morbidity. Very little work, however, refers specifically to old age. Despite their illuminating qualities, one of the basic difficulties with this literature is that it is largely based on the experience of the United States and is restricted to a narrow epidemiological focus, for example, individual risks rather than population based studies that enhance our knowledge of the impact of social factors on gender and health state. The risk factor approach has led to an excessive concern with ill health, frailty, and disability as the dominant paradigm of ageing, particularly in the eyes of policy makers worldwide.[1-4]

Narrow focus

The narrow regional focus and unidisciplinary mode limit the generalisability of information on health status, health seeking behaviour, and differences in the patterns of health care utilisation. Emerging evidence from the United Kingdom, on the other hand, has had a broader focus with greater attempts to merge existing, albeit limited, health data with the social and structural determinants of health status in later life. Factors such as class, occupational category, and the impact of earlier life material inequalities on gender and health in later life assume greater significance than in the literature from the United States.[5]

Despite these fundamental problems, this chapter will try to provide a global overview by drawing upon some of the key issues raised from the divergent and conflicting evidence available. It will endeavour to answer some of the basic dilemmas facing researchers and policy makers: Why do women live longer yet in poorer health than men? What are the health service and policy implications of such differences in life chance and health state for both developed and developing countries?

Mortality differences

At a global level, as data on mortality is more readily available, sex differences in mortality have often been a starting point for exploring differences in overall health states between men and women.

In all developed countries male mortality rates are higher than those of females, but in all countries for which data are available women report more acute illness than men and make greater use of health services.[67] The contrast between male excess mortality and female excess morbidity—"women get sick and men die"—was apparently observed in England as early as 1927 but has been the cause of only sporadic comment since that time.[8] More recent evidence from the United Kingdom and the United States suggests that whilst women experience substantially more disability than men they die from the same causes.[57]

Life expectancy and sex composition: the global picture

Longevity has increased considerably in the twentieth century. Improvements in life expectancy and health status are associated with the expansion of public health measures, disease eradication programmes, and reduced death rates, mainly among infants and children in developed countries. In developing countries, despite differences in rates, there have been substantial gains in life expectancy over a compressed period in time.

Gender differentials are a major feature of the trends in life expectancy and mortality. As tables 22.1 and 22.2 illustrate, women outlive men in all the countries of Europe and North America. Subsequently sex differences in absolute increments are most apparent at the oldest ages. Hence the observation that health and socioeconomic problems in later life are by and large problems of elderly women, despite the fact that the past two decades have witnessed a decline in women's advantage in longevity.[5]

Developed countries

Gender differentials in developed countries became evident during the 1950s when the male–female increases in life expectancy from the first half of the century developed divergent paths; female life expectancy continued to rise in all countries, whilst male gains began to slow down between 1950 and 1970. After this period of stagnation male life expectancy began to rise again except in the former eastern European block.[8]

According to the US Bureau of Census in 1900, the European and North American gender gap in life expectancy was typically 2–3 years. Currently, however, women outlive men in most developed countries by

211

Table 22.1   Life expectancy (years) and gender gap (years) in selected countries worldwide

	Life expectancy* for men	Life expectancy* for women	Gender gap†
Sweden	73	79	4
Australia	71	78	7
Former Soviet Union	64	74	10
China	62	66	4
Japan	73	79	4
Philippines	59	62	3
Indonesia	49	51	3
India‡	46	45	−1
Egypt	54	56	2
Mauritania	41	44	3
Guinea-Bissau	39	43	4
Ethiopia	38	41	3

* The average number of years a person may expect to live.
† The difference in years between female and male life expectancy.
‡ Note that in India, unlike any other country listed, average female life expectancy at birth is less than that of males.
From *UN demographic yearbook*. Washington: UN, 1980; or latest year available of *The new state of the world atlas*. New York: Kidron and Segal, 1987.

5–9 years. Women have lower mortality than men in every age group and for most causes of death. Average female life expectancy currently exceeds 80 years in many developed countries and is approaching a threshold in many others.[8]

Developing countries

In developing countries there are smaller differences in life expectancy between males and females, as illustrated by table 22.1. In some Asian and Middle Eastern countries the trends may be reversed as a result of sociocultural factors, such as son preference and female foeticide as well as life threatening conditions facing women during the reproductive period.[8]

In assessing sex differentials in mortality from a global perspective, Lopez and Ruzicka[9] suggest that death rates interact closely with levels of development; in predominantly rural countries any female biological advantage is reduced as a consequence of higher maternal mortality, inadequate nutrition, and limited access to education and health care.

In more urbanised regions improved sanitation and public health measures coupled with a relatively better standard of living reduce some of the social and environmental disadvantages that exist in the rural areas. This tends to reduce social and environmental risks and strengthen the natural biological and genetic advantages in longevity that females have historically exhibited over males to the extent where female life expectancy exceeds that of males.[9]

Table 22.2   Longevity and sex differences in mortality in selected countries

Region/Country	Circa 1900		Circa 1950		Circa 1990	
	Male	Female	Male	Female	Male	Female
United States	48·3	51·1	66	71·7	72·1	79
Western Europe						
England/Wales	46·4	50·1	66·2	71·1	73·3	79·2
France	45·3	48·7	63·7	69·4	73·4	81·9
Germany	43·8	46·6	64·6	68·5	73·4	80·6
Italy	42·9	43·2	63·7	67·2	74·5	81·4
Sweden	52·8	55·3	69·9	72·6	74·7	80·7
Southern and eastern Europe						
Greece	38·1	39·7	63·4	66·7	75	80·2
Hungary	36·6	38·2	59·3	63·4	67·2	75·4
Poland			57·2	62·8	28·2	76·7
Other						
Canada			66·4	70·9	74	80·7
Japan	42·8	44·3	59·6	63·1	76·4	82·1
New Zealand			67·2	71·3	72·2	78·4

Adapted from Kinsella[8]: 21.

Linking sex differentials in mortality with levels of social and economic development concurs with the analysis of mortality data from 24 developed countries undertaken by Nathanson.[10] This suggests that the strongest predictor of female life expectancy is reflected by the level of affluence in a particular country, thereby reinforcing an emergent perspective that in both low and high mortality countries sex differentials are likely to vary geographically and by material factors.

Reasons for sex composition and differences in mortality

Sex composition is affected by a complex interaction of factors over the life span: the sex ratio at birth, mortality rates through life, the nature and patterns of migration, and crises such as wars. Between 1900 and 1970 the increase in the sex differential was attributable to decreasing mortality rates for diseases affecting only women (maternal mortality and cancer of the uterus) and increasing mortality rates for diseases principally affecting men (cancer of the lung and cardiovascular diseases).[4]

Although sex differences in health and mortality have existed throughout the twentieth century, the reasons for the differences continue to be debated.[7] There are a number of perspectives: one suggestion is that particular social and environmental factors act to the detriment of men and higher male mortality is therefore essentially a function of lifestyles. Another set of views is more biologically grounded in claiming that women have greater constitutional resistance to degenerative conditions than men

213

and this is reflected in lower mortality. There are also hypotheses that suggest that existing differentials arise from a combination of genetic factors coupled with risks acquired during life, complemented by attitudes that influence perception of symptoms and health seeking behaviour that follows. In terms of acquired risks it seems likely that smoking habits have had a major impact on male mortality since the 1950s. Although men's overall risk appears to be higher than that of women, there is still a need for more detailed information about specific risk factors that cause male disadvantage.[10]

Methodological issues

Many methodological issues are raised when dealing with cause of death. The quality of death data is affected by underreporting, lack of precise information on cause, and variations in diagnosis, as well as sociocultural factors, which affect both diagnosis and recording. Of particular relevance to developing countries are the additional problems of underlying causes; these often relate to anaemia and nutritional deficiencies, especially with regard to older men and women.

Many developing countries do not collect or publish health data either by sex or by age. A United Nations survey in the early 1980s found that, among 76 developing countries responding to a UN inquiry on the issue, less than one half (38%) collected and published health statistics separately by sex, and even fewer had any data on the specific health problems of older women.[11]

Mortality differentials

It appears that constitutional and environmental factors are closely intertwined in affecting sex differences in mortality and any disaggregation of such factors would inevitably be misleading.[9] While the boundary between social and biological factors influencing death remains indistinct, gains made by both sexes in terms of life expectancy in the past three to four decades suggest major environmental influences. Nathanson[10] extends this positive outcome in life expectancy to support the hypothesis that women's social status is a key indicator of life expectancy; the greater the degree of gender equality in a particular social formation, the lower the level of female mortality.[9 10] This is supported by Gibson's overview of older women, life style, and health status from a comparative perspective.[12]

The tentative suggestions from current evidence are that, while women display greater intrinsic genetic robustness, men's lifestyles and acquired behaviours generate greater risk of mortality; however, women have higher incidence rates for most non-fatal diseases.[7 9 11] Higher incidence coupled with longer life means that women would therefore typically live longer with more non-fatal conditions.

214

This, however, leaves unanswered the question of the role of socioeconomic factors in mortality differentials; few studies assess the role of class differences on mortality at older ages owing to both methodological problems, such as the effect of selection upon survival, and substantive issues such as definition of social status in terms of location and context—who does one compare with whom? The absence of detailed studies in both developed and developing countries means that such issues are particularly controversial when applied to later life. Emerging evidence from the United States and the United Kingdom has suggested that socioeconomic status plays a critical role in perceived health status[5]; however, whether class differences in health status in later life are greater than gender differences remains a critical point for further discussion. In addition, the more conclusive evidence of mortality differentials among adults by occupational status and living circumstances needs to be applied and analysed for older ages.[13]

Gender differences in the patterns of morbidity

Methodological issues

If the evidence on the causes for sex differences in mortality is inconclusive, the information on morbidity remains more controversial. We are enmeshed in problems, both methodological and contextual.[2 9–11] Recent interpretations of the patterns of gender differentials in morbidity have also been beset by gender role stereotyping. These have often affected the nature and context of investigations, for example timely interventions, and therefore the outcome of particular illnesses are attributed to "feminine traits", such as having more access to leisure time and a better ability to communicate with physicians.[11 14]

A number of other methodological issues prevaricate; for example, it is widely acknowledged that data collection on morbidity is not uniform.[2 15 16] The use of proxy interviewers, particularly for elderly people, is regarded as problematic. Among associated difficulties highlighted by American health surveys is the relationship between interviewer and respondent where chronic conditions are often understated.[4]

It has also been suggested that where gender differentials are concerned health statistics based on physician attendance alone do not reflect the true burden of morbidity because many non-fatal chronic conditions are excluded.[16]

Methodological dilemmas on morbidity are aggravated by the way in which health status is determined; these are often subjective measures (self reported health) that ascertain functional ability. Such measures are imbued with a wide range of social, cultural, and material factors that ultimately affect the expression of quality of life.[7]

Exploring gender differences in morbidity

Health status

The methodological dilemmas of ascertaining health status are compounded by the exclusion of older people from many large scale studies. This reluctance to study health status in later life is in part due to the multiplicity of pathological conditions likely to exist in old age[2 7 9 10 13 16] but also to ageism.

The American evidence on morbidity differentials classifies differences into a number of categories: (a) risks associated with biological/physiological factors; (b) risks acquired over a lifetime; and (c) risks associated with reporting behaviour. The relative impact of each appears to depend upon particular disciplinary perspectives.[9] As suggested previously, there has been a tendency to seek exclusively behaviouristic explanations as opposed to structural ones for existing differentials. Thus analyses of data are undertaken on the basis of individual differences rather than on any association of individual mortality or morbidity with social and structural factors, such as race and class.

A threefold classification has been created by Verbrugge to determine morbidity differentials in later life, which provides an overview to this approach.[17]

Biological risk approach

A considerable volume of current literature supports the biological hypothesis resting on genetic causality as explanatory variables for existing differentials in mortality and morbidity. These suggest that men are less durable biologically than women and that this is offset only during women's reproductive years by pregnancy related mortality and morbidity.[3 4 11] It holds that women have better genetic resistance and are therefore more resistant to some X chromosome related diseases, and as a consequence women (up to the time of menopause) are better protected than men from cardiovascular morbidity by specific sex hormones. It is also suggested that the pathology of some diseases and their developmental course may be different for men and women. In sum, the biological risk approach claims that women are biologically better able than men to cope with morbidity and mortality and especially so beyond the reproductive years.

Acquired risks

There is a growing volume of literature touching upon risks acquired over a lifetime that affect patterns of disease in later life. The American literature in particular is, however, based on traditional divisions of male productive and female reproductive work, their associated risks, and how they are likely to transform over time as women acquire male "bad" habits;

216

for example, men are attributed with "type A" behaviour, which is described as aggressive and reckless, and as generating an array of self imposed stresses.[10 15] Women, on the other hand, are said to be more able to take self care and therapeutic actions that work to their advantage.[17 18] Some of this gender role stereotyping has been questioned in recent years, and it is suggested that social status and financial autonomy rather than acquired behaviours play a much greater role in determining levels of morbidity and mortality in both men and women.[10 19]

Psychosocial aspects of morbidity differentials

The psychosocial perspectives are concerned with illness behaviour and the perception of symptoms. The prevailing hypotheses suggest that women are more aware of physical symptoms; a myriad of explanations are provided for this apparent gender difference in perceptions of illness and in reporting behaviours. These range from greater contact with health services during childbirth and child rearing periods to differences in patterns of behaviour. In this context it is claimed that men are often unable to come to terms with illnesses and are thus less able than women to acknowledge symptoms. Women apparently do not suffer from such a stigma and in this view are able to deal with symptoms earlier and avail themselves of better care. Thus for authors such as Mechanic the apparent sex differential in morbidity is related almost entirely to gender related definitions and perceptions of sickness rather than to actual differences.[14]

This is not, however, supported by more recent work by a number of authors, including Wingard,[4] who argues that, despite a mortality advantage, women experience more illness than men. For Wingard, while morbidity differentials reflect in part women's greater utilisation of services, including patterns of physician diagnosis, the differences appear to persist when physical examinations are used for assessment in population based samples; women do appear to have higher rates of conditions that rarely cause death (such as rheumatoid arthritis), whereas men have more fatal conditions (such as coronary heart disease).[29 17]

Developing countries

There is little empirical information available in developing countries on gender differentials in health status in later life. Only a handful of local studies are available from Asia, Africa, and Latin America, and as part of research where gender differentials in health status have been incidental.[20 21] The absence of empirical data on morbidity is reinforced by the methodological dilemmas of validity and appropriateness already mentioned for developed countries. There is, in addition, the issue of a narrow focus on the reproductive years, specifically on fertility behaviour. A recent review on women's health by Koblinsky et al suggests, for example, that women's health in these regions has been too narrowly defined by fertility regulation;

this has created a very narrow conceptualisation bounded by the reproductive years of 15–45 years.[22] They call for a broader definition of health that incorporates a life cycle perspective, taking into account the effects upon health of workload, nutrition, migration, and stress events, such as wars.

There is much greater consistency of interpretation of existing evidence. In part related to the paucity of information, there is, however, greater acknowledgement of the interaction of health, environment, and social status on patterns of gender morbidity.[6 7 12 16 18] There is much less emphasis on a biomedical or disease oriented approach. The findings from these studies suggest that many of the health problems affecting older women in developing countries are directly linked to their environment and circumstances of life. Thus while there are gynaecological problems created by repeat pregnancies during reproductive years, other conditions such as disfunctional hips and joints are emphatically associated with a lifetime of arduous labour and with poverty. Such factors, coupled with poor nutritional and social status, are universally acknowledged as aggravating factors for poor health in later life.[12]

The cumulative and interactive effects of infectious diseases, repeat pregnancies, heavy workload, and psychological stress would have their effects on the health of older women. There is common agreement that an overriding feature of the health of women in developing countries is the context of poverty.[19 22]

Recent evidence from the more developed regions suggests that lifestyle related illnesses typically found in industrialised countries, such as coronary heart disease, are increasing in both men and women.[16] The four leading causes of death of women between the ages of 45 and 64 years in Latin America and the Caribbean are, for example, heart disease, cancers, strokes, and diabetes.[21]

There are increasing similarities between developed and developing regions for women with mental disorders, such as dementia and depression, which may be increasing in prevalence among older women.[16 23] Depression is linked to stresses from the double shifts of work outside and inside the home.[16 23] For many, the primacy of caring for children and separation from them in mid-life can lead to a sudden sense of loss and powerlessness, which is reinforced by economic dependency. For others, caring for surviving relatives or partners well into later life remains largely unrecognised and often taxing on both physical and mental health. The effect of caring roles on women's health requires much greater documentation. Despite a higher prevalence of depression among women, Western studies highlight greater levels of social networking and strategies of coping among women than among men.

Policy implications

The health challenges of gender facing policy makers throughout the world vary in accordance with trends in demographic and epidemiological transitions taking place. It is universally clear, however, that the largest proportion of survivors into later life are older women. Despite this there is a considerable gap in research into the health needs of older women throughout the world. Assessing current and future needs for health care necessitates a clearer direction and an interdisciplinary mode. The purpose of this would be to improve the collection of data, incorporating more older women in current research but also ensuring that it does not focus exclusively on a medical model and involves interdisciplinary collaboration.

Despite differences, however, there is much in common in the health and social needs of women worldwide. These relate to the need to ensure that both research and policy are premised upon a life cycle approach without excluding the possibilities of targeted interventions in later life. It is only through such a careful and motivated strategy that one would be better able to plan for future needs of older men and women at a personal as well as a social level.

1 Kramer M. The rising pandemic mental disorders and associated chronic diseases and disabilities. *Acta Psychiatr Scand* 1980;**62**(suppl 285):382–92.
2 Manton KG. Changing concepts of morbidity and mortality in the elderly population. *Milbank Mem Fund Q* 1982;**60**:183–244.
3 Waldren I. Why do women live longer than men? *Soc Sci Med* 1976;**10**:349–62.
4 Wingard DL. The sex differential in morbidity, mortality and lifestyle. *Am Rev Public Health* 1984;**5**:433–58.
5 Arber S, Ginn J. *Gender and later life: a sociological analysis of resource and constraints.* London: Sage Publications, 1991.
6 Verbrugge LM. Female illness rates and illness behaviour: testing hypotheses about sex differences in health. *Women and Health* 1979;4:61–79.
7 Verbrugge LM. Gender, ageing and health. In: Kyriakos S, Markides K, editors. *Ageing and health perspectives on gender, race, ethnicity and class.* Newbury Park: C A Sage Publications, 1989:23–79.
8 Kinsella K, Taeuber CM. *An aging world II.* Washington: US Department of Commerce Bureau of the Census, 1993.
9 Lopez AD, Ruzicka LT. *Sex differentials in mortality: trends, determinants and consequences.* Canberra: Department of Demography, Australian National University, 1983. (Miscellaneous series, No 4.)
10 Nathanson CA. Premature adult mortality in developed countries: from description to explanation. In: Lopez A, Caselli G, Volkanen T, editors. *Adult mortality in developed countries.* Oxford: OUP, 1995.
11 Waldren I. What do we know about causes of sex differences in mortality? A review of the literature. *Popul Bull UN* 1985;**18**:59–76.
12 Gibson MJS. *Older women around the world.* Washington: International Federation on Ageing, 1985.
13 Moser KA, Pugh H, Goldblatt PO. Inequalities in women's health: looking at mortality differentials using an alternative approach. *BMJ* 1988;**296**:1221–4.
14 Mechanic D. Sex, illness behaviour and the use of health services. *Soc Sci Med* 1978;12B:207–14.
15 Heikkinnen E, Waters WE, Brzeninski ZJ. *The elderly in eleven countries: a sociomedical survey.* Copenhagen: WHO, 1983. (Public health in Europe 21.)
16 Sennot-Miller L. The health and socio-economic situation of mid-life and older women in Latin America and the Caribbean. In: Pan American Health Organisation and the American Association of Retired Persons. *Midlife and older women in Latin America and the Caribbean.* Washington: PAHO/AARP, 1989:1–121.
17 Verbrugge LM. Females and illness, recent trends in sex differences in the United States. *J Health Soc Behav* 1985:Sep 26:156–82.

18 Jordanova LJ. Natural facts: a historical perspective on science and sexuality. In: MacCormack C, Strathern M, editors. *Nature, culture and gender.* New York: Cambridge University Press, 1980:42–69.

19 Vallin J. Can sex differentials in mortality be explained by socioeconomic differentials? In: Lopez A, Caselli G, Volkanen T, editors. *Adult mortality in developed countries.* Oxford: OUP, 1995.

20 World Health Organization. *Ageing in the western Pacific: a four country study.* Manila: WHO Regional Office for the Western Pacific, 1986.

21 Pan American Health Organisation. *Toward the well-being of the elderly.* Washington: PAHO, 1985.

22 Koblinsky M, Timyan J, Gay J, editors. *The health of women: a global perspective.* Boulder, CO: Westview Press, 1993.

23 Paltiel F. *Mental health of women in the Americas.* Washington: WHO, 1992. (Pan American Health Organisation scientific publications, No 5451.)

23 Quality of life

ANN BOWLING

Success in the West is usually determined by economic achievement and occupational status. In the developed world, with the emphasis on affluence and with the increasing longevity of populations, there is a general interest in knowledge about how to find the "goodness" of life, sometimes called life satisfaction or quality of life. Quality of life research spans a range of topics, from quality of life in the last year of life to quality of life in urban environments. The concept of quality of life has a usage across many disciplines—in geography, literature, philosophy, health economics, advertising, health promotion, and the medical and social sciences.

Purchasing debates in health care have been focusing on health care costs in relation to broader "health gains" or "benefits" (that is, health related quality of life) from the treatments and interventions that are being contracted for. In public health and in social services, quality of life is increasingly incorporated into criteria for the assessment of people's needs for effective services. The emphasis of research and audit is on the measurement of health outcomes in its broadest sense. Treatment and care need to be evaluated in terms of whether they are more likely to lead to an outcome of a life worth living in social, psychological, and physical terms.

Definitions

Health status is often referred to as quality of life, and, in order to narrow down its operationalisation in research studies, quality of life is increasingly referred to as health related quality of life. Health related quality of life is a subjective concept and essentially relates to the perceived effects of health status on the ability to live a fulfilling life.

From a health care perspective, quality of life can be said to refer to the social, emotional, and physical wellbeing of patients following treatment, thus mirroring the World Health Organization's definition of health: a "state of complete physical, mental and social wellbeing and not merely the absence of disease or infirmity."[1] WHO has since added "autonomy" to this list.[2] More precisely, health related quality of life is thus the achievement of optimum levels of mental, physical, role (for example, work, parent, carer, etc), and social functioning, including relationships,

221

and perceptions of health, fitness, life satisfaction, and wellbeing. It should also include some assessment of the patient's level of satisfaction with treatment, outcome, and health status and with future prospects.

Psychologists, sociologists, and social gerontologists carried out most of the early empirical social research on quality of life in studies in the United States that attempted to estimate wellbeing, satisfaction, or happiness, and what people meant by "the good life". Lawton first proposed a theoretical model of quality of life as "the good life", defined as psychological wellbeing, perceived quality of life, behavioural competence, and the "objective" environment.[3] Andrews argued that quality of life is the extent to which pleasure and satisfaction have been obtained.[4] The gerontological literature on the topics of "successful ageing", "positive ageing", and "quality of older age" has focused largely on life satisfaction and morale,[5] and more recently on feelings of control and motivation.[6] Ultimately, however, the question of what is quality of life remains philosophical.

WHO has under its umbrella a working party on quality of life that is undertaking a 10 country study of health related quality of life. The WHO Quality of Life (WHOQOL) Group has provided a definition of quality of life that also takes individual perception and relationship to the environment into account:

> Quality of life is defined as an individual's perception of their position in life in the context of the culture and value systems in which they live and in relation to their goals, expectations, standards and concerns. It is a broad ranging concept affected in a complex way by the person's physical health, psychological state, level of independence, social relationships, and their relationships to salient features of their environment.[7]

This definition underpins the WHOQOL—this is an instrument being developed for measuring quality of life that can be used in a variety of cultural settings.[7] It is being developed as a core instrument and modules are being planned that will be specific to certain population groups (cancer patients, elderly people, etc). Extensive piloting of the instrument is currently underway. The WHOQOL is designed to be self administered; it contains five broad domains: physical health (bodily states and functions), psychological health, level of independence, social relationships, and environment. Each domain contains several facets (for example, physical health includes pain and discomfort, vitality and fatigue, and sensory functions). Care is being taken to make the questions sensitive to individual cultures, while measuring the same domains across cultures. The resulting instrument should be suitable for use in clinical and population settings.

Measurement scales

In choosing a health status measure or set of measures, key questions to consider are whether a disease specific and/or a generic measure is needed, and whether either requires supplementation with single domain measures (for example, depression) that are of importance to the study aims.

Disease specific measures

Clearly criteria for assessing outcome of care will vary for different disease syndromes. A universal questionnaire to elicit the relevant information for a number of conditions would require one of enormous length. Disease specific quality of life scales are needed, not simply for greater brevity but to ensure sensitivity to sometimes small but clinically significant changes in health status and levels of disease severity.

Single domain measures

Domain specific areas of interest will vary according to how the condition and its treatment affect the patient and the aims and scope of research. Thus for some diseases and conditions measures of psychiatric status will necessitate the inclusion of a memory test as well as a depression scale. The measurement of physical functioning may be restricted to crude scales with global categories, ranging from fully functioning to bed bound for more dramatic conditions and interventions where great changes are expected, but may need to be more refined and sensitive (that is, at the "less restrictive" end of the scale) in the case of more moderate cases. Other domains of potential relevance may include other physical effects (such as pain), social role functioning (including maintenance of social relationships and activities), psychological wellbeing (including happiness/satisfaction), achievement of personal goals and aspirations, personal control, adjustment and coping ability (modifying variables), wellbeing, self concept and esteem, body image, and satisfaction with care and treatment.

Generic measures

Comprehensive measures that implicitly or explicitly aim to tap health related quality of life are usually referred to as broader measures of health status. They should encompass the dimensions of physical, mental, and social health. Investigators have tended to supplement generic health status measures with specific disease items. They have used generic measures in order to make comparisons with other conditions, to broaden their outcome indicators, and because of the slow development of disease specific questionnaires.

The most popular generic measures include the Rand batteries, in particular the increasingly used SF-36,[8] the Sickness Impact Profile,[9] the Nottingham Health Profile,[10] and the McMaster Health Index Questionnaire.[11] A popular and promising generic measure that is being developed for use in primary medical care is the Dartmouth Coop Function Charts.[12]

Who should rate quality of life?

In health care the debate sometimes revolves around whether the quality of life assessment should be made by the patient or by a health professional (such as a doctor). Objections to physician ratings include the argument that, while a particular patient may judge their quality of life to be low, he or she may nevertheless value life as precious. Some clinicians object to patients' ratings on the grounds of their subjectivity. This subjectivity, as it reflects the patient's point of view, should be viewed as their strength. The implication is that patients should complete questionnaires about their health status themselves or the questionnaire should be administered to them by a trained interviewer. "Significant others" (for example, relatives) and health care professionals should only complete ratings where their perspective is *also* required.

Measuring the health related quality of life of elderly people

Apart from any disease specific measures that may be regarded as important, the domains that require measurement among older people include health problems that can cause handicap, as well as those that are also potentially remediable. The measurement of social support is essential, as its existence can be a key factor in the maintenance of independent living in the community. A multidimensional approach to assessment is needed and this requires the separate (rather than aggregated) measurement and analysis of physical, mental, and social health.

Appropriate scales

Among the appropriate measures of life satisfaction and self esteem, Lawton's Philadelphia Geriatric Morale Scale is the most psychometrically robust and the most popular[13]; of the brief mental status tests, the Abbreviated Mental Test is frequently used.[14] In relation to measures of physical functioning, the functioning subsection of the Older Americans Resources and Services Schedule is judged to be superior to most scales for use with elderly people.[15] The full instrument covers physical, social, and psychological wellbeing; it is lengthy, although a short version has been developed. A scale for measuring depression and anxiety that does not include somatic items, such as the Hospital Anxiety and Depression Scale,[16] is also appropriate for use with older people. A range of scales appropriate for measuring intergenerational support were reviewed by Kane and Kane,[17] and another more recent scale for measuring supportive relationships generally is the Rand Medical Outcomes Study Social Support Questionnaire.[18]

Recommended scales

A working group representing the Royal College of Physicians and the British Geriatrics Society identified a set of assessment scales for use with elderly patients that they recommended for the evaluation of care and outcome of care.[19] Their recommended battery for use in community settings included the broad instrument Sickness Impact Profile[9] or its British version—the Functional Limitations Profile[20]—and the Philadelphia Geriatric Center Morale Scale.[13] As the working group pointed out, these scales will also need supplementing with a measure of cognitive function, memory, and depression.

The Royal College of General Practitioners has developed a package of appropriate assessment scales for use by general practitioners in Britain in their annual health checks on patients aged 75 and over. Its national distribution is at the planning stage.[21] The scales have to be concise for use in practice settings. The scales in the pack include the Abbreviated Mental Test,[14] the Geriatric Depression Scale,[22] and the Barthel Functional Assessment Scale.[23]

Lack of consensus

There is, however, no consensus on recommended packages, which is inevitable when numerous scales are available from which to choose. While international opinion agrees that the Philadelphia Geriatric Center Morale Scale[13] is the instrument of choice for measuring life satisfaction and morale (its psychometric properties are slightly superior to other existing scales), there is disagreement over the other recommended scales. A major disadvantage of the popular Sickness Impact Profile/Functional Limitations Profile[9 20] is its length. A major British study of outcomes of asthma and diabetes in general practice has discarded the last named because of its ceiling effects and because item non-response was so high (95 of the 136 items were endorsed by less than 10% of the respondents).[24] Additionally, the use of such a long scale means that the researcher has little opportunity to add other batteries of interest, whereas other shorter scales, such as the SF-36, permit the addition of several other scales. The SF-36 requires further testing with elderly people because its appropriateness has not been fully established.

A multicentre standardised assessment of the elderly study was carried out alongside the production of the report of the British Geriatrics Society and Royal College of Physicians. The assessments that were used included the Barthel Index,[23] the Abbreviated Mental Test,[14] the Geriatric Depression Scale,[22] the Philadelphia Geriatric Center Morale Scale,[13] and several questions on communication and social circumstances; however, this choice of a battery is also open to debate. Several investigators have criticised the use of the Barthel Index in community settings (it is a severe and limited measure appropriate to institutional settings). It can be used in the community, but with more appropriate adaptations for use in this setting.

The unsatisfactory length of the Sickness Impact Profile and the insensitivity of the Barthel Index when used in community settings and for global use (as opposed to disease specific—for example, stroke) illustrate the crude state of existing screening instruments for use with older people. Far more research is needed into the development and use of health status and functional ability scales for older people living at home.

Disease specific and/or generic scales?

The assessment of older people requires the use of scales that are specific and are sensitive to the needs and problems of this age group (such as functional ability scales). It should not, however, be forgotten that the majority of the chronic diseases prevalent in both developed and developing countries are the diseases of "old age"—for example, cancers, arthritis and rheumatism, stroke, and heart disease—and disease specific scales are also appropriate with this age group. Moreover, only a small proportion of people over retirement age are severely disabled or in need of long term care, a fact which further emphasises the need for non-ageist but "age sensitive" philosophies of treatment and care[25] and the assessment of outcome. The methodological difficulty is the existence of multiple pathology among very elderly people, and it may not be practical or desirable to apply several disease specific scales to the same group of elderly patients. There is no easy solution to this problem and it needs to be considered in relation to the individual clinical problem or research issue.

Disease specific measures need to be supplemented with scales appropriate for older people, particularly for functional ability. Functional ability and self rated health status measures have been reported to be better predictors of service needs and use than traditional disease oriented assessments.[26] Assessments and interventions that focus on functional ability are often judged to be likely to improve outcomes. These judgements are not, however, based on studies that determine the effectiveness of functional status assessment in real life clinical practice, partly as a result of the scarcity of data. A recent trial of functional disability screening in clinical practice showed no significant differences in outcome between experimental and control groups in relation to functional or health status.[27]

In sum, although multidimensional measures are essential elements of any assessment with this age group, disease specific scales *are also* appropriate in relation to specific conditions; for example, older people as well as younger people can suffer from breathlessness in various situations when they suffer from coronary and respiratory disease, and they also suffer from the toxic effects of any treatments that they may receive. It is just as desirable to measure these effects in order to assess need for and outcome of care of older people as it is in younger people, particularly with the increase in the numbers of people in their late 70s to mid-80s and the emphasis on positive ageing and equal rights to appropriate treatments among all age groups.

1 World Health Organization. *Official records of the WHO, No 2*. Geneva: Interim Commission: United Nations, WHO, 1948:100.
2 World Health Organization. The uses of epidemiology in the study of the elderly: report of a WHO scientific group on the epidemiology of ageing. *Tech Rep Ser* 1984:706.
3 Lawton MP. Environment and other determinants of well-being in older people. *Gerontologist* 1983;**23**:349–57.
4 Andrews FM. Social indicators of perceived life quality. *Soc Indic Res* 1974;**1**:279–99.
5 Palmore E. Predictors of successful aging. *Gerontologist* 1979;**19**:427–43.
6 Baltes PB, Baltes MM. *Successful aging: perspectives from the behavioural sciences*. New York: Cambridge University Press, 1990.
7 WHOQOL. *Measuring quality of life. The development of the World Health Organization Quality of Life Instrument (WHOQOL)*. Geneva: WHO Division of Mental Health, 1993.
8 Ware JE. Measuring patient's views: the optimum outcome measure. *BMJ* 1993;**306**: 1429–30.
9 Bergner M, Bobbitt RA, Pollard WE, *et al*. The Sickness Impact Profile: validation of a health status measure. *Med Care* 1976;**14**:57–67.
10 Hunt SM, McEwan J, Mckenna SP. *Measuring health status*. London: Croom Helm, 1986.
11 Chambers LW, Sackett DL, Goldsmith CH, *et al*. Development and application of an index of social function. *Health Serv Res* 1976;**11**:430–41.
12 Nelson E, Wasson J, Kirk J, *et al*. Assessment of function in routine clinical practice: description of the Coop chart method and preliminary findings. *J Chronic Dis* 1987; **40**(suppl):55–63S.
13 Lawton MP. The Philadelphia geriatric morale scale: a revision. *J Gerontol* 1975;**30**:85–9.
14 Hodgkinson HM. Evaluation of a mental test score for assessment of mental impairment in the elderly. *Age Ageing* 1972;**1**:233–8.
15 Fillenbaum GG, Smyer MA. The development, validity and reliability of the OARS Multidimensional Functional Assessment Questionnaire. *J Gerontol* 1981;**36**:428–34.
16 Zigmond AS, Snaith RP. The hospital anxiety and depression scale. *Acta Psychiat Scand* 1983;**67**:361–70.
17 Kane RA, Kane RL. *Assessing the elderly*. Lexington, MA: Lexington Books, 1988.
18 Sherbourne CD, Stewart AL. The MOS social support survey. *Soc Sci Med* 1991;**32**: 705–14.
19 British Geriatrics Society/Royal College of Physicians. *Standardised clinical instruments and measurement scales for elderly patients. Working party report*. London: RCP, 1992.
20 Charlton J, Patrick D, Peach H. Use of multivariate measures of disability in health surveys. *J Epidemiol Community Health* 1983;**37**:296–304.
21 Wallace P. Health checks for people aged 75 and over in general practice. An international package for assessment [abstract]. *Fam Pract* 1994;**10**:477.
22 Yesavage JA, Brink TL, Rose TL, *et al*. Development and validation of a geriatric depression screening scale—a preliminary report. *J Psychiatr Res* 1983;**17**:37–49.
23 Mahoney FI, Barthel DW. Functional evaluation: the Barthel Index. *Md State Med J* 1965;**14**:61–5.
24 McColl E, Steen IJ, Meadows K, *et al*. Developing outcome measures for ambulatory care: an application to asthma and diabetes. *Soc Sci Med* (in press).
25 Fentiman IS, Tirelli U, Monfardini S, *et al*. Cancer in the elderly: why so badly treated? *Lancet* 1990;**335**:1020–2.
26 Waters WE, Heikkinen E, Dontas AS, editors. *Health, lifestyles and services for the elderly*. Copenhagen: WHO, 1989. (Report from the WHO Regional Office for Europe. Public health in Europe, No 29.)
27 Rubenstein LV, Calkins DR, Young RT, *et al*. Improving patient function: a randomised trial of functional disability screening. *Ann Intern Med* 1989;**111**:836–42.

24 Functional ability

GERDA G FILLENBAUM

Measurement: impairment, disability, handicap

Within the context of the International Classification of Impairments, Disabilities, and Handicaps,[1] impairment is defined as "any loss or abnormality of psychological, physiological, or anatomic structure or function"; disability is defined as "any restriction or lack (resulting from an impairment) of ability to perform an activity in the manner or within the range considered normal for a human being"; and handicap is defined as "a disadvantage for a given individual, resulting from an impairment or a disability, that limits or prevents the fulfilment of a role that is normal . . . for that individual."

There is a logical but not invariable progression from impairment to disability and from disability to handicap. Functional ability falls within the general context of disability. It is assessed by determining whether common everyday tasks can be performed. Impairments, such as reduction in vision, hearing, understanding, or capacity to move, may result in increased difficulty in performing common tasks (getting around, taking care of oneself) and create problems in becoming, or remaining, a fully participating member of society (that is, they result in a handicap).

Assessment of functional ability

As age increases, there tends to be a concomitant increase in the presence and number of chronic conditions; in consequence attention must turn away from cure to alleviation of symptoms and maintenance of personal independence. Information on functional ability is critical because it permits focus and concentration on those activities basic to continued independent living.

Functional ability is typically assessed in terms of tasks subsumed under the general heading of "activities of daily living" (ADL). These activities have been classified into three types: mobility (the ability to get around), instrumental activities of daily living (IADL) (complex activities needed for daily living), and physical activities of daily living (PADL) (sometimes called personal self maintenance tasks or basic activities of daily living because they focus on basic bodily needs).[2]

228

Measures of functional ability may be designed for very specific purposes, such as to identify the impact of intervention in rehabilitation[3] or to assess level of dementia,[4][5] or they may be more broadly applicable. Our focus here is on the latter, on representative, broadly used, carefully evaluated measures that provide information on functional abilities and in consequence the services needed to maintain personal wellbeing and independence.

Physical activities of daily living

Physical (basic) activities of daily living include tasks that must be performed if a physically healthy life is to be maintained. These activities tend to be relevant in all cultures and to be independent of gender. Perhaps the best known and one of the most widely used assessments is the six item index of independence in activities of daily living.[6] The items, in hierarchical order of difficulty (which also reflects the order of acquisition in childhood, retention in old age, and reacquisition with rehabilitation), are feeding, continence, transfer (moving in and out of bed or chair), attending to self at the toilet, dressing, and bathing. This particular order has been questioned and evidence for alternative hierarchies has been presented. There is also some question as to whether continence should remain a part of this hierarchy or whether it should be assessed independently; independent assessment is currently favoured.

On this measure performance may be scored on either a two point scale (independent v dependent functioning) or a three point scale (independent v receives some help v receives considerable help or is unable to perform the activity). In either case the steps of the scale are carefully described. It may be as well to note here that three levels may be the maximum that most respondents can distinguish reliably.

Table 24.1 indicates by gender and age group the percentage of American community residents reporting difficulty with selected PADL.

Instrumental activities of daily living

IADL are more complex tasks, the performance of which is necessary to remain a participating member of society. These tasks may not be independent of gender or relevant in all cultures, indeed bias may be appropriate. The Older Americans Resources and Services (OARS) IADL scale,[8] which was designed to be a gender free modification of the original sex specific scales developed by Lawton and Brody,[9] focuses on seven activities, which are (in increasing order of difficulty): being responsible for own medicine, using the telephone, handling personal finances, preparing meals, shopping, travelling out of walking distance, and doing housework. Each item is scored on a three point scale (can perform unaided/needs help/totally unable to do). Factor analysis indicates that this scale is multidimensional, the items on responsibility for own medicine and use of

229

Table 24.1   Percentage of US community residents 65 years of age and over who report difficulty in performing selected physical activities of daily living

Age (years)	Eat	Transfer	Toilet	Dress	Bathe	Walk
Men						
65–69	1·7	4·7	2·3	4·1	5·3	11·5
70–74	1·4	5·0	2·4	4·9	6·1	14·9
75–79	2·3	4·7	2·7	6·7	7·8	15·6
80–84	3·0	8·7	5·6	8·5	12·3	24·2
85 +	4·3	12·7	10·0	14·1	23·1	32·2
All 65 +	2·0	5·6	3·1	5·8	7·6	15·5
Women						
65–69	0·9	5·7	2·2	3·7	5·1	12·9
70–74	1·0	8·6	3·4	4·8	9·1	17·8
75–79	3·3	9·3	5·0	6·2	11·1	22·2
80–84	3·4	14·3	9·0	10·2	19·2	31·4
85 +	4·4	27·2	15·9	17·7	30·1	43·3
All 65 +	1·7	9·7	5·1	6·5	11·2	20·9

From Dawson and Hendershot.[7]

the telephone falling on one dimension and the remaining five items falling on another.

Table 24.2 indicates the percentage of American community residents reporting difficulty in performing some of these tasks.

Mobility

While both the Katz and the OARS scales include items on mobility (such inquiry is implicit in the Katz toileting item and explicit in the OARS travel item), an extensively used three item abbreviated version of the Rosow–Breslau scale[10] of physical health functioning includes two items that may straddle the gap between the Katz and OARS mobility items. These items inquire about ability to walk half a mile and to climb a flight of stairs.

Single hierarchical scales

Serious attempts have been made to develop single hierarchical scales that include information on mobility, IADL, and PADL.[11][12] Although, in general, problems with mobility precede problems in other areas, success has been limited. This may in part reflect limitations of available statistical software. The advantage of a strongly hierarchical measure is that it permits more rapid assessment; inability to perform any one item indicates that items below it in the hierarchy cannot be performed either. So far, however, no scale has been developed that is so powerful. The disadvantage of hierarchical measures is that they do not provide, and indeed may mask,

230

Table 24.2   Percentage of US community residents 65 years of age and over who report difficulty in performing instrumental activities of daily living

Age (years)	Telephone	Manage money	Meals	Shops	Housework	
					Heavy	Light
Men						
65–69	3·0	2·6	2·6	4·1	9·8	3·5
70–74	4·3	3·1	3·6	5·3	13·0	3·4
75–79	6·3	5·2	5·1	7·6	14·6	5·2
80–84	11·3	5·8	7·8	13·9	18·9	8·2
85 +	18·4	19·0	18·5	26·8	33·3	15·2
All 65 +	5·6	4·4	4·7	7·3	13·7	4·9
Women						
65–69	1·3	1·4	4·2	6·4	21·8	4·0
70–74	2·8	2·3	5·5	9·4	27·3	6·2
75–79	4·1	5·2	8·3	14·5	33·2	8·4
80–84	6·0	9·3	14·0	24·7	41·7	14·0
85 +	17·1	26·2	29·5	41·6	54·2	27·4
All 65 +	4·2	5·5	8·7	14·1	30·8	27·4

From Dawson and Hendershot.[7]

unique profiles of functional ability, for there is increasing evidence that different physical disorders have a differential relationship to aspects of functional status.

Manner of gathering information

Information is typically obtained from the person being assessed or from someone who knows that person well (an attendant or family member). These alternative sources do not, however, provide equivalent information.[13][14] Furthermore, the manner in which an item is phrased may influence the response obtained,[15] making comparison across studies problematic. Performance based measures (observing execution of the task) have sometimes been recommended in the interests of increased objectivity but their advantages may have been overestimated.[16]

Level of ability to perform a task is typically rated on a two or three point scale. The scale may be extended to include information on whether a device or another person is needed to provide help (if help is needed), with use of a device typically seen as indicating greater independence than is help received from another person. Clarification as to whether difficulty in performance is due to physical or mental problems is increasingly sought.

Variation

Time

With increase in life expectancy, the question has arisen as to whether the onset of chronic disease and accompanying disability has been delayed or whether time spent with illness and disability has increased. The former seems to be the case. Review of American data indicates that in 1989 as compared with 1982 a smaller percentage of the older population (65 years and older) was disabled, those who were disabled in general had fewer disabilities, and a smaller proportion entered nursing homes. Importantly, improved status became more obvious as age increased.[17] Comparable findings have been reported from Sweden and the United Kingdom. Gender, education, and income have been found to be related to disability, as have selected medical treatments. As the education and income levels of persons entering the older years increase, and medical treatments and health habits improve, further gains can be expected.

Place

While the prevalence of PADL problems is comparable across developed countries, the prevalence of mobility and IADL problems differs from country to country and by gender, probably reflecting social roles and expectations.[18] There are particular problems in applying measures standardised in developed countries to the elderly in developing countries. Certain kinds of facility (for example, banks, telephones) may be irrelevant for part of the population; other tasks (for example, food preparation) may require quite different skills. Furthermore, while they are respected, minimal performance and social involvement may be expected of the elderly. Under such circumstances assessment using measures developed elsewhere may provide inaccurate information.[19] Attempts to develop more appropriate measures, particularly for selected Asian populations, are underway and some success has been achieved.[20 21]

Person

The prevalence of problems with physical functioning increases with age and may vary as a function of sex, race, and socioeconomic status. Progression, however, is not invariably in the direction of increased disability. The fewer the number of problems and the less basic the activity the greater the likelihood of improvement when disability is present.

Associations and causal links with disease

While there is an association between morbidity, disability, and mortality, all health conditions do not necessarily result in disability. Nevertheless, certain types of health conditions have been found to be associated with certain types of ADL problems. Of a variety of chronic conditions common to the elderly, stroke, dementia, low vision, and arthritis/rheumatism are likely to be associated with a larger number of ADL disabilities.[22] More specifically, those with impaired IADL performance (difficulty using the

232

telephone, handling money, taking medication) are more likely to have diagnoses indicative of poor cognitive functioning (arteriosclerosis, "senile") or have problems with vision. Conditions such as diabetes and circulatory disease are reported by persons who only have PADL problems, while those who are not disabled have been found to have few serious medical problems.[23]

While there is a marked association between severe cognitive impairment and ability to perform IADL tasks (such that it has been appropriate to develop IADL measures to assess dementia),[45] in general there is no close link between a specific health condition (or the severity of that condition) and ability to perform a specific activity.

Intervention

The intervention that is offered should be such as to compensate for the functional disability while maintaining the individual at that preferred level of independence commensurate with appropriate conventionally accepted standards of health and safety. In addition to determining the remedial and rehabilitative care that is needed it is also necessary to determine which basic maintenance and supportive services are required. Alternative approaches to doing this (two will be described here) have been developed. Each identifies the activities for which compensation is needed. The OARS approach[8] focuses on the specific services needed, while the approach of Isaacs and Neville[24] identifies the type of service provider and the length of time during a 24 hour day that somebody should be present. OARS ascertains the precise services needed by identifying those ADL that cannot be performed adequately and determines whether the needs they represent are already being addressed (and if so, the likelihood that they will continue to be addressed), so permitting selection of appropriate supplementary services. The aim is not to bring everybody up to the same level of functioning but to make sure that the individual is physically maintained, and then to provide those additional compensatory services from which the individual can benefit.

The Isaacs and Neville approach also begins by determining functional ability and extent of help received, as well as the feasibility of that help continuing. Based on this information people are grouped into three classes according to the length of time they can safely be left alone (cannot be left alone safely; some care, preferably scheduled, needed each day; care needed, but not each day), and into four categories according to whether they are alone at night, and for how long they are alone during the day. This information, in combination, permits assessment of the amount of additional service needed and the level of skill required of a provider—the longer the hours per day, the greater the level of skill needed.

Ultimately intervention to compensate for problems in functional ability must be tailored to individual conditions. Planning for service needs can, however, be done on a population basis. In some cases intervention can be population based, resulting in improvements for the able bodied as well. Good examples of this are legislated transportation and architectural requirements, which, intended to make access easier for those who have problems with mobility, make access and use easier for all.

Health policy

Ideally health policy requires the allocation of services to the elderly based on the need for those services and their relevance. As a result alternative ways of determining need have been explored. These range from full scale epidemiological surveys of the older population to determine their functional abilities, to estimating status based on demographic information. The latter approach, when linked to sound data, provides reasonable information in a cost effective manner.

Much of the maintenance and supportive service received by the elderly is provided by family and friends. Increasingly provision to make this possible is being made by the workplace. Where mobility (for example, helping with transportation) and IADL tasks (for example, shopping, housekeeping, cooking) are concerned, in-home receipt, even if paid, is cheaper than institutional care. Where PADL tasks are concerned, particularly if constant supervision is needed, the cost of in-home care when estimated on the basis of agency level reimbursement may become more than that of institutional care. In addition, the feasibility of providing adequate care may require resources that are not readily available. Thus while the elderly are discouraged from entering institutions (and typically prefer to remain at home) there are times when this is an appropriate and may even be a preferred choice.

The aim of health policy is to increase active life expectancy by reducing the length of time disabled. To do this it will be necessary to improve general socioeconomic status, encourage the development of good health habits in the younger years and their maintenance with increasing age, and promote the use of evaluated preventive treatment (for example, oestrogen for women to delay or prevent osteoporosis, aspirin to reduce recurrent stroke) at the appropriate time. Thus a multifaceted approach to maintaining functional ability and to providing needed services is in order.

1 World Health Organization. *International classification of impairments, diseases and handicaps.* Geneva: WHO, 1980.
2 Katz S. Assessing self-maintenance: activities of daily living, mobility and instrumental activities of daily living. *J Am Geriatr Soc* 1980;**31**:721–7.
3 Linacre JM, Heinemann AW, Wright BD, Granger CV, Hamilton BB. The structure and stability of the functional independence measure. *Arch Phys Med Rehabil* 1994;**75**:127–32.
4 Loewenstein DA, Amigo E, Duara R, *et al.* A new scale for the assessment of functional status in Alzheimer's disease and related disorders. *J Gerontol* 1989;**44**:114–21.
5 Mahurin RK, DeBettignies RH, Pirozzolo FJ. Structured assessment of independent living skills: preliminary report of a performance of functional abilities in dementia. *J Gerontol* 1991;**46**:58–66.

6 Katz S, Akpom CA. A measure of primary socio-biologic functions. *Int J Health Serv* 1976;**6**:493–507.

7 Dawson D, Hendershot G, Fulton J. Aging in the eighties: functional limitations of individuals age 65 years and over. Advancedata No. 133, June 10, 1987.

8 Fillenbaum GG. *Multidimensional functional assessment of older adults: the Duke Older Americans Resources and Services procedures*. Hillsdale, NJ: Erlbaum, 1988.

9 Lawton MP, Brody EM. Assessment of older people: self-maintaining and instrumental activities of daily living. *Gerontologist* 1969;**9**:179–86.

10 Rosow I, Breslau N. A Guttmann health scale for the aged. *J Gerontol* 1966;**21**:556–9.

11 Spector WD, Katz S, Murphy JB, Fulton JP. The hierarchical relationship between activities of daily living and instrumental activities of daily living. *J Chronic Dis* 1987;**40**: 481–9.

12 Kemper GIJM, Suurmeijer TPBM. The development of a hierarchical polychotomous ADL-IADL scale for non-institutionalized elders. *Gerontologist* 1990;**30**:497–502.

13 Dorevitch MI, Cossar RM, Bailey FJ, *et al*. The accuracy of self and informant ratings of physical functional capacity of the elderly. *J Clin Epidemiol* 1992;**45**:791–8.

14 Rubenstein LZ, Schairer C, Wieland GD, Kane R. Systematic biases in functional status assessment of elderly adults: effects of different data sources. *J Gerontol* 1984;**39**:686–91.

15 Wiener JM, Hanley RJ, Clark R, van Nostrand NF. Measuring the activities of daily living: comparisons across national surveys. *J Gerontol* 1990;**45**:S229–37.

16 Myers A, Holiday PJ, Harvey KA, Hutchinson KS. Functional performance measures: are they superior to self-assessment? *J Gerontol Med Sci* 1993;**48**:M196–206.

17 Manton KG, Corder LS, Stallard E. Estimates of change in chronic disability and institutional incidence and prevalence rates in the US elderly population from the 1982, 1984, and 1989 National Long Term Care Survey. *J Gerontol* 1993;**48**:S153–66.

18 Fillenbaum GG. Development of a brief, internationally usable screening instrument. In: Maddox GL, Busse EW, editors *Aging: the universal human experience. Highlights of the 1985 International Congress of Gerontology*. New York: Springer, 1987.

19 Andrews GR, Esterman AJ, Braunack-Mayer AJ, Rungie CM. *Aging in the Western Pacific*. Manila: World Health Organization, 1986.

20 Jitapunkul S, Kamolratanakul P, Ebrahim S. The meaning of activities of daily living in a Thai elderly population: development of a new index. *Age Aging* 1994;**23**:97–101.

21 Chandra V, Ganguli M, Ratcliff G, *et al*. Studies of the epidemiology of dementia: comparisons between developed and developing countries. *Aging Clin Exp Res* 1994;**6**: 307–21.

22 Ford AB, Folmar SJ, Salmon RB, Medalie JH, Roy AW, Galazka SS. Health and function in the old and very old. *J Am Geriatr Soc* 1988;**36**:187–97.

23 Manton KG, Soldo BJ. Dynamics of health changes in the oldest old: new perspectives and evidence. *Milbank Mem Fund Q* 1985;**63**:206–85.

24 Isaacs B, Neville Y. The needs of old people: the "interval" as a method of measurement. *Br J Prev Soc Med* 1976;**30**:79–85.

25 Social networks and support

EMILY GRUNDY

Social ties have long been recognised as an important constituent of, and contributor to, the health and wellbeing of people of all ages. Most older people are not socially isolated but events that are both stressful and deplete the social environment, such as bereavement, are common in later life. Older people, particularly those with disabilities, are also likely to rely on support networks for practical help. For these reasons the quantity and quality of social support available to the older population should be considered by the planners and providers of health and welfare services. While there is a rapidly growing literature on this topic,[1] our understanding of, for example, how and why social ties influence health, remains incomplete and a number of seemingly conflicting results have been reported.[2] This is partly due to the confusion or ellipsis of demographic, social network, and social support variables used in some studies and the wide range of instruments used to measure each. As the definition of key concepts is important, these are outlined below.

Social networks have been defined as sets of linkages among identified groups of people, the characteristics of which have some explanatory power. These characteristics (of networks rather than of the individuals within them) include factors such as size, geographic dispersion, the proportion of relatives within the network, and the "density" of the network. Dense, or integrated, networks are those in which most members know most other members. There is some evidence that integrated networks function better than looser ones as sources of coordinated support for elderly people, particularly in times of crisis.[3] Looser networks, however, may allow older people greater freedom to "shop around" for the most appropriate type of contact or assistance.

Social support has been conceptualised as the interactive process through which emotional, instrumental, and informational aid is received from one's social network. Emotional support includes the sense of being loved and valued and may be particularly important for morale and as a buffer to the adverse effects of stress.

Instrumental support includes services such as help with shopping, food preparation, and personal care. This type of support is obviously very

236

important for disabled older people unable to carry out essential daily activities unaided. A wide range of studies have shown that close relatives provide the most help with activities of daily living, particularly personal care, and the most help in times of illness.[4] Social networks built around relatives may thus be the most effective for the provision of instrumental support, particularly if a great deal of assistance is required.

Friends and more distant relatives, however, may help with domestic tasks, such as shopping. There is also evidence that friendships are particularly important for morale.

The third element of social support, *guidance* and information, may include advice on obtaining help from formal services. As a number of studies have shown that many older people have unmet informational needs, the importance of this type of support should not be underestimated.

There is some evidence that perceptions of whether support is available or adequate may be as important for wellbeing as actual levels of support.[5] One study of depression in elderly New Zealand women[6] found that there was no difference in the availability of support and extent of social integration between cases and non-cases; however, those with depression *perceived* their social relationships and activities as inadequate. Clearly perceptions of the adequacy of support are likely to be influenced by factors such as personality and indeed by conditions such as depression, so it is difficult to draw strong conclusions from this and similar findings other than the obvious one that individuals' support needs vary considerably.

Size of social networks

Studies from diverse localities suggest that the size of most older people's social networks ranges between five and seven.[7] Older women tend to have larger networks than men and, not surprisingly, relatives and friends rather than former workmates feature more prominently in them. Social networks are built up over the life course and so, although they may change with time, longstanding sociodemographic, cultural, and personality factors are important influences. It is known, for example, that social class and education are associated with different patterns of interaction and with differences in migration, an important influence on the geographic dispersion of a social network.[8][9] Very few elderly people lack any contact with friends or relatives. Data from the European Observatory of Older People suggest that among those over 60 the proportion lacking any contact with friends or relatives ranged from less than 2% in Nordic countries to just over 6% in Greece.[10]

Changes in network size

Data from longitudinal studies show changes in network size over time with, in general, decreases in size being more usual than increases. Results from a longitudinal study of very old people living in Hackney, inner London, for example, showed that 42% of survivors experienced a decrease in the size of their social network over a three year follow up period, while only 16% had a larger network at follow up than at baseline. While only 1% lacked any social network at baseline, at follow up this applied to 14%.[7]

Declines in network size may not necessarily imply declines in available support as remaining members may increase their contribution, although, particularly in the case of family members providing care, this may be at some personal cost. Advancing age and increasing disability may also change the nature of existing social relationships. In the 1985 British general household survey nearly half of those aged 85 or over reported never going out to visit family and friends, instead relying on being visited. Increasing support needs may breach established norms of reciprocity and so change, and sometimes jeopardise, the pre-existing relationship. The loss of friends may have particularly important consequences for the emotional wellbeing of older people as a number of studies suggest that, while relatives provide most practical help, friends are more important for morale and emotional wellbeing.[11] Size and characteristics of social networks have been shown to vary with location. Bowling and Farquhar found that 65–84 year old inhabitants of a semirural area of Essex had larger social networks than an equivalent group living in Hackney in inner London.[12] Differences between the social networks of old people living in rural Wales and those living in Liverpool have also been reported.[13]

Social networks and health

House et al,[14] in a review of the evidence on links between social relationships and health, commented that this evidence "increasingly approximates the evidence in the 1964 [US] Surgeon General's report that established smoking as a cause or risk factor for mortality and morbidity from a range of diseases."

This conclusion was based on a review of the relative risks of poor social integration on age adjusted mortality reported in five large prospective studies, together with evidence from a range of other investigations in both human and animal populations. A recent review of 12 large prospective studies of social ties and mortality in middle aged and elderly people concluded that, although the evidence was highly suggestive of a link between social ties and mortality, the results were not unequivocal.[2] In part this was thought to reflect the range of measures used, a problem referred to earlier. Another difficulty is deducing the causal direction of any association; even in longitudinal studies it is possible that the effects of social ties on health (or vice versa) may predate the point of baseline measurement, a particular problem in elderly populations whose characteristics are influenced by selective survival. As noted earlier, social support is hypothesised to influence health mainly as a buffer to stress.

238

The biological mechanisms whereby support may buffer the effects of stress are thought to lie in stimulation of appropriate neuroendocrine and immunological functions.[15] Cassel[16] proposed that stressors affect general susceptibility to disease and so lead to elevated mortality from a range of causes. Results from studies, including the Honolulu heart study, have, however, led some to question this, as these results suggested a weak link with mortality from heart disease but not with other or all causes of mortality. It may be that emotional support is associated with the prognosis rather than the aetiology of certain diseases. Several studies have shown striking differences in the outcome of men with acute myocardial infarction according to available emotional support.[17] Similarly, social support has been linked with the prognosis rather than the aetiology of breast cancer.[18]

A number of studies have shown that social participation, rather than or as well as social support, is associated with mortality and other indicators of health. Most well known are the results from the Alameda County study in the United States, which showed a negative association between church membership and mortality (after controlling for variations in health status and health related behaviours).[19] In the longitudinal study of very old people in Hackney, inner London, referred to earlier, club membership was associated with lower mortality among women.[2] Again it is difficult to deduce causality (as the socially active undoubtedly differ from "non-joiners" and poor health restricts opportunities for participation) but such a link seems biologically plausible both because of the effects of participation on morale and because such participation may involve activities such as physical exercise, which are known to be beneficial.

The relationship between instrumental support and health has been surprisingly little studied but help with shopping, cooking, and personal care might be expected to lead to better health by improving nutrition and hygiene. Guidance and information may also be hypothesised to influence health by, for example, the promotion of a healthier lifestyle and appropriate referral to medical services.

Social support and use of formal services

It might seem obvious that the availability of a supportive network of family and friends would reduce the use of formal services and indeed many studies suggest that this is the case[4]; however, informal networks may also act as a bridge to formal services, particularly specialised ones such as medical care, that cannot easily be provided by family or friends.[20] Moreover, while close relatives may tend to provide help themselves rather than seeking assistance from formal services, neighbours and friends may be more likely to make referrals to formal agencies.[21] One recent study of formal service use among a sample of elderly people in New York state found that those who received help from children were less likely to use community based services than others, while receiving help from friends was positively associated with service use.[22]

Several studies have shown differences between the social networks of service users and general elderly populations. Wenger, for example, found that 40% of a sample of social services clients had a very limited social network, classified as "private restricted," compared with 10–15% of general samples of elderly people.[23] Wenger and her colleagues have also argued that the most appropriate type of intervention depends to some extent on the type of social network an older person belongs to, and that an assessment of network type should be included in assessments for services.

Health policy

The European Office of the World Health Organization included the following among its "Targets for Health for All":

> By 1990 all member states should have specific programmes which enhance the major roles of the family and other social groups in developing and supporting healthy lifestyles.[24]

Despite this and the evidence reviewed above, which suggests that the promotion of social ties and activities should be considered part of any health promotion intervention, well designed studies to test the effect of appropriate interventions are lacking. To a large extent this reflects the difficulty involved in establishing any such intervention and defining suitable outcome measures.

Friendship, love, and supportive relatives cannot be prescribed (although many practitioners would argue that skilled interventions may help maintain them). Possibly beneficial community wide interventions, such as designing public space to facilitate social interaction, are similarly hard to implement and assess. The effect of other potentially valuable interventions, such as drop in centres or befriending schemes, generally have not been assessed in any rigorous way. Given the strength of the evidence linking social relationships with health, it is time that the promotion of good social relationships was more fully recognised as an objective and that imaginative research designs were employed to test the effect of various interventions.

1 Minkler M. Social support and health of the elderly. In: Cohen S, Syme SL, editors. *Social support and health.* New York: Academic Press, 1985:199–216.
2 Grundy E, Bowling A, Farquhar M. Social support, life satisfaction and survival at older ages. In: Caselli G, Lopez A, editors. *Health and mortality among elderly populations.* Oxford: Clarendon Press (in press).
3 Walker K, Macbride A, Vachon MLS. Social support networks and the crisis of bereavement. *Soc Sci Med* 1977;11:34–41.
4 Stoller E, Earl L. Help with activities of daily life: sources of support for the non-institutionalized elderly. *Gerontologist* 1983;23:64–70.
5 Krause N. Satisfaction with social support and self-rated health in older adults. *Gerontologist* 1987;27:301–8.
6 Walton VA, Romans-Clarkson SE, Mullen PE, Herbisohn GP. The mental health of elderly women in the community. *Int J Geriatr Psychiatry* 1990;5:257–63.

7 Bowling A, Farquhar M, Grundy E. Changes in network composition among older people living in Inner London and Essex. *Health and Place* 1995;**1**:149–66.

8 Willmott P. *Friendship networks and social support.* London: Policy Studies Institute, 1987.

9 Clark RL, Wolf DA. Proximity of children and elderly migration. In: Rogers A, editor. *Elderly migration and population redistribution.* London: Belhaven Press, 1992:77–96.

10 Commission of the European Communities. *Age and attitudes: main results from a Eurobarometer Survey.* Brussels: Commission of the European Communities, Directorate-General V, 1993.

11 Lee GR. Kinship and social support of the elderly: the case of the United States. *Ageing Soc* 1985;**5**:19–38.

12 Bowling A, Farquhar M. Associations with social networks, social support, health status and psychiatric morbidity in three samples of elderly people. *Soc Psychiatry Psychiatr Epidemiol* 1991;**26**:115–26.

13 Wenger GC. *A comparison of urban with rural support networks: Liverpool and North Wales—Working Paper 3.* Bangor: Centre for Social Policy Research and Development, University of Wales, 1992.

14 House JS, Landis KL, Umberson D. Social relationships and health. *Science* 1988;**241**: 540–5.

15 Berkman LF. The changing and heterogenous nature of aging and longevity: a social and biomedical perspective. *Ann Rev Gerontol Geriatr* 1988;**8**:37–68.

16 Cassel J. The contribution of the social environment to host resistance. *Am J Epidemiol* 1976;**104**:107–23.

17 Berkman LF, Leo-Summers L, Horowitz RI. Emotional support and survival after myocardial infarction. *Ann Intern Med* 1992;**117**:1003–9.

18 Vernon SW, Jackson GL. Social support, prognoses and adjustment to breast cancer. In: Markides KS, Cooper GL, editors. *Aging, stress and disease.* New York: Academic Press, 1989:165–98.

19 Berkman LF, Syme SL. Social networks, host resistance, and mortality: a nine year follow-up study of Alameda county residents. *Am J Epidemiol* 1979;**109**:186–204.

20 Sussman M. The family life of old people. In: Binstock R, Shanas E, editors. *Handbook of aging and the social sciences.* New York: Van Nostrand Reinhold, 1976.

21 Ward RA, Sherman S, LaGory M. Informal networks and knowledge of services for older persons. *J Gerontol* 1984;**39**:216–23.

22 Logan JR, Spitze G. Informal support and the use of formal services by older Americans. *J Gerontol* 1994;**49**:S25–34.

23 Wenger GC. *Support networks of older people: a guide for practitioners.* Bangor: Centre for Social Policy Research and Development, University College of Wales, 1994.

24 World Health Organization. *Targets for Health for All.* Geneva: WHO European Office, 1986.

Part III
Diseases and problems

26 Hypertension

JOHN M STARR, CHRIS J BULPITT

Measurement

In 1733 Stephen Hales first measured blood pressure directly by inserting a glass tube into a horse's carotid artery. Thankfully, over the successive two centuries less invasive methods were developed, but these have led to some confusion about what is meant by arterial blood pressure. Firstly, it is important to know the site at which blood pressure is measured: brachial artery pressures may be very different from those of a digital artery. Secondly, values obtained using a cuff may rarely be considerably higher than those acquired by direct cannulation if there is reduced compliance of the arterial wall; a phenomenon known as "pseudohypertension". Thirdly, the widely used auscultatory methods rely on the propagation of a blood pressure wave along the artery. The wave depends to some extent on the properties of the arterial wall and, owing to wave reflection, on how close to the periphery measurements are taken. These problems would be daunting enough for a static parameter but the variation of arterial blood pressure over time introduces even more complicated methodological issues.

Variation: time, place, and person

The introduction of relatively non-invasive methods of intermittent ambulatory blood pressure measurement increased awareness that isolated blood pressure values are often a poor reflection of 24 hour blood pressure control. In health, blood pressure increases physiologically with exercise, and stress also has a significant effect on blood pressure. This together with activity partly explains the diurnal variation observed in most people, with "dipping" of blood pressure during sleep at night. The loss of diurnal variation may be associated with greater end organ damage as manifested by left ventricular hypertrophy.[1] Stress may also explain the so called "white coat" effect leading to higher readings and, similarly, home blood pressure values may be lower than those found in the clinic. As well as these relatively short term stress effects, long term stress may exert significant influence on blood pressure, partly explaining variations with time. Kenyans who migrated from the country into a presumably more stressful urban environment and a different diet were found to have higher systolic and diastolic pressures compared with controls who remained in rural areas.[2]

These observations, together with those from the British Department of the Environment study,[3] suggest an interaction between a stressful lifestyle, perhaps acting through increased sympathetic drive, and salt load.

Despite all these potential causes of variation the greatest error in blood pressure measurement is often associated with untrained observers. These include the tendency to round values to the nearest 5–10 mm Hg, the use of too small an inflatable cuff, deflating the cuff too quickly, and not allowing the subject to rest for long enough.[4] In old age extra attention is needed because lying blood pressures may be considerably greater than standing pressures, and pressure differences may also be observed between hemiplegic and non-hemiplegic limbs.

These methodological issues would be a great problem if we were to search for some "true" arterial blood pressure. Fortunately most now pragmatically accept the view that as long as we use the same methods to measure blood pressure as were employed in a study establishing an association between blood pressure, morbidity, and mortality, then the results are relevant. This is why adherence to widely accepted guidelines is of the utmost importance.

Age trends

A healthy individual's blood pressure tends to increase with age. In addition, a phenomenon, known as "tracking", means that if blood pressure lies in the top 5% of the distribution at six weeks of life, it is likely to do so at six years and in middle age. Such tracking is consistent with epidemiological data relating low birth and high placental weights to high adult blood pressure,[5] and suggests that events in early life are important determinants. It is in middle age that treatment, disease, and death are most likely to intervene for those with the highest pressures, so that the elderly hypertensive can be considered a survivor. Furthermore, hypertension is far more common in the old. Over the age of 50 years a dissociation between systolic and diastolic pressures occurs, with diastolic pressures relatively lower than systolic pressures due to the reduced arterial compliance partly associated with atheromatous arterial disease. This relationship holds even in advanced age when a reduction in cardiac output occurs. Environmental risk factors, such as smoking, diet and urban residence, predispose to both large vessel atheroma and coronary atherosclerosis. The risk for any individual probably relates to which lesions are most critical. Epidemiological studies suggest that neither a high systolic nor a high diastolic pressure are risk indicators for cardiovascular or total mortality in men aged over 75 years or women aged over 85 years. Indeed the very elderly hypertensive lives longer than his or her normotensive counterpart. Of course, such epidemiological data cannot tell us whether or not we should treat hypertensive old people. This is an important question because the tendency for blood pressure to increase with age combined with preferential survival means that the prevalence of casual systolic hypertension (systolic blood pressure greater than 159 mm Hg on a single reading) in the United States increases dramatically from 19% in men aged 60 years to 41% in men aged 80 years. The prevalence of casual systolic hypertension also increases for women, from 27% at 60 years to 50% at 80 years. By contrast, casual diastolic hypertension (a single reading greater than 89 mm Hg) falls from 43% in men aged 60 to 21% at 80, and from 41% for women at 60 to 20% at 80 years of age.[6]

Associations and causal links

Hypertension is a good example of the difference between a diagnosis and a disease. By invoking mechanical explanations, elevated blood pressure may be considered a risk factor for cardiovascular events in its own right; however, in the old it may often be a manifestation of an underlying disease state, usually associated with insulin resistance.[7] Thus high blood pressure may not necessarily comprise part of the causal chain between that disease state and adverse events. Insulin resistance is associated with a cluster of overlapping abnormalities that, together with hypertension, includes diabetes mellitus, hyperlipidaemia, central obesity, and chronic renal impairment. There is usually increased activity of the sympathetic nervous system. The increased sympathetic drive may interact with a high salt load and contribute firstly by central nervous system mediated actions integrating baroreflex and other neuronal inputs, secondly by effects on hormonal systems, such as vasopressin, the renin–angiotensin system, and atrial natriuretic peptide, and thirdly more directly on cell membrane ion channels.[8]

Thus paradigms of hypertension have shifted from systemic disease through organ specific effects to trophic and ionic events on a molecular level. Of course, sodium, potassium, and other ions have long been recognized as significant in the aetiology of hypertension, but the contribution of ion fluxes to intracellular signal transduction, and hence to cell growth and differentiation, was not appreciated until fairly recently. Consequently therapies can be considered to act by reducing systemic blood pressure, but other aspects, for example the protection of specific end organs against damage such as the preferential regression of left ventricular hypertrophy, may also be important. It is perhaps too early to consider the implications of the more recent molecular biological discoveries on antihypertensive treatment but these will inform future epidemiological models of hypertension that focus on gene–environment interactions.

Intervention

Broadly speaking, interventions can be divided into pharmacological and non-pharmacological. The non-pharmacological interventions follow logically from the aetiological considerations above. They include weight loss, reduced salt intake, and stress reduction. The INTERSALT study, which did not include elderly subjects, found that trials of sodium restriction in targeted individuals generally show an effect similar to that predicted by cross-sectional population data and that this increases with age. The effects of community based salt restriction are less clear and may depend on other genetic and environmental factors typical of the particular community; for example, salt restriction lowered blood pressure more in Portugal than in Belgium.[9] Reducing alcohol intake may also decrease blood pressure but there is evidence in hypertensive subjects that moderate alcohol intake, possibly wine rather than beer, confers some protection against cardiovascular disease.[10] Conversely the non-drinkers at higher risk may have stopped drinking as a result of illness and this, rather than the lack of alcohol, may explain the findings.[11] This concept is hotly debated. Naively, non-pharmacological therapies might be considered without risk, so that everyone would benefit to some extent, however small, from their adoption. Figure 26.1 depicts the theoretical situation where any individual on the blood pressure curve should reduce their risk with a lowering of pressure. This is the basis of the population approach where large numbers are at a small risk and stand to benefit from general measures. In fact the adverse effects of non-pharmacological treatments, if any, have not been defined. For this reason some caution should be exercised, not only because patients may complain about dietary restrictions but also interventions such as lowering lipids, for example, may be associated with unexpected adverse outcomes.[12] A small fixed risk might be represented as in fig 26.2 but this is still likely to be lower than the risks of pharmacological agents. Such comparisons of benefit with risk can be altered by other factors, such as smoking, which might indicate intervention at lower pressures (fig 26.3).

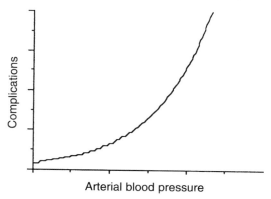

Fig 26.1   Risk of cardiovascular complications associated with arterial blood pressure. This approximates to an exponential function.

The use of pharmacological agents is not without the risk of unwanted side effects, especially in the elderly. Moreover, there is very little experimental

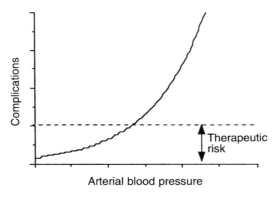

Fig 26.2   Theoretical benefit:risk curve for antihypertensive treatment. Treatment is indicated at pressures above the intersection of the curve of the complication rate from blood pressure with the therapeutic risk.

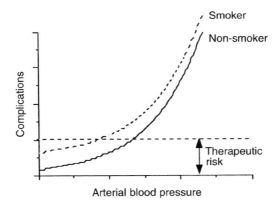

Fig 26.3   Theoretical benefit:risk curve for antihypertensive treatment of a smoker compared with a non-smoker. Treatment may be indicated at lower blood pressure levels for smokers.

evidence to support their use in the over 80s, although benefit in the younger elderly is now well established. Demographic changes mean that an urgent answer is required as to whether treating the "old" old is beneficial. In England and Wales, for instance, the population aged 65–74 years fell minimally by 0·03% between 1982 and 1992, whereas those aged over 85 years rose by 51% to nearly 800 000 during the same period. At present we have only three trials to guide us (table 26.1). The numbers over 80 years in the European Working Party on High Blood Pressure in the Elderly (EWPHE)[13] and the Swedish Trial in Old Patients with Hypertension (STOP)[14] trials were too few to exclude either a large benefit or large adverse effect of treatment. The American Systolic Hypertension in the Elderly Programme (SHEP)[15] found a 45% reduction in stroke incidence; however, the trial was concerned with subjects with isolated

249

systolic hypertension and only 10% of the strokes were fatal. The adverse consequences of treatment also require further clarification. Both the SYST-EUR[16] and the SYST-CHINA[17] trials should inform us further about the treatment of isolated systolic hypertension in those over 80 years, and the Hypertension in the Very Elderly Trial (HYVET),[18] only recently started, will provide data on combined systolic and diastolic hypertension. These trials illustrate the gradual move from older antihypertensives with considerable side effects, such as methyldopa in the EWPHE trial, to newer agents with fewer side effects and better quality of life profiles, such as the angiotensin converting enzyme inhibitors, selective calcium antagonists, and diuretics.

Table 26.1   Summary of results of antihypertensive treatment trials in subjects aged over 80 years

Trial	Blood pressure criteria (mm Hg)	Number >80 years	Result of active treatment
EWPHE	160–239/90–119	155	No benefit (low power)
STOP-hypertension	180–230/90–120 or <180/105–120	269	No benefit (low power)
SHEP	160–219/<90	649	45% reduction in stroke incidence

Evaluations of efficacy

The large trials are able to consider the efficacy of a drug in terms of major end points such as death and stroke. Although treatment may reduce such events by the same percentage in both young and old adults, because the incidence of these events is far higher in old people the absolute efficacy in terms of number of strokes prevented is far greater in the elderly.[19] Smaller studies consider surrogate variables—for example, blood pressure reduction—as a measure of efficacy. Such indices may only correlate weakly with primary outcomes for the aetiological reasons set out above. Some antihypertensives may lower blood pressure, but at the expense of increasing lipids and impairing glucose tolerance. Furthermore, in clinical practice a drug which brings down blood pressure but impairs the sense of wellbeing will be less popular. This clinical observation is supported by data from the Medical Research Council trial in the elderly[20] and raises two further points: firstly, the central nervous system actions of antihypertensive agents are of particular importance; secondly, psychological wellbeing may be improved but not functional abilities. Such a dissociation means that drug adverse effects and benefits need to be evaluated by appraisal of multidimensional outcomes. The values in table 26.2, taken from the EWPHE trial, illustrate that benefits are often bought at a price; however, large benefits are worth the cost, whereas small benefits are easily

250

outweighed by small adverse effects. In the MRC trial a small benefit from lowering stroke rate with atenolol as first line treatment was negated by undetermined factors so total mortality was not reduced.

Table 26.2 Benefits and risks observed in the EWPHE trial

Benefit	No/1000 per year	Risk	No/1000 per year
Cardiac deaths	−11	Gout	+4
Cerebrovascular deaths	−6	Mild hypokalaemia	+71
Non-fatal cerebrovascular events	−11	Elevation of serum creatinine	+23
Severe congestive cardiac failure	−8	Diabetes	+9
Severe retinal changes	−4	Dry mouth	+124
Need for β blocker	−4	Diarrhoea	+71
		Need for hypoglycaemic drugs	+7
		Need for peripheral vasodilators	+7

Health policy

An individual's response to a drug is very different from the reduction of the mean blood pressure of a population. A minor population decrease may reduce stroke incidence substantially, as a slightly high pressure is very prevalent and associated with an increased risk. Population based non-pharmacological actions, such as encouraging less salt in the diet and stopping smoking, are potentially powerful interventions. Nevertheless, the population approach, if instituted, must be supplemented by the treatment of individual high risk patients.

The population approach gains importance in the light of the relative ineffectiveness of targeting individuals. This has improved recently so that the "rule of halves" has now become "the rule of thirds". Many studies demonstrate that about a third of people who fulfil treatment criteria are undetected. Of those recognized as hypertensive a third remain untreated, and of those who receive medication a third fail to have their blood pressure adequately controlled.[21] In view of this, blood pressure measurement is now an important component of health screening in the elderly. Such screening may be enhanced by assessment of end organ damage in an attempt to identify a putative subgroup who are at greater risk and who require lower treatment thresholds. The evidence suggests that usual hypertensive thresholds should be set at a systolic level greater than 160 mm Hg or a diastolic greater than 95 mm Hg in subjects under 80 years. These readings should be sustained over at least three months and maintained both sitting and standing. Until we have further data from trials such as SYS-EUR, SYS-CHINA, and HYVET, the question as to whether the increasing numbers of patients over 80 years should be treated cannot, however, be answered.

1 Verdecchia P, Schillaci G, Guerrieri M, *et al.* Circadian blood pressure changes and left ventricular hypertrophy in essential hypertension. *Circulation* 1990;**81**:528–36.
2 Poulter NR, Khaw KT, Hopwood BEC, *et al.* The Kenyan Luo migration study: observations on the initiation of a rise in blood pressure. *BMJ* 1990;**300**:967–72.
3 Staessen J, Poulter NR, Fletcher AE, *et al.* Psycho-emotional stress and salt intake may interact to raise blood pressure. *J Cardiovasc Risk* 1994;**1**:45–51.
4 Petrie JC, O'Brien ET, Littler WA, De Swiet M. Recommendations on blood pressure measurement. *BMJ* 1986;**293**:611.
5 Barker DJP, Bull AR, Osmond C, Simmonds SJ. Fetal and placental size and risk of hypertension in adult life. *BMJ* 1990;**301**:259–62.
6 US Department of Health, Education and Welfare. *Blood pressure levels of persons 6–74 years, United States, 1971–1974.* Washington: DHEW, 1978. (Vital and health statistics series II, No 203, DHEW Publication No HRA 78-1648.)
7 Shen DC, Shieh SM, Fuh MT, Wu DA, Chen YDI, Reaven GM. Resistance to insulin stimulated glucose uptake in patients with hypertension. *J Clin Endocrinol Metab* 1988; **66**:580–3.
8 Starr JM, Whalley LJ. *ACE inhibitors: central actions.* Raven Press, New York, 1994.
9 Elliott P. The INTERSALT study: an addition to the evidence on salt and blood pressure, and some implications. *J Hum Hypertens* 1989;**3**:289–98.
10 Stampfer MJ, Colditz GA, Willett WC, Speizer FE, Hennekens CH. A prospective study of moderate alcohol consumption and the risk of coronary heart disease and stroke in women. *N Engl J Med* 1988;**319**:267–73.
11 Shaper AG, Wannamethee G, Walker M. Alcohol and mortality in British men: explaining the U-shaped curve. *Lancet* 1988;**ii**:1267–73.
12 Smith GD, Pekkanen J. Should there be a moratorium on the use of cholesterol lowering drugs? *BMJ* 1992;**304**:431–4.
13 Fletcher AE, Amery A, Birkenhager W, *et al.* Risks and benefits in the trial of the European Working Party on High Blood Pressure in the Elderly. *J Hypertens* 1991;**9**:225–30.
14 Dahlof B, Lindholm LH, Hansson L, Schersten B, Ekbom T, Webster P-O. Morbidity and mortality in the Swedish trial in old patients with hypertension (STOP-Hypertension). *Lancet* 1991;**338**:1281–5.
15 SHEP Cooperative Research Group. Prevention of stroke by antihypertensive drug treatment in older patients with isolated systolic hypertension: final results of the systolic hypertension in the elderly program (SHEP). *JAMA* 1991;**265**:3255–64.
16 Amery A, Birkenhager W, Bulpitt CJ, Clement D, De Leeuw P, Dollery C, *et al.* SYST-EUR. A multicentre trial on the treatment of isolated systolic hypertension in the elderly: objectives, protocol, and organisation. *Aging* 1991;**3**:287–302.
17 Systolic Hypertension in the Elderly's Collaborative Group Coordinating Center. Systolic hypertension in the elderly: Chinese trial (Syst-China)—interim report. *J Cardiol* 1992; **20**:270–5.
18 Bulpitt CJ, Fletcher AE, Amery A, *et al.* The hypertension in the very elderly trial (HYVET). *J Hum Hypertens* 1994;**8**:631–2.
19 Beard K, Bulpitt CJ, Mascie-Taylor H, O'Malley K, Sever P, Webb S. Management of elderly patients with sustained hypertension. *BMJ* 1992;**304**:412–6.
20 MRC Working Party. Medical Research Council trial of treatment of hypertension in older adults: principal results. *BMJ* 1992;**304**:405–12.
21 Strasser T, Wilhelmsen L, editors. *Assessing hypertension control and management.* Copenhagen: WHO Regional Publications, 1993.

27 Ischaemic heart disease

MICHAEL MARMOT

Definition

The major recognised clinical manifestations of ischaemic heart disease (IHD) are:

- Angina pectoris
- Acute myocardial infarction
- Sudden death, with or without a history of previous infarction and/or preceding chest pain.

These have been defined for epidemiological purposes and a large body of data exists using these definitions.[1] In addition, especially in the elderly, there may be other manifestations that lend themselves less readily to precise definition appropriate for epidemiological study but may be major causes of morbidity and mortality, such as congestive cardiac failure.

IHD arises because of shortage of blood to the myocardium due to a combination of atherosclerosis and thrombosis. The overwhelming majority of cases with clinical IHD have atherosclerosis leading to narrowing of the coronary arteries. Most myocardial infarctions probably result from thrombosis at the site of rupture of an atherosclerotic plaque.

Doctors who fill in death certificates know that these are of variable quality and of doubtful uniformity. They are often, therefore, among the first to question whether international differences in IHD death rates represent true differences. This has been studied among middle aged people, 35–64, using the 38 population based registries of myocardial infarction that are part of the World Health Organization MONICA Project.[2] Figure 27.1 shows IHD death rates for each of the 38 centres based on strictly defined and applied criteria used by special teams of investigators, and for comparison national IHD death rates based on routine vital statistical data. There is close agreement. MONICA data also show a high correlation between incidence of non-fatal disease and mortality rates. This suggests that conclusions, based on vital statistical data, of marked difference in the occurrence of IHD are likely not to be artefacts resulting from variations in recording and classification of cause of death.

Although there may be less accuracy of death certificates in the very old, evidence suggests that international variations at age 65–74, for example, are similar to those at younger ages.

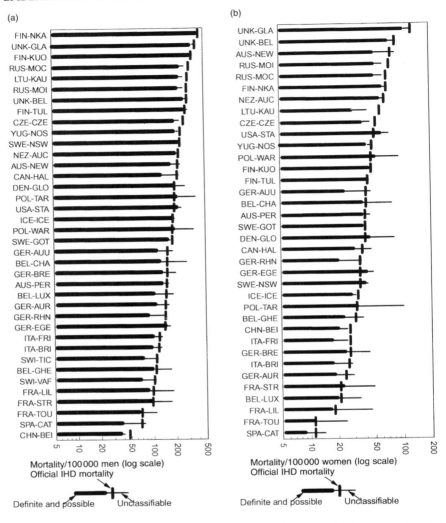

Fig 27.1   Ischaemic heart disease death rates for (a) men and (b) women from 38 population based registries.

Magnitude of the problem

In the United Kingdom in 1990 IHD accounted for 30% of deaths in men and 23% of deaths in women. IHD is important as a cause of death in both middle aged and older persons. It accounts for 24% of all years of life lost up to age 75 in males in England and Wales; in addition, 83% of deaths occurring from IHD were in people over 65.

It is also a major cause of morbidity. In England and Wales, for example, at age 65–74, 8% of men and 4% of women consult their general practitioner for IHD in one year.[3] At the same age the prevalence of angina in the

254

general population is 7%, and 12% report a history of chest pain suggestive of myocardial infarction.[4]

In the United Kingdom IHD costs the health service about the same amount each year as stroke. Whereas the great bulk of the stroke costs are for inpatient care, for IHD the major part of the cost is for pharmaceuticals. About 1% of the cost is for primary prevention. Similarly, in the United States medical costs of coronary heart disease are high.[5]

Variation

Place

Figure 27.1 shows marked variation in IHD mortality internationally: high in Finland, the United Kingdom, and central and eastern European countries; low in Spain, France, Switzerland, Italy, and China. MONICA data suggest that less than 25% of this variation in IHD mortality can be explained by variations in smoking, blood pressure, and plasma total cholesterol level.[6]

There are substantial regional variations in IHD mortality in the United Kingdom: higher in Scotland, particularly western Scotland, and the north of England; lower in the south east and East Anglia.[7 8]

Time

Figure 27.2 shows substantial variations across Europe in time trends in IHD mortality.[9] Many of the countries of western Europe show substantial declines in mortality rates. In stark contrast are the countries of central and eastern Europe, where rates have risen sharply. The declines in countries of western Europe now approach those of the United States, Canada, and Australia where the drop in IHD mortality rates began somewhat earlier. Interestingly Japan, which has the lowest IHD rate of any industrialised country, also shows a steep decline in IHD mortality rates over the last two decades.[10]

In the United States, where the decline in IHD mortality has been studied most assiduously, the decline appears to affect all age groups at about the same time, that is, it is not a cohort effect that could be related to earlier life experiences affecting different cohorts differentially. It appears more likely to be the result of changed circumstances acting with fairly short lag time. Treatment may have made some contribution to this. Reduction in incidence rates is likely to have been a major contributor, presumably reflecting changed levels of risk factors.

Person

At younger ages there is a large body of evidence relating the "classical" risk factors to IHD incidence. Levels of plasma cholesterol, blood pressure,

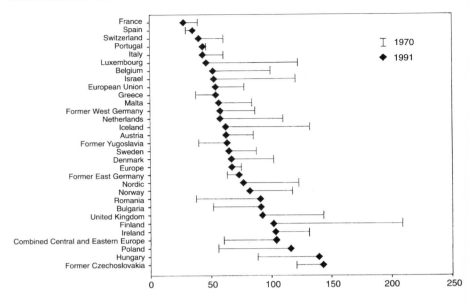

Fig 27.2 Mortality (/100 000) from ischaemic heart disease in males 0–64 years, in 1970 and 1991, age standardized.

and smoking show independent and graded associations with subsequent incidence of IHD. The evidence suggests that the association between these three factors and subsequent IHD is causal but, as indicated above, they do not account for all variations in occurrence of IHD. The geographic variations within the United Kingdom and across Europe must have some other basis.

In the United Kingdom and other countries there are marked social variations in IHD mortality: higher rates in those of lower socioeconomic status. This appears to have changed over time.[11] In the 1930s and up to the 1950s IHD mortality was more common in those of higher social class. With a faster increase in lower socioeconomic groups and a levelling off and subsequent decline in higher socioeconomic groups the social class distribution changed, leading to the present situation of a higher rate in lower socioeconomic groups. This was confirmed in the Whitehall study of British civil servants which showed a clear inverse association between grade of employment and mortality from IHD and from a range of other causes of death. Only about a quarter of this gradient could be accounted for by differences in plasma cholesterol, blood pressure, or smoking.[12]

Nevertheless, these factors are important predictors of risk in individuals. Most of the data, however, come from studies in middle aged people. There is a persistent rumour that the effect of these factors on subsequent risk declines with age. There are at least two issues here: the appropriate measure of effect, and the age at which the risk factor is measured.

256

Table 27.1 comes from an analysis of pooled data from a number of longitudinal studies. It shows that in men and women plasma total cholesterol and low density lipoprotein (LDL) cholesterol, and in women high levels of high density lipoprotein (HDL) cholesterol, continue to predict disease at ages 65 years or over[13]; however, the relative risk declines. This may be a sign that the aetiological force of these risk measures does decline at older ages. This does not mean that their importance either to individuals or to public health declines. A declining relative risk is applied to a greater absolute risk as age increases. Figure 27.3 from the Whitehall study shows that, although relative risk of IHD associated with a given difference in plasma cholesterol concentration declines with age, the absolute difference increases.[14]

Table 27.1   Predictive power of cholesterol fraction for prospective ischaemic heart disease (IHD) risk

Age (years)	Women	Men
Total cholesterol		
Relative risk of fatal IHD comparing >6·2 mmol/l *v* <5·2 mmol/l		
<65 years	2·44*	1·73*
≥65 years	1·12*	1·32*
HDL cholesterol		
Relative risk of fatal IHD comparing <1·3 mmol/l *v* >1·6 mmol/l		
<65 years	2·13*	2·31*
≥65 years	1·75*	1·09
LDL cholesterol		
Relative risk of fatal IHD comparing >4·1 mmol/l *v* <3·6 mmol/l		
<65 years	3·27*	1·92*
≥65 years	1·13	1·51*

* Relative risk greater than 1·0: $p < 0.05$.
Relative risk compares undesirable and desirable levels of cholesterol fraction on the basis of the US National Cholesterol Education Program cut points. Measurement taken before and after age 65.

The second issue relates to the age at which cholesterol or other risk factors are measured. Figure 27.4 reproduces data from the 18 year follow up of Whitehall.[15] Standardising for age at death, the longer the time interval between cholesterol measurement and IHD death, the stronger was the association. This means the younger the age at which cholesterol was measured the more predictive it is. A single measurement of plasma total cholesterol in middle aged men continues to predict well into old age. A measurement taken at older age is less predictive. It implies that for a given age at measurement the power to predict does not decline appreciably with age.

Determinants of IHD

There are well described genetic abnormalities related to increased risk of IHD. The best worked out of these is familial hypercholesterolaemia,

257

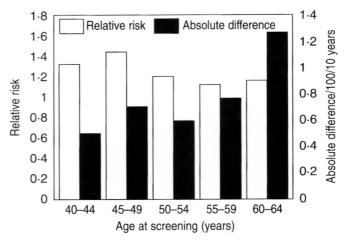

Fig 27.3   Relationship of age to relative risk of death from ischaemic heart disease and absolute difference.

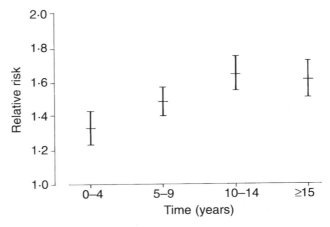

Fig 27.4   Relationship between risk of death from ischaemic heart disease (IHD) and time between cholesterol measurement and death from IHD.

in which high levels of plasma LDL cholesterol are associated with absence of LDL receptors on cell membranes. Such genetic abnormalities by themselves are probably responsible for a small proportion of IHD occurring after the age of 50.

As with most major disease problems, there are likely to be environmental as well as genetic components in causation. Three observations point to the importance of environmental factors: the rapid time changes; the fact that when people migrate their risk changes from that of the old country toward that of the new; and the fact that studies of individual risk factors show that these are manipulable, with subsequent change in risk.

Examples of possible gene–environment interactions are shown by the variable individual response of plasma cholesterol level to changes in dietary fat intake.[7] There is much work in progress aimed at determining genetic markers of susceptibility. The fact that having a close relative with IHD is associated with increased risk may be the result of both shared genes and environment.

Risk factors can be divided into: *inherent biological traits* such as age and sex that cannot themselves be altered; *physiological characteristics* that predict future occurrence of IHD, such as blood pressure, serum lipids, fibrinogen and factor VII concentration, weight/height², central adiposity, and factors connected with insulin resistance such as high plasma insulin; *behaviours*, such as diet, smoking, physical inactivity, and non-drinking, that may be linked with the physiological characteristics listed; *social characteristics*, such as social class or ethnic group; and *environmental features*, which may be physical (temperature, soft water), biological, or psychosocial.[16] These are interrelated.

A significant new body of evidence suggests that important determinants of adult cardiovascular risk may have their origins early in life: in utero or the first year of life.[17] Thinness at birth and low weight at one year are related to IHD risk factors and IHD mortality in middle age.

Intervention

Primary prevention

These risk factors have different implications for prevention. A physiological characteristic such as blood pressure may be lowered by drugs irrespective of the determinants of high blood pressure; or the intervention point could be behaviour—for example, tobacco smoking or changes in diet that affect blood pressure. If risk factors differ by social characteristics, prevention should deal with the social distribution of factors. An appropriate response to an environmental cause, such as cold, will be to protect against it; the response to an adverse psychosocial environment might be to change the environment.

In general the evidence both from trials and observational studies suggests that it is possible to reduce levels of risk factors; and reducing risk factors reduces risk.

Secondary prevention

A number of interventions appear to reduce recurrence rates of IHD in the first year or two after myocardial infarction: β blockers, aspirin, and possibly other antiplatelet agents. In the longer term there is likely to be benefit from reducing risk factors, such as cholesterol, blood pressure, and smoking.

Treatment

This is a rapidly changing field. Until recently there was little evidence that treatment of the acute myocardial infarction had any appreciable impact on overall mortality from IHD in the population. This may change. The so called clot busting drugs, tissue plasminogen activator (tPA) and streptokinase, have a clear impact on reducing the case fatality of acute myocardial infarction.

Coronary artery bypass grafting reduces symptoms of angina and, at least in people with more severe atherosclerosis, appears to reduce mortality rates.

Health policy

About 40% of myocardial infarctions are fatal in the first year after the attack. Of these fatalities about half occur in the first two hours, the majority before access to medical care is feasible. Although prompt effective treatment will continue to be of crucial importance, major reductions in morbidity and mortality must come from reductions in incidence, that is, new occurrences of disease.

The implications of the discussion on determinants is that the time to start prevention of IHD in the elderly is before people become elderly. If cholesterol measured in middle age is a better predictor of disease in the elderly than cholesterol measured later, it might follow that interventions to lower cholesterol might have greater impact if started earlier in life. The suggestion from Barker's work is that in principle intervention should begin with the very beginnings of life.

This should not imply that time has run out for those currently elderly. Risk factors still predict and the absolute differences in risk between high and low risk groups may be greater in the elderly. There is evidence that lowering blood pressure in the elderly, for example, reduces overall cardiovascular mortality,[18] and also has greater absolute benefits than at younger ages.[19]

There has been much debate about the relative merits of a high risk strategy of prevention compared with one that attempts to lower risk in the whole population.[20] Given the generally high level of risk factors in the elderly an approach that calls for screening, identification, and pharmacological treatment of those at high risk would cover a high proportion of the population and would have far reaching economic implications. It is unlikely to be affordable even if the benefits of intervention were shown to outweigh the disadvantages. This means that lifestyle and environmental change will be the main strategies of prevention.

A major challenge for the future is to determine the most appropriate strategy for reduction both of socioeconomic differences in IHD mortality and of the differences across Europe.

1 Rose G, Blackburn H, Gillum RF, Prineas RJ. *Cardiovascular survey methods*. Geneva: WHO, 1982.
2 Tunstall-Pedoe H, Kuulasmaa K, Amouyel P, Arveiler D, Rajakangas AM, Pajak A. Myocardial infarction and coronary deaths in the World Health Organization MONICA project. Registration procedures, event rates, and case-fatality rates in 38 populations from 21 countries in four continents. *Circulation* 1994;**90**:583–612.
3 Office of Population Censuses and Surveys. *Morbidity statistics from General Practice 1991–1992*. London: HMSO, 1994. (OPCS Monitor MB5.)
4 Murabito JM, Anderson KM, Kannel WB, Evans JC, Levy D. Risk of coronary heart disease in subjects with chest discomfort: the Framingham heart study. *Am J Med* 1990; **89**:297–302.
5 Wittels EH, Hay JW, Gotto AM. Medical costs of coronary heart disease in the United States. *Am J Cardiol* 1990;**65**:432–40.
6 World Health Organization Monica Project. Ecological analysis of the association between mortality and major factors of cardiovascular disease. *Int J Epidemiol* 1994;**23**:505–16.
7 Committee on Medical Aspects of Food Policy. *Nutritional aspects of cardiovascular disease*. London: HMSO, 1994:1–186.
8 Shaper AG, Pocock SJ, Walker M, Phillips AN, Whitehead TP, Macfarlane PW. Risk factors for ischaemic heart disease: the prospective phase of the British regional heart study. *J Epidemiol Community Health* 1985;**39**:197–209.
9 Bobak M, Marmot MG. East–West health divide and potential explanations. In: *Proceedings of the European Health Policy Conference*; 1994, Copenhagen, 1995.
10 Marmot MG. Coronary heart disease: rise and fall of a modern epidemic. In: Marmot MG, Elliott P, editors. *Coronary heart disease epidemiology. From aetiology to public health*. Oxford: Oxford University Press, 1992:3–19.
11 Marmot MG, Adelstein AM, Robinson N, Rose GA. Changing social class distribution of heart disease. *BMJ* 1978;**ii**:1109–12.
12 Marmot MG, Shipley MJ, Rose G. Inequalities in death—specific explanations of a general pattern. *Lancet* 1984;**i**:1003–6.
13 Manolio TA, Pearson TA, Wenger NK, Barrett-Connor E, Payne GH, Harlan WR. Cholesterol and heart disease in older persons and women: review of an NHLBI workshop (June 1990). *Ann Epidemiol* 1992;**2**:161–176.
14 Rose G, Shipley M. Plasma cholesterol concentration and death from coronary heart disease: 10 year results of the Whitehall study. *BMJ* 1986;**293**:306–8.
15 Shipley MJ, Pocock SJ, Marmot MG. Does plasma cholesterol concentration predict mortality from coronary heart disease in elderly people? 18 year follow up in Whitehall study. *BMJ* 1991;**303**:89–92.
16 Marmot MG, Poulter NR. Primary prevention of stroke. *Lancet* 1992;**339**:344–7.
17 Barker DJP. *Fetal and infant origins of adult disease*. London: BMJ Publishing Group, 1992: 1–343.
18 Insua J, Sacks H, Lau T, *et al*. Drug treatment of hypertension in the elderly: a meta-analysis. *Ann Intern Med* 1994;**121**:355–62.
19 Beard K, Bulpitt C, Mascie-Taylor H, *et al*. Management of elderly patients with sustained hypertension. *BMJ* 1992;**304**:412–6.
20 Rose G. *The strategy of preventive medicine*. Oxford: Oxford University Press, 1992.

28 Stroke

SHAH EBRAHIM

Definitions and diagnostic criteria

Stroke is a clinical diagnosis and is defined using the following World Health Organization criteria: "focal or global neurological impairment of sudden onset lasting longer than 24 hours (or leading to death)" and of presumed vascular aetiology.[1]

A major problem in stroke epidemiology is that the pathological damage that leads to a stroke is not a single process. Thrombosis of arteries, platelet emboli from the carotid arteries, fibrin emboli from the atrium, increased viscosity of blood, or rupture of microaneurysms of intracerebral arteries all lead to remarkably similar clinical presentations. Much of our understanding of variation, association and causation, intervention and health policy is weakened because stroke is treated as a single disease.

Comparability between stroke incidence studies has been weakened by inclusion of first and subsequent strokes, use of different age groupings, and incomplete years of observation.[2] For the purposes of incidence surveys it is advisable to use WHO criteria described for the MONICA study,[3] which overcome many of these problems.

The accuracy of clinical diagnosis of stroke is reasonably good (sensitivity 90%, specificity 97%) when compared with large autopsy series[4]; however, accuracy in diagnosis of specific types of stroke (for example, haemorrhage, thrombosis, or embolus) is poor. Computed tomography (CT) is able to make a clear diagnosis in about 70% of cases when carried out in community surveys,[5] although about a third of patients with symptoms do not have any lesion on CT. Doctors with good clinical skills working with younger patients in hospital or specialist stroke services will achieve the highest accuracy. In older people it is sometimes very difficult to determine whether a stroke has occurred, particularly in the presence of comorbidity.

Diagnostic scores differentiating haemorrhagic from thrombotic stroke have a role in epidemiological studies and have not been widely used. They are not sufficiently accurate for clinical purposes.

Risk

The incidence of stroke is usually measured using the number of first strokes as the numerator and person years at risk as the denominator.

Stroke shows a dramatic increase in risk with age (fig 28.1), which means that great care must be taken in comparing crude mortality or incidence rates between populations that may differ in age structure.

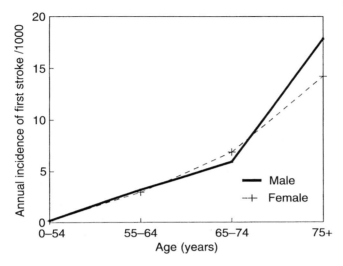

Fig 28.1   Stroke and age.

In general, incidence and mortality rates are closely related, which allows routine mortality data to be used as a reasonable proxy for the true burden of disease.

Magnitude of the problem

Stroke is a major cause of mortality and morbidity in most countries of the world. Crude incidence rates are around two per 1000 a year in Western countries, which equates to about 100 000 first strokes in Britain each year.[6] Three out of four strokes occur in people aged over 65 years. Demographic trends will lead to an ageing population, which will result in increases in the numbers of strokes as stroke risk is strongly related to increasing age.

About a third of stroke patients die within six months of the event and the majority of deaths occur in the first month.

Stroke is an expensive disease for health services. In the NHS approximately 4% of the budget is spent on stroke services each year.[7] The bulk of this spending is on hospital care, with a small fraction spent on subsequent community care.

263

Variation

Time

Stroke has shown major secular decline over this century in many Western countries, with reductions in mortality of about 1% a year at all ages for both men and women since the early 1900s. Rates of decline have accelerated in more recent times to about 2% a year; however, the increased elderly population at risk of stroke has led to increases in the absolute numbers of strokes that must be treated and cared for in the community. Figure 28.2 shows the death rates from stroke for England and Wales (1901–91).

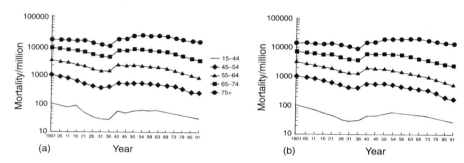

Fig 28.2   Stroke death rates in (a) men and (b) women in England and Wales 1901–91.

In eastern and central Europe stroke rates have increased, particularly among men (fig 28.3). The explanation for these differential trends is not clear but environmental and socioeconomic factors are likely to be important.

It is likely that the decline in mortality is mirrored by a decline in incidence.[8] Although it is possible that changes in diagnostic fashion and coding may have played a part in the decline, it is generally accepted that this is a real phenomenon. Explanations for the decline in stroke include reductions in stroke and hypertension risk factors and better primary prevention.[9]

Place

Stroke mortality rates vary widely throughout the world and are particularly high in Portugal and eastern and central Europe (fig 28.4). Studies of incidence are beset with problems of diagnostic criteria, poor case ascertainment, defining the population at risk, inadequate sample size, incomplete year of observation, and non-standard presentation of rates.

Within the United Kingdom stroke mortality varies at least twofold but the explanation for geographical variation remains unclear. Certainly it is not explained by differences in classical cardiovascular risk factors.

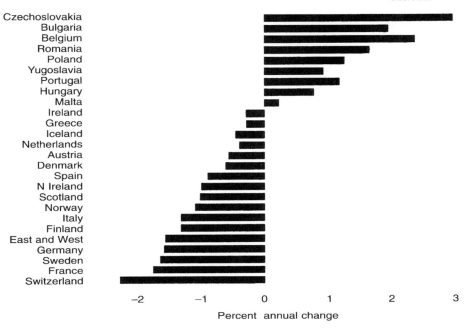

Fig 28.3   Trends in stroke mortality in men aged 35–64: Europe 1955–9 to 1975–9.

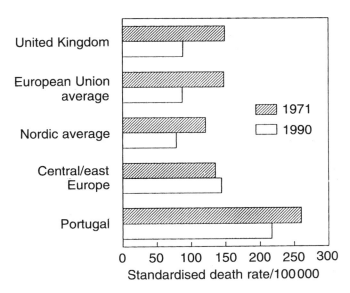

Fig 28.4   Standardised death rates (SDR) for stroke in different countries (1971 and 1990).

265

Person

Family, ecological, and twin studies have demonstrated that early life influences have an impact on subsequent risk of stroke; however, with the exception of homocystinurea, genetic factors do not appear to be very important in stroke.

Many factors influence the chance of having a stroke: male sex, increased age, high blood pressure, smoking, body build, alcohol, ischaemic heart disease and atrial fibrillation, previous transient ischaemic attacks, diabetes, lower social class, raised lipids, polycythaemia, physical inactivity, various medications (antihypertensives, oestrogens), diet. The relative risk of these factors is shown in table 28.1.

Table 28.1   Risk factors for stroke

Risk factor	Relative risk
Age (55–64 *v* 75 + years)	5
Blood pressure (160/95 + mm Hg)	7
Smoking (current status)	4*
Body build (30 kg/m²)	1–2
Ischaemic heart disease	3
Heart failure	5
Atrial fibrillation	3–7
Past transient ischaemic attack	5
Diabetes mellitus	2
Social class (I *v* V)	1·6
Blood triglycerides (6·5 mmol/l +)	2·4*
Raised haematocrit	2
Physical activity (little *v* light/heavy)	2·5
Oral contraceptives (ever use)	9
Postmenopausal oestrogens	0·53
Alcohol (acute intoxication)	5*

* Men only.
From Ebrahim.[9]

In terms of population attributable risk, raised blood pressure, smoking, and physical inactivity may explain about a third of strokes.

Many of the studies quoted did not study the people most at risk of stroke—those over 75 years. The importance of hypertension declines with increasing age. Intervention studies have, however, demonstrated benefits from treating high blood pressure up to the age of 80 years (see chapter 26).

Determinants of stroke

High blood pressure, smoking, physical inactivity, and pre-existing ischaemic heart disease are major explanations for stroke risk in populations and individuals. Determinants of secular and geographic variability remain obscure and are not fully explained by these factors. It is likely that stroke incidence is susceptable to variation in socioeconomic status but the mechanisms by which this occurs are not understood.

Intervention

Primary prevention

Blood pressure, smoking, obesity, diabetes, inactivity, heart disease, atrial fibrillation, transient ischaemic attacks, polycythaemia, alcohol abuse, and raised blood lipids might be considered treatable. The benefits of treating blood pressure even at mildly raised levels have been demonstrated (see chapter 26). The impact of reducing other risk factors is not known from empirical studies but it is assumed that reductions in smoking and activity will lead to benefits.

Secondary prevention

The use of aspirin after transient ischaemic attack and mild stroke is of benefit in preventing further attacks and strokes.[10] Treatment of diabetes and polycythaemia are not of proven benefit in reducing the risk of stroke. Smoking, obesity, alcohol abuse, and inactivity are all personal behaviours that should be modified for many reasons, but on present evidence only smoking can be singled out as being justified on the basis of reducing the risk of stroke.[11 12]

There is now strong evidence from randomised controlled trials that carotid endarterectomy is effective in reducing the risk of stroke[13]; however, the indications for operation are very specific (between 70 and 99% stenosis) and there is mounting concern that surgeons are carrying out many inappropriate procedures.[14] Furthermore, the risk:benefit ratio is dependent on the skill of the surgeon. Many surgeons do not perform enough operations to acquire the necessary skills and there is a strong case for limiting the procedure to a small number of regional specialist centres.

Anticoagulants have a role in reducing stroke risk in people with atrial fibrillation.[15] There are risks of bleeding from anticoagulants and it is probable that older people are at greater risk of the bleeding complications of this treatment. The quality of anticoagulant control is the major determinant of bleeding risk and, in centres where this is adequate, age should not be a barrier to treatment.

Acute treatment

There is no acute treatment available that will reduce the mortality or limit brain damage due to stroke. Hospital case fatality has declined markedly over the last 20–30 years but it is not clear whether this is due to better supportive treatment or reduced severity of strokes in patients admitted to hospitals. The latter explanation is plausible as it is likely that the ratio of haemorrhagic (which has a poor prognosis) to thrombotic stroke has declined over the same time.

Rehabilitation

Several randomised controlled trials of stroke units have demonstrated their benefits in reducing both mortality and disability.[9 16] Stroke units are associated with shorter lengths of hospital stay as well as better outcomes.

Health policy

Burden of stroke

Stroke is an avoidable disease that presents a major burden for health and social services and families. The size of this burden is not well described by numbers of deaths, or even numbers of non-fatal cases, as the outcome for survivors is very variable. Disability adjusted life years attributed to stroke demonstrate that it ranks as one of the greatest burdens (see chapter 5) and, as it is avoidable, should receive high priority for prevention and control. Table 28.2 shows the disability adjusted life years lost as a result of stroke in different regions of the world.[17]

Table 28.2 Disability adjusted life years (DALYs) attributed to stroke and as a percentage of all DALYs lost

Region	Females (× 100 000)		Males (× 100 000)	
	DALYs	%	DALYs	%
Sub-Saharan Africa	25·3	1·8	17·4	1·0
India	35·0	2·3	27·5	1·8
China	58·1	5·9	68·4	6·6
Latin America	14·0	3·1	13·2	2·3
Middle East	18·5	2·6	15·5	2·1
Former socialist Europe	29·7	11·9	21·8	6·7
Established market economies	26·6	6·4	23·1	4·4
World	229·0	3·5	203·1	2·8

Prevention

Primary prevention would appear to be the most attractive option for reducing the burdens associated with stroke but estimates of the costs and benefits (in terms of disability adjusted life years) suggest that detection and treatment of mild to moderate hypertension is expensive. Depending on the economic estimates made and the level of development of primary health care, costs are between about £1000 and £30 000 per disability adjusted life year.[18]

Secondary prevention by means of reducing recurrent stroke by aspirin treatment stands out as an extremely cost effective strategy. This is because the target population is relatively easy to define, the treatment is extremely cheap and requires little monitoring, and, most importantly, the treatment is very effective in a population at extremely high risk of recurrence.

Treatment

The benefits of stroke units are large and it might be expected that all health districts should ensure they have comprehensive stroke services established. In addition to the benefits associated with better outcomes, it is likely that the efficiency savings would be sufficient to pay for the service.

1 World Health Organization. Cerebrovascular disease: a clinical and research classification. *WHO Offset Publ* 1978:43.
2 Malmgren R, Warlow C, Bamford J, Sandercock P. Geographical and secular trends in stroke incidence. *Lancet* 1987;**ii**:1196–9.
3 World Health Organization. MONICA (monitoring trends and determinants in cardiovascular disease) project: objectives and design. *Int J Epidemiol* 1989;**18**(suppl 1): S29–37.
4 Heasman MA, Lipworth L. *Accuracy of certification of cause of death*. London: HMSO, 1966:23–4. (Studies on medical and population subjects, No 20.)
5 Sandercock P, Molyneux A, Warlow C. The value of CT scanning in patients with stroke: Oxford community stroke project. *BMJ* 1985;**290**:193–6.
6 Bamford J, Sandercock P, Dennis M, *et al*. A prospective study of acute cerebrovascular disease in the community: the Oxfordshire community stroke project. 1. Methodology, demography and incident cases of first-ever stroke. *J Neurol Neurosurg Psychiatry* 1988; **297**:126–8.
7 Office of Health Economics. *Stroke*. London: OHE, 1988.
8 Garraway WM, Whisnant JP, Furlan AJ, *et al*. The declining incidence of stroke. *New Engl J Med* 1979;**300**:449–52.
9 Ebrahim S. *Clinical epidemiology of stroke*. Oxford: Oxford University Press, 1990.
10 Antiplatelet Trialists' Collaboration. Secondary prevention of vascular disease by prolonged antiplatelet treatment. *BMJ* 1988;**296**:320–31.
11 Medical Research Council Working Party. Stroke and coronary heart disease in mild hypertension: risk factors and the value of treatment. *BMJ* 1988;**296**:1565–70.
12 Bonita R, Scragg R, Stewart A, Jackson R, Beaglehole R. Cigarette smoking and risk of premature stroke in men and women. *BMJ* 1986;**293**:6–8.
13 European Carotid Surgery Trialists' Collaborative Group. MRC European carotid surgery trial: interim results for symptomatic patients with severe (70–99%) or with mild (0–29%) carotid stenosis. *Lancet* 1991;**337**:1235–43.
14 Winslow CM, Solomon DH, Chassin MR, *et al*. The appropriateness of carotid endarterectomy. *New Engl J Med* 1988;**318**:721–7.
15 Gustafsson C, Asplund K, Britton M, Norrving B, Olson B, Marke L. Cost effectiveness of primary stroke prevention in atrial fibrillation: Swedish national perspective. *BMJ* 1992; **305**:1457–60.
16 Langhorne P, Williams BO, Gilchrist W, Howie K. Do stroke units save lives? *Lancet* 1993;**342**:395–8.
17 World Bank. *World Development Report 1993*. Washington: World Bank.
18 Drummond M, Coyle D. Assessing the economic value of antihypertensive medicines. *J Hum Hypertens* 1992;**6**:495–501.

29 Alzheimer's disease

ALBERTO SPAGNOLI

Definitions and diagnostic criteria

Alzheimer's disease (AD) "is a brain disorder characterised by a progressive dementia that occurs in middle or late life," and by "degeneration of specific nerve cells, presence of neuritic plaques, and neurofibrillary tangles."[1]

The core phenomenon of AD is the degeneration of nerve cells, usually starting from the limbic association cortex. This has two levels of clinical expression, cognitive impairment and behavioural functioning disorders, which characterise the dementia syndrome. Dementia is "the decline of memory and other cognitive functions in comparison with the patient's previous level of function"[1] caused by several disorders of the brain. Early in the course of dementia, work and social activities are significantly impaired, but patients can still live independently. In the late phases, activities of daily living are also impaired so that continuous supervision and help are required.

Using the NINCDS-ADRDA (National Institute of Neurological and Communicative Disorders and Stroke–Alzheimer's Disease and Related Disorders Association) diagnostic criteria[1] a clinical diagnosis of possible or probable AD can be made. For definite AD the clinical diagnosis of probable AD requires histopathological confirmation. When probable AD is diagnosed by doctors experienced in the evaluation of dementia examining a standardised set of medical records, the following reliability[2] and validity[3] indices can be achieved: interrater reliability 0·64 (κ), sensitivity 0·92, specificity 0·65, negative predictive value 0·84, positive predictive value 0·82. A diagnostic accuracy of 84% has been obtained using the NINCDS-ADRDA clinical diagnostic criteria and a somewhat different protocol for postmortem assessment.[4]

The 10th revision of the International Classification of Diseases (ICD-10)[5] distinguishes the dementia in AD with early onset (before the age of 65) from that with late onset (after 65). The former usually causes wider impairment of cognitive functions early in its course. It is not known whether this difference indicates separate disease processes, and epidemiologists have generally adopted a unitary view of AD.

The above features imply some major problems in AD epidemiology. The pathological lesions of AD are also seen in a variety of conditions,

270

such as normal ageing, head trauma, chromosomal abnormalities, viral diseases, and metabolic disorders, so they are not specific to AD, suggesting the possibility of multiple aetiological mechanisms. Since the clinical diagnosis of AD is one of exclusion, misclassification is possible. Complex procedures increase diagnostic accuracy but limit the feasibility of large field studies. The AD patient's memory impairment makes informant reports necessary (for example, in case–control studies). Furthermore, as it is difficult to date the onset, the time relation between the occurrence of putative risk factors and the disease onset may be unclear, making it difficult to distinguish the effects from the causes.

Magnitude of the problem

Because of the changing age structure of the population, differences in age structure between populations, and the strong association between AD and age, crude estimates (for example, 60 +) of prevalence and incidence are of limited value. Age specific prevalences[6] and incidences[7] for AD are reported in table 29.1.

Table 29.1   Prevalence and incidence of Alzheimer's disease (AD)

Age (years)	Total	Men	Women
A Prevalence (percentage and 95% CI) of AD (NINCDS-ADRDA or equivalent criteria)[6]			
30–59	0·02 (0–0·05)	0·0	0·03
60–69	0·3 (0·1–0·6)	0·3	0·4
70–79	3·2 (2·4–4·0)	2·5	3·6
80–89	10·8 (9·0–12·0)	10·0	11·2
B Cumulative five-year incidence (rates per 1000 and 95% CI) of probable AD (NINCDS-ADRDA)[7]			
65–69	3·5 (0–8·4)	5·0	2·7
70–74	15·7 (3·2–28·2)	14·1	16·8
75–79	30·0 (9·5–50·6)	21·8	34·0
80–84	53·5 (14·8–92·1)	40·9	59·9
85–89	72·8 (0–154·4)	83·3	69·3

A recent Swedish study[8] confirmed the high prevalence (12·9%) of AD in people aged 85. The few available incidence studies show large differences in the absolute values and wide confidence intervals. Table 29.1 presents the findings of one of the most reliable studies.

The median survival from symptom onset is 9·3 years (range 1·8 to more than 16 years).[9] AD reduces life expectancy both in the early onset form (by 10 years after onset, 15% observed survival v 85% expected in subjects without dementia)[10] and in 85 year old patients (three year survival: observed 58%, expected 77%).[8] Suggestions of an improvement in case survival in recent decades lacks convincing evidence.

Over periods up to four years the rate of cognitive decline is slower in AD patients with mild cognitive impairment at initial evaluation than it

271

is in those with severe impairment.[11] The effects of sex, age at onset, disproportionate or early aphasia or apraxia, EEG abnormalities, extrapyramidal signs, and a number of psychiatric symptoms (for example, aggressive behaviour, hallucinations) on the rate of cognitive and functional decline are unclear.

Information on rates of institutionalisation is scant. One study found that 37·5% of patients aged 85 with AD lived in institutions, compared with 1·7% of subjects without dementia.[8] Other studies[12 13] report rates of institutionalisation of demented patients from 6 to 14%. In any event up to 80%[14] of residents in geriatric institutions suffer from dementia.

Care of the average AD patient costs between $16 000 and $47 000 a year, depending on the severity of the disease, the setting (nursing home, home), the country, and the method employed to assess formal and informal support in monetary terms.[15 16] Informal care amounts to three quarters of the cost of patients living at home. Current limitations of services and financing systems put a tremendous burden on the families.

Variation in time, place, and person

A possible rise in the incidence of AD over the years is open to discussion. Surveys from Europe, the United States, and Japan do not show major geographic differences in age specific prevalences of AD.[6] This can reflect small differences in incidence or risk, given a comparable mean survival time, or differences in incidence with an inverse correlation between incidence and survival. Data on survival of AD patients suggest that the first hypothesis is the most plausible. Limited international differences in the incidence of AD are borne out by incidence studies.

The homogeneity of prevalence and incidence contrasts with geographical differences in genetic and environmental factors possibly related to AD. The major role of age as a risk factor may conceal the effects of other weaker factors.

Prevalence and incidence rise steeply with age (table 29.1), at least up to age 90. Age specific prevalences of AD tend to be higher for women, while sex differences (women>men) in incidence are less consistent or even absent. This may reflect longer survival of women or lack of statistical power to detect a difference because sample sizes are limited.

Determinants

Table 29.2 presents the risk factors for which the evidence is most convincing.[17–23] Apart from age, a family history of dementia or AD in first degree relatives is a major risk factor; 47% of AD patients have a family history of dementia among first degree relatives, and 39% of AD.[19] The odds ratio for a family history of dementia decreases with increasing age at AD onset in the patients and is significantly lower in patients who have

272

one first degree relative with dementia than in those with two or more affected relatives.[17]

Table 29.2   Risk and protective factors for Alzheimer's disease (AD)

Factor	Odds ratio (95% CI)
Sociodemographic characteristics	
Age	See table 29.1
Female sex	See table 29.1
Familial or genetic factors	
Family history of dementia	3·5 (2·6–4·6)[17]*
(first degree relatives)	3·64 (2·10–6·33)[18]
	2·21 (1·17–4·18)[19]
	7·50 (1·55–36·32)[20]
	4·36 (1·55–12·3)[21]
Family history of AD (first degree relatives)	4·27 (2·34–7·80)[18]
	2·12 (1·08–4·17)[19]
	4·69 (1·58–13·9)[21]
Family history of Down's syndrome	11·33 (1·19–68·1)[18]
	2·7 (1·2–5·7)[17]*
Previous illness or trauma	
Head trauma	1·82 (1·26–2·67)[22]
Prior treatments	
Anti-inflammatory drugs	0·25 (0·07–0·74)[23]

* Pooling and reanalysis of data from 11 case–control studies.

Nearly all individuals with Down's syndrome develop the neuropathological features of AD in middle and old age, with an average onset of dementia at 54 years.[24] Case–control studies suggest that a family history of Down's syndrome is a risk factor for AD.

The role of family history as an indicator of genetic factors in the development of AD is supported by reports of some families in which AD is transmitted in an autosomal dominant pattern and by the discovery of at least three AD loci on chromosomes 14, 19, and 21; however, there are monozygotic twins discordant for AD and in the majority of late onset cases it is difficult to discern a pattern of inheritance. These observations suggest that an alteration in one of several genes, or in more than one gene, can cause AD, and that environmental factors play a crucial role in its pathogenesis, raising questions about putative neurotoxins, the duration of exposure, and the delay between exposure and the onset of symptoms.

Head trauma may be related to AD as a consequence of neural damage and decrease in the functional reserve of the brain or of membrane destruction and production of neurotoxic compounds (for example, amyloid, free radicals).

A recent study (cotwin control study)[23] suggests an inverse association between prior treatment with anti-inflammatory drugs (steroids, adrenocoticotrophic hormone, non-steroidal anti-inflammatory drugs) and

AD. Neurobiological investigations provide a rationale for this observation (plaques and tangles in AD brains are immunopositive for several complement component proteins) and support the suggestion that chronic inflammatory activity sustained by altered immune responses may be involved in the pathogenesis of AD. Thus, anti-inflammatory drugs could prevent or delay the disease.

It has also been suggested that education may play a protective role[25] but evidence is contradictory and it is hard to interpret the positive findings. Education could operate through factors related to lifestyle and occupational exposures, or by providing a greater resistance to the effects of dementing diseases (greater cognitive or synaptic reserve); however, the association could also reflect a diagnostic bias because performance in cognitive tests correlates with education and the level of education may influence selection in studies.

Very recently the analysis of genetic polymorphisms at the apolipoprotein E (Apo E) locus on chromosome 19 has shown an increased frequency of the E4 allele in sporadic and familial late onset AD. Apo E is a protein which plays an important role in plasma cholesterol and triglyceride metabolism. Inheritance of the E4 allele is a major risk factor for late onset AD, while inheritance of the relatively rare E2 allele seems to be protective in most ethnic groups, and the risk with the most common E3 allele lies in the middle. The risk increases with the number of E4 alleles inherited, so that the mean age of onset is 15 years earlier in persons with two E4 rather than two E3 alleles.[26] In a case–control study[27] of 113 postmortem cases of sporadic AD and 77 control brains, the estimated odds ratio for carrying at least one copy of the E4 allele in the AD cases compared with the controls was 15·5 (95% CI 6·2–38·5). The population attributable risk was 0·53, suggesting that about half of AD in this population was associated with the presence of at least one copy of the E4 allele. Electron micrographic imaging tests have shown that Apo E can be found in some neurones and in vitro studies suggest that Apo E4 promotes β amyloid fibril formation.[28]

E4 allele is not necessary for developing AD; it increases the risk and lowers the age of onset. Because about 1–2% of the population inherits Apo E4/4, whereas about 50% is Apo E3/3, there will be large numbers of Apo E3/3 patients. It has been suggested that at present the use of Apo E genotyping for persons that are symptom free has insufficient epidemiological support to be useful, while E4 allele could be a strong predictor of which patients with mild memory problems will later develop AD.

Intervention

At present AD appears to be related to genes controlling brain ageing, specific genes related to AD, and a poorly understood range of environmental factors. Because of the uncertainty about the aetiology and pathogenesis, and because ageing and familial factors are the major established risk factors, primary prevention based on modification of risk factors is necessarily limited to head trauma, to which only a small proportion is exposed. More research is needed to confirm the protective role of anti-inflammatory drugs.

In view of the multifactorial aetiology of AD, it is arbitrary to attribute a given proportion of incident cases to any single risk factor, implying automatically an avoidable fraction. Thus the direct public health implications of findings from case–control studies are limited.

Hopes for effective therapeutic measures are also limited, given the biological complexity of the disease and the results of many drug trials. At best these show a slower rate of progression, of dubious short term clinical value, for selected patients not identifiable a priori. There are sometimes appreciable adverse reactions (for example, tacrine).

The possibility of restoring or maintaining lost functions through rehabilitation schemes needs proper controlled trials.

Health policy

The ageing of the population will produce an increase in the prevalence of AD. If this is indeed an age related disease, varying in incidence with age but not related to the ageing process, prospects for valuable and specific medical intervention are theoretically open; however, if it is an age dependent disease, meaning it is an intrinsic part of ageing, such prospects will depend on our understanding of brain ageing and we may have to be content with delaying its onset. The burden of terminal AD would, however, still exist.

The present lack of specific therapeutic measures does not mean that nothing can be done. On the contrary, much can and must be done. Health care has been biased toward acute hospital services for adults and children, subdivision into clinical specialties, and a separation between medical and social services. AD patients require services that, regardless of how they are organised in different national contexts, must be integrated and coordinated as regards to health and social sectors and settings (home, community, hospital, residential care). Each component of the network is necessary but not enough on its own.

The limits to our understanding of a disease often make us say that "more research is needed", usually meaning research on aetiology and diagnosis; however, in terms of desired outcomes, while the study of the disease *processes* pertains to the level of impairment, the study of health care *projects* refers to disability and handicap. More services, higher standards of practice, and more active promotion of evaluative research are needed, especially in view of preliminary evidence of the beneficial effects of some model services.[29 30]

The relationships between AD patients, their informal and formal carers, and the spatial organisation of their physical environment are key factors that need further investigation.

Demographic and epidemiological changes have led to increasing demand for extrahospital services (home, community, residential) to meet the needs for rehabilitation and long term care. Thus services are also now in a state of transition in many countries. These changes clearly imply a cultural shift, with more active participation of patients and carers in the processes of decision making choices, such as where to live for years of long term care. This is especially true for AD, in view of the practical help and emotional support provided by families, neighbours, and friends. About four out of five caring relatives are spouses or adult children, most of them women.[29]

At the core of the health problems there are now people with disability, AD being one of the leading causes of disability in the elderly, whose main feature is the combination of medical and psychosocial needs. Health care for AD differs both from the typical acute disorders and from chronic disorders needing long term care after the acute phase (for example, stroke, spinal cord lesions). AD of itself presents neither an acute nor a post-acute phase requiring intensive care followed by post-acute rehabilitation. Patients need prompt detection of those functional impairments that can be successfully treated or at least slowed in their progressive course and the management of additional problems such as delirium, adverse drug reactions, depression, and problem behaviours.

Though the importance of efficient use of funds and cost containment in the delivery of health care is beyond dispute, the efficacy of specific medical interventions, such as drugs and rehabilitation, needs a more rigorous approach. The needs of patients and care givers and the formal

---

Box 29.1—Main types of intervention in health care for patients with Alzheimer's disease

- Diagnosis and staging of the disease (for example, early identification, follow up)
- Comprehensive assessment and review (for example, comorbidity, psychosocial information, strain of the carer)
- Management of intercurrent medical and psychosocial events
- Initiation or change of therapies (drugs, rehabilitation)
- Change to a different care setting (home, community services, institution, hospital)
- Help and support for principal carers or families (for example, home help, respite care, information on available services, information on the disease, advice on care-giving activities and techniques)

---

and informal support measures must be described and understood better to draw a clearer picture of goals, expectations, and costs.

Box 29.1 proposes six general types of intervention, which should be properly described and evaluated. Each type of intervention can be performed at several levels of service (for example, home care, day hospital), with possibly differing outcomes depending on the relationships between targets attained and costs.

For patients with severe AD the valuable anti-institutional strategies and culture produced by social psychiatry need to be reframed, and the points of assent and distance need to be defined, especially regarding the value of the patient's independence and the dignity of disability, involvement in an active life and the "respect of apathy", efforts toward resocialisation, and the difficult and dynamic balance between stimulation and protection, for example, from hyperstimulation or abuse.

This work was supported by the Consiglio Nazionale delle Ricerche (CNR), Convenzione Psicofarmacologia.

1 McKhann G, Drachman D, Folstein M, Katzman R, Price D, Stadlan EM. Clinical diagnosis of Alzheimer's disease: report of the NINCDS-ADRDA work group under the auspices of Department of Health and Human Services Task Force on Alzheimer's disease. *Neurology* 1984;**34**:939–44.
2 Kukull WA, Larson EB, Reifler BV, Lampe TH, Yerby M, Hughes J. Interrater reliability of Alzheimer's disease diagnosis. *Neurology* 1990;**40**:257–60.
3 Kukull WA, Larson EB, Reifler BV, Lampe TH, Yerby MS, Hughes JP. The validity of 3 clinical diagnostic criteria for Alzheimer's disease. *Neurology* 1990;**40**:1364–69.
4 Mirra SS, Heyman A, McKeel D, *et al*. The Consortium to Establish a Registry for Alzheimer's Disease (CERAD). Part II. Standardization of the neuropathologic assessment of Alzheimer's disease. *Neurology* 1991;**41**:479–86.
5 World Health Organization. *The ICD-10 classification of mental and behavioural disorders: clinical descriptions and diagnostic guidelines*. Geneva: WHO, 1992.
6 Rocca WA, Hofman A, Brayne C, *et al*. Frequency and distribution of Alzheimer's disease in Europe: a collaborative study of 1980–1990 prevalence findings. *Ann Neurol* 1991;**30**: 381–90.
7 Bachman DL, Wolf PA, Linn RT, *et al*. Incidence of dementia and probable Alzheimer's disease in a general population: the Framingham study. *Neurology* 1993;**43**:515–19.
8 Skoog I, Nilsson L, Palmertz B, Andreasson LA, Svanborg A. A population-based study of dementia in 85-year-olds. *N Engl J Med* 1993;**328**:153–8.
9 Walsh JS, Welch HG, Larson EB. Survival of outpatients with Alzheimer-type dementia. *Ann Intern Med* 1990;**113**:429–34.
10 Jorm AF. *The epidemiology of Alzheimer's disease and related disorders*. London: Chapman and Hall, 1990.
11 Morris JC, Edlund S, Clark C, *et al*. The Consortium to Establish a Registry for Alzheimer's Disease (CERAD). Part IV. Rates of cognitive change in the longitudinal assessment of probable Alzheimer's disease. *Neurology* 1993;**43**:2457–65.
12 Kay DWK, Beamish P, Roth M. Old age mental disorders in Newcastle upon Tyne. *Br J Psychiatry* 1964;**110**:146–58.
13 Rocca WA, Bonaiuto S, Lippi A, *et al*. Prevalence of clinically diagnosed Alzheimer's disease and other dementing disorders: a door-to-door survey in Appignano, Macerata Province, Italy. *Neurology* 1990;**40**:626–31.
14 Murphy E. A more ambitious vision for residential long-term care. *Int J Geriatr Psychiatry* 1992;**7**:851–2.
15 Keen J. Dementia: questions of cost and value. *Int J Geriatr Psychiatry* 1993;**8**:369–78.
16 Max W. The economic impact of Alzheimer's disease. *Neurology* 1993;**43**(suppl 4):S6–10.

17 Van Duijn CM, Clayton D, Chandra V, *et al.* Familial aggregation of Alzheimer's disease and related disorders: a collaborative re-analysis of case–control studies. *Int J Epidemiol* 1991;**20**:S13–20.

18 Broe GA, Henderson AS, Creasey H, *et al.* A case–control study of Alzheimer's disease in Australia. *Neurology* 1990;**40**:1698–707.

19 Graves AB, White E, Koepsell TD, *et al.* A case–control study of Alzheimer's disease. *Ann Neurol* 1990;**28**:766–74.

20 Li G, Shen YC, Li TY, Chen CH, Zhau YW, Silverman JM. A case–control study of Alzheimer's disease in China. *Neurology* 1992;**42**:1481–88.

21 Prince M, Cullen M, Mann A. Risk factors for Alzheimer's disease and dementia: a case–control study based on the MRC elderly hypertension trial. *Neurology* 1994;**44**: 97–104.

22 Mortimer JA, Van Duijn CM, Chandra V, Fratiglioni L, Graves AB, Heyman A, *et al.* Head trauma as a risk factor for Alzheimer's disease: a collaborative re-analysis of case–control studies. *Int J Epidemiol* 1991;**20**:S28–35.

23 Breitner JCS, Gau BA, Welsh KA, Plassman BL, McDonald WM, Helms MJ, *et al.* Inverse association of anti-inflammatory treatments and Alzheimer's disease: initial results of a co-twin control study. *Neurology* 1994;**44**:227–32.

24 Lai F, Williams RS. A prospective study of Alzheimer disease in Down syndrome. *Arch Neurol* 1989;**46**:849–53.

25 Katzman R. Education and the prevalence of dementia and Alzheimer's disease. *Neurology* 1993;**43**:13–20.

26 Roses AD, Strittmatter WJ, Pericak-Vance MA, Corder EH, Saunders AM, Schmechel DE. Clinical application of apolipoprotein E genotyping to Alzheimer's disease. *Lancet* 1994;**343**:1564–5.

27 Nalbantoglu J, Gilfix BM, Bertrand P, *et al.* Predictive value of apolipoprotein E genotyping in Alzheimer's disease: results of an autopsy series and an analysis of several combined studies. *Ann Neurol* 1994;**36**:889–95.

28 Ma J, Yee A, Brewer B Jr, Das S, Potter H. Amyloid-associated proteins α1-antichymotrypsin and apolipoprotein E promote assembly of Alzheimer β-protein into filaments. *Nature* 1994;**372**:92–4.

29 Levin E. Carers-problems, strains, and services. In: Jacoby R, Oppenheimer C, editors. *Psychiatry in the elderly.* Oxford: Oxford University Press, 1991:301–12.

30 Harrison S, Sheldon TA. Psychiatric services for elderly people: evaluating system performance. *Int J Geriatr Psychiatry* 1994;**9**:259–72.

30 Depressive illness

MARTIN BLANCHARD

Definitions and diagnostic criteria

The term "depression" has a broad range of meanings. It is generally viewed as a subjective experience involving feelings, some of which can be described as sadness, lowness in spirits, hopelessness, dejection, unhappiness, and loneliness. While it is accepted that depression involves a lowering of mood, the depressed individual needs to display certain morbid mental phenomena, a particular level of mood change, and a minimum duration of symptoms in order to attain the concept of clinical status or depressive illness. Depression can be classed as a clinical entity and a serious mental health problem, an illness with a biological basis quite separate and distinct from the reactive mood changes experienced by everybody from time to time. The boundaries of "normal" sadness may not, however, always be clear and it is also argued that depressed mood in otherwise normal people may only be quantitatively but not qualitatively different from the depression found in patients referred for psychiatric care. Any additional features of depression are then said to arise when low mood becomes prolonged or intensified.

The features of depression can be divided into four spheres: emotional, motivational, cognitive, and vegetative. Emotional manifestations include sadness, anxiety, irritability, anger, and anhedonia. The concept of anhedonia, the loss of ability to experience pleasure, has been regarded as critical in the distinction between depression as an illness and depressive symptoms within the community.[1] Some people with depression can, however, deny sadness, and instead feel inhibited in their feelings.

Motivational aspects manifest as inertia, difficulty in functioning, and sometimes in even performing the most basic daily activities. In severe depression this appears as "psychomotor retardation".

Cognitive features have been considered by some researchers and theorists[2] to be causal in depression, whereas many see them as manifestations of an underlying disorder. Depressed people view themselves, the world around them, and the future in negative, pessimistic terms. They see themselves as inadequate and perceive little hope for change to the better. Occasionally they will express the wish to die or to end their own existence. As well as these "negative cognitions" the depressed person may have slow thoughts and complain of difficulty in concentrating and difficulty and uncertainty in making decisions.

The presence of vegetative symptoms is sometimes taken to indicate the presence of a "clinical" depression. These features are believed to reflect biological changes and therefore are believed to be more amenable to pharmacological manipulation. They include fatigue, sleep disturbance (difficulty getting off to sleep, restless sleep, early morning wakening, and occasionally excessive sleeping), and appetite disturbance (usually a decrease in appetite and enjoyment of food with occasional evidence of weight loss but sometimes an increase in eating with concomitant weight gain). There may be associated nausea and constipation, loss of sexual interest and enjoyment, non-specific somatic symptoms including headaches, and a decreased tolerance of any minor ailments.

Classification systems

At the present time a variety of classification systems have evolved based on phenomenology, response to treatment, and prognosis, that is until the "ignorance of aetiology of depression" is removed.[3]

The contemporary psychiatric diagnostic approach to depression has developed from Kraepelin, who separated psychopathology into the two broad syndromes of dementia praecox and manic depressive illness (affective disorders) the latter being episodic in nature, Leonhard proposed the now widely accepted differentiation of affective disorders between bipolar depression (with manic episodes) and unipolar depression (in the absence of manic episodes). Within the latter group there is a debate between a categorical approach to classification—the concept that there is a discrete population of people who can be regarded as depressed—and a dimensional approach—the assumption that depression is a continuum and that the disease state is dependent on how much depression an individual has. The situation is similar to the controversy over the diagnosis of hypertension and the difficulties in defining a discrete "diseased" group.

The simplest classification is based upon a continuity of depression: the construction of a list of symptoms, and assignment of a particular depression score according to the number of symptoms present. "Caseness" or need for clinical concern may be arbitrarily defined by definition of a cut point on any particular scale. Examples of such depression scales are the Beck Depression Inventory,[4] the Center for Epidemiologic Studies Depression Scale (CES-D),[5] the Geriatric Depression Scale (GDS),[6] and the SELFCARE (D) questionnaire.[7]

The major nosological systems that have lately been developed internationally are, however, categorical systems: the Diagnostic and Statistical Manual of Mental Disorders of the American Psychiatric Association (DSM-IIIR)[8] and the International Classification of Diseases, currently undergoing its 10th revision (ICD-10) (box 30.1).[9] The DSM-IIIR classification system separates mood disorders into bipolar and depressive disorders depending upon whether or not a manic episode, as defined in the manual, has been present. Depressive disorders are then classified as (a) major depressive episodes—depressed mood for at least two weeks with at least five other symptoms from a list given (with or without melancholia); (b) dysthymia—depressed mood for more days than not over a two year period plus two from a list of symptoms; or (c) depressive disorder not otherwise specified (DNOS). The ICD-10 classification system lists affective disorders as (a) manic episodes with or without psychotic symptoms; (b) depressive disorders; (c) bipolar affective disorders; (d) recurrent depressive disorders; (e) persistent affective disorders; and (f) other mood disorders. Groups (b)–(d) are separated according to degree of severity (mild, moderate, or severe) and presence or absence of psychotic symptoms. As an example, the criteria for mild depressive episode are symptoms, as listed, severe enough to cause distress and usually to be noticed by other people for a minimum of two weeks.

Box 30.1—Criteria for depressive disorders in DSM-IIIR and ICD-10

DSM-IIIR

- *Major depressive episode*
  Two weeks duration
  Five out of nine:
  1 Depressed mood most of day, nearly every day
  2 Markedly diminished interest
  3 Weight loss or weight gain (5% body weight in a month) or decrease or increase in appetite
  4 Insomnia or hypersomnia
  5 Agitation or retardation
  6 Fatigue
  7 Worthlessness or excessive guilt
  8 Depressed ability to think or concentrate
  9 Recurrent morbid thoughts

  Mild:minor impairment

  Moderate:intermediate

ICD-10

- *Mild depressive episode*
  Can continue to function
  About two weeks duration
  Two out of three:
  1 Lowered mood
  2 Decreased interest
  3 Increased fatigue

  and two out of seven:
  1 Decreased concentration
  2 Lowered selfesteem
  3 Ideas of guilt
  4 Bleak outlook on the future
  5 Ideas of self harm
  6 Disturbed sleep
  7 Decreased appetite

- *Moderate depressive episode*
  Difficulty continuing to function

Box continued

Box continued

DSM-IIR	ICD-10

DSM-IIR

Severe:marked interference

With or without psychotic features

Single or recurrent episodes

Melancholic subtype—five out of nine:
1 Diminished interest
2 Lack of reactivity
3 Diurnal variation of mood
4 Early morning wakening
5 Objective retardation or agitation
6 Anorexia or weight loss
7 No significant personality disorder prior to onset
8 ≥ one previous episode with close to recovery or recovery
9 Previous good response to adequate antidepressants

- *Bipolar disorder*
Current mixed
Current manic
Current depressed

- *Dysthymia*
Depressed mood for two years
Never without for more than two months, plus two out of six:
1 Poor appetite
2 Insomnia
3 Decreased energy
4 Lowered self esteem
5 Decreased concentration
6 Hopelessness

- *Cyclothymia*
Two years duration
Hypomania plus mild depression not without for more than 2 months

- *Depression not otherwise specified*

ICD-10

Two out of three above and 3–4 out of seven of above

- *Severe depressive episode*
Unlikely to be able to function
Three out of three of above and four out of seven above

- *Severe with psychotic features*
Optional subtype: with or without somatic symptoms
≥ four out of seven of:
1 Diminished interest
2 Diminished reactivity
3 Early morning wakening
4 Diurnal variation of mood
5 Objective retardation or agitation
6 Weight loss
7 Loss of libido

- *Recurrent depressive disorder*
Subtypes as above

- *Bipolar affective disorder*
Current mixed
Current manic
Current depressed

- *Persistent affective disorders*
Dysthymia
Longstanding depression, not severe enough for recurrent diagnosis
Cyclothymia
Persistent instability of mood, mild depression and elation

- *Other affective disorders*

Modifications for older people

There are specific difficulties in the assessment and classification of depression in older people. (1) There may be clinical differences in the presentation of depression when older people are compared with younger people. (2) There is an increase in physical illness and disability in old age, both of which have an interactive relationship with depression. (3) It can be difficult to distinguish depression from the cognitive deficits of dementia, an increasingly prevalent condition with advancing age. (4) There is a "grey" area between depression requiring intervention and the state of demoralisation, which is often felt to be part of the ageing process.

To help overcome some of these difficulties assessment measures with accompanying classification systems have been designed specifically for older people. One is the Comprehensive Assessment and Referral Evaluation (CARE), which detects among other things "pervasive depression".[10 11] This concept of depression acknowledges that levels of depression, less severe than, for instance, DSM-IIIR major depression, may still have detrimental effects on emotional, social, cognitive, and physiological functioning in older people and may also benefit from clinical intervention. The Geriatric Mental State–AGECAT system (GMS-AGECAT) consists of a clinical interview schedule, the GMS, and a computer programme, the AGECAT, which are available on laptop computers for use in epidemiological surveys. The GMS assesses depression as a continuum from non-caseness through subcaseness to "neurotic" or milder cases and "psychotic" or severer cases. As with levels on depressive symptomatology the instrument is able to gauge a level on seven other symptom clusters (organicity, manic symptoms, schizophrenia/paranoid related symptoms, anxiety, phobias, obsessive/compulsive symptoms, and hypochondriasis). The AGECAT programme can therefore provide a hierarchically determined diagnostic classification and a descriptive picture of a depression.[12]

Magnitude of the problem

Prevalence surveys of depression among older people have measured morbidity at three levels: community, primary care, and hospital clinic. These results are not comparable because passage between these levels is not free. Large hidden morbidity is discovered among the older population in the community sample; a large number of cases never reach specialist mental health resources from primary care, and severe and resistant cases tend to accumulate in clinics. In addition, all published prevalence studies have their own idiosyncrasies of case definition, sample frame, and means of assessment that make differences between results hard to interpret.

Depressive symptoms appear to be more frequent with increasing age and its concomitant disability but results from the National Institute of Mental Health/Epidemiological Catchment Area (NIMH/ECA), which focused on DSM-IIIR diagnoses, reported DSM-IIIR major depression at a rate of 1·1% (six month period prevalence rate), which was 2–3 times less prevalent than amongst younger age groups. The prevalence of bipolar disorder was 0·1% and dysthymia 2·4%—also substantially lower in older people.[13] Similarly a recent study in Australia also discovered a rate of 1·0% for DSM-IIIR major depression in a community survey of people aged 70 years or older but there was evidence of a high level of depressive symptoms.[14] These depressive symptoms correlated with poor physical health, disability, and a history of previous depression.

Thus, although the majority of older adults may not fit DSM-III criteria for major depression but rather have depressive symptoms associated with physical illness and/or adjustment to life stress, it is important to stress that *"any health policy based on the prevalence of major depressive disorders will be ineffective if the loss of social, emotional, physiological, and cognitive function is associated with depressive symptoms that are substantial and widespread but not congruent with a diagnosis of a major disorder."*[15]

In contrast the CARE instruments assessing the concept of "pervasive depression" yielded very similar rates of depression in New York (13%) and London (12·9%). Similarly the "psychiatrist" definition of caseness as developed for the GMS schedule demonstrated rates of 3·0% "psychotic" or more severe depression and 8·3% "neurotic" or milder depression among the older Liverpool community. From the results of a three year follow up the incidence of GMS depression caseness was estimated as 23·7/1000 per year.[16]

Variation

Time

Sir Aubrey Lewis in 1945 analysed the admission data for "first attacks" of psychiatric illnesses of older people, demonstrating that between 1907 and 1937 the rate of admission for men fell from 109 to 79 per 100 000, but for women there was a less dramatic fall of 91 to 77 per 100 000. This fall in admissions began just after the first world war years and continued until 1932. It probably reflected the use of general hospital beds and the increasing numbers of older mentally ill being inappropriately cared for in public assistance institutions rather than a reflection of a true decline in the incidence of mental illness.

There has been little information since then concerning the changing prevalence rate of depression among older people over time; however, the important cultural change has been an appreciation of the significant yet remediable detrimental effect depression may have upon quality of life.

Place

The prevalence of depression is higher among older attenders at primary care practices[17] and also among hospitalised patients[18] than in the community. There is also a higher prevalence rate among people in residential homes, but this was more marked in London than in New York, Mannheim, or Milan.[19]

Person

Certain aspects of an individual's constitution seem to affect the propensity to depression. Depression is more common among women by a ratio of about 2:1.

A study from Los Angeles using the CARE instrument suggested that there is a higher prevalence of depression (26%) among the older Hispanics in the city.

Family studies have indicated that patients with earlier onset depression have more relatives with earlier onset depression and a greater risk for affective disorder amongst their relatives.[20] Whether this difference is due to the incomplete penetrance of genes in later onset depression or the fact that a genetic form of disorder manifests itself earlier in life is as yet unknown.

Certain subgroups of older people with depression may show specific abnormalities of brain structure, hypothalamic–pituitary–adrenal function, and neurotransmitter status. These people may have a "biological propensity" towards onset and/or poor prognosis of depression.[21-23]

A strong association between depression and physical ill health amongst older people has been consistently reported. Certain illnesses may have a direct aetiological role in depression, either through physiological or cognitive means, whereas others may act as maintaining factors.[15] Alzheimer's disease is also associated with an increased rate of depression as observed by a trained clinician.[24] The phenomenology of the depression associated with physical illness and disability is, however, characteristic more of dysthymia than "major" depression.[25] In patients who have suffered a stroke, major depression appears to be strongly associated with left frontal or left basoganglial lesions.[26]

Bereavement may greatly increase the risk of depression and dysphoria. Bereaved subjects with depression report significantly fewer symptoms of guilt compared with the non-bereaved with depression.[27] Community studies tend to use shorter measures of social factors than studies of hospital based populations, and also relate these to severity of depressive symptoms rather than to the presence of clinical case level depression. Nevertheless, there is evidence that social factors can influence onset and course of depression among older people in terms of life events, difficulties, and intimacy status,[28] social class, size and homogeneity (sex, age, and religion) of the social network, marital conflicts, and source of primary confiding.[29 30] It must, however, be borne in mind that depressive symptoms may themselves affect social support. (1) They may discourage support. (2) They may make the person unable to effect the necessary social behaviours

285

in order to keep a network. (3) They may alter a person's view as to how available and adequate the available support is. Longitudinal studies to examine the outcome effect of social variables on the onset of depression and its subsequent course are necessary.

Determinants of depressive illness

A past history of depression, a family history of depression, physical illness/disability, institutionalisation, bereavement, major non-health life events and difficulties (including socioeconomic, marital, and filial), and lack of emotional support are all associated with depression in later life. These interrelated factors may only increase the risk of depression a small amount. Absence of specific factors cannot be taken as evidence to exclude depression.

Intervention

Primary prevention

Attempts should be made to encourage a healthier more active lifestyle and to minimise the effects of physical ill health when it occurs. Support and counselling targeted at critical times of loss or crisis, when none is readily available, may be of benefit. An increased economic provision for older people may enable them to obtain a better quality of life as a result of expanded social and leisure opportunities.

Secondary prevention

Several studies have indicated that, although older people are frequent visitors to their general practitioners, much of their depression is either not recognised or misdiagnosed. Thus there is a lack of diagnostic accuracy.

A consultation may be adversely affected by doctor and patient characteristics, including ageism, "understandability" of depressive symptoms, anxieties about treatment, stigmatisation, and somatisation.

Improvement of recognition within the primary care setting could involve the training of practitioners in better interview techniques, screening questionnaires as indicators of morbidity, and the education of all primary care staff to increase sensitivity to depressive symptomatology and to facilitate questioning to elicit such symptoms.

Tertiary prevention

Initial studies appeared to show a poor overall prognosis among the more severe cases of depression but further research has indicated that the reality may not be quite so gloomy. Between 30 and 60% remain well or have a further episode(s) followed by full recovery, whereas 7% suffer continuous depressive symptoms.

Male sex, poor physical health at presentation or developing subsequently, the severity of the initial illness and the presence of psychotic symptoms, duration of illness, and severe life events in the follow up year are the main predictors of poor outcome. The presence of an intimate relationship does not appear to help prevent relapse in the face of continuing life stressors.

Later onset depressives (60 years or older) are more likely to remain completely well during follow up and less likely to have frequent or disabling relapses. Treatment compliance, long term follow up, and maintenance antidepressant therapy are associated with favourable outcome.[31-34]

Medication may also be used to maintain improvement in mental state and therefore influence overall prognosis.[35] Electroconvulsive therapy (ECT) is an important treatment for severe depressive states in late life. The additional risk involved in the use of ECT in physically ill people is not great when compared with that of continued depression or the side effects of alternative treatments. The side effects of ECT are not felt to be a major problem. The features of depression that should have a good outcome when treated with ECT are symptoms of guilt, increased severity, agitation (unlike the younger depressed), loss of interest, and duration of illness.[36]

There is no reason to assume that findings in the behaviour and cognitive therapy literature are not applicable to older people. Behavioural, cognitive, or brief psychodynamic therapies when compared with a six week treatment delayed control group have been demonstrated to produce a significant decline in depression score. There was very little evidence of spontaneous remission among the control group. Cognitive behavioural therapy may lead to a more effectively maintained improvement at one year treatment free follow up.[37 38]

Health policy

Burden

Depressive illness is a common yet in no way inevitable condition of old age. It is a treatable illness and it is associated with increased use of health and social services, increased mortality, and reduced quality of life for sufferers and carers.

287

Prevention

Primary prevention involves complex issues, including improved management of physical illnesses associated with old age, careful prescribing, crisis support, and increasing economic provision for older people to enable greater social and leisure activities.

Secondary prevention requires a primary care initiative of improved recognition and coordinated care management strategies; because of the large morbidity, this will involve primary care workers other than the general practitioner and these workers will require training.

Treatment

Apart from the benefits in reduction of mortality and improved quality of life it is hoped that correct treatment of depression will reduce the extra use of health and social services by depressed older people. Because of the strong association with the physical illnesses of old age, the management of depression should be seen as an integral part of the multifaceted management practised in health care services for older people.

1 Snaith P. The concepts of mild depression. *Br J Psychiatry* 1987;**150**:387–93.
2 Beck A. *Depression: clinical, experimental and theoretical aspects.* New York, Harper and Row, 1967.
3 Kendall R. The classification of depressions: a review of contemporary confusion. *Br J Psychiatry* 1976;**129**:15–28.
4 Beck A, Ward C, Mendelson M, Mock J, Erbaugh J. An inventory for measuring depression. *Arch Gen Psychiatry* 1961;**4**:561–71.
5 Radloff L. The CES-D scale: a self-report depression scale for research in the general population. *Appl Psychol Meas* 1977;**1**:385.
6 Yesavage J, Rose T, Lum O. Development and validation of a geriatric depression screening scale: a preliminary report. *J Psychiatr Res* 1983;**17**:37–49.
7 Bird A, Macdonald A, Mann A, Philpott M. Preliminary experience with the SELFCARE (D): a self-rating depression questionnaire for use in elderly, non-instutionalised subjects. *Int J Geriatr Psychiatry* 1987;**2**:131–8.
8 American Psychiatric Association. *Diagnostic and statistical manual of mental disorders,* 3rd ed, revised. Washington: APA, World Health Organization, 1987.
9 World Health Organization. *ICD-10 classification of mental and behavioural disorders. Clinical descriptions and diagnostic guidelines.* Geneva, WHO, 1992.
10 Gurland B, Copeland J, Kuriansky J, *et al. The mind and mood of aging.* London, Croom Helm, 1983.
11 Kay D, Henderson A, Scott R, Wilson J, Rickwood D, Grayson D. Dementia and depression amongst the elderly living in the Hobart community: the effect of the diagnostic criteria on the prevalence rates. *Psychol Med* 1985;**15**:771–8.
12 Copeland J, Dewey M, Griffiths-Jones H. A computerized psychiatric diagnostic system and case nomenclature for elderly subjects: GMS and AGECAT. *Psychol Med* 1986;**16**:89–99.
13 Weissman M, Myers J, Tischler G, *et al.* Psychiatric disorders (DSM-III) and cognitive impairment among the elderly in a US urban community. *Acta Psychiatr Scand* 1985;**71**:366–79.
14 Henderson AS, Jorm AF, Mackinnon A, *et al.* The prevalence of depressive disorders and the distribution of depressive symptoms in later life: a survey using draft ICD-10 and DSM-IIIR. *Psychol Med* 1993;**23**:719–24.

15 Kennedy G, Kelman H, Thomas C, *et al.* Hierarchy of characteristics associated with depressive symptoms in an urban elderly sample. *Am J Psychiatry* 1989;**146**:220–5.

16 Copeland J, Davidson I, Dewey M, *et al.* Alzheimer's disease, other dementias, depression and pseudodementia: prevalence, incidence and three-year outcome in Liverpool. *Br J Psychiatry* 1992;**161**:230–9.

17 Macdonald A. Do general practitioners "miss" depression in elderly patients? *BMJ* 1986;**292**:1365–7.

18 Koenig HG, Meador KG, Cohen HJ, Blazer D. Depression in elderly hospitalised patients with medical illness. *Arch Intern Med* 1988;**148**:1929–36.

19 Ames D, Ashby D, Mann AH, Graham N. Psychiatric illness in elderly residents of part III homes in one London borough: prognosis and review. *Age Ageing* 1988;**17**:249–56.

20 Maier W, Lichtermann D, Minges J, Heun R, Hallmayer J, Klingler T. Unipolar depression in the aged: determinants of familial aggregation. *J Affective Disord* 1991;**23**:53–61.

21 Jacoby R, Dolan R, Levy R, Baldy R. Quantitative computed tomography in elderly depressed patients. *Br J Psychiatry* 1983;**143**:124–7.

22 Krishnan KRR, McDonald WM, Doraiswamy PM, *et al.* Neuroanatomical substrates of depression in the elderly. *Eur Arch Psychiatry Clin Neurosci* 1993;**243**:41–6.

23 Leake A, Charlton BG, Lowry PJ, Jackson S, Fairbairn A, Ferrier IN. Plasma N-POMC, ACTH and cortisol concentrations in a psychogeriatric population. *Br J Psychiatry* 1990;**156**:676–9.

24 Burns A, Jacoby R, Levy R. Psychiatric phenomena in Alzheimer's disease. III. Disorders of mood. *Br J Psychiatry* 1990;**157**:81–5.

25 Bruce ML, McNamara R. Psychiatric status among the homebound elderly: an epidemiologic perspective. *J Am Geriatr Soc* 1992;**40**:561–6.

26 Starkstein SE, Robinson RG. Affective disorders and cerebral vascular disease. *Br J Psychiatry* 1989;**154**:170–82.

27 Bruce ML, Kim K, Leaf PJ, Jacobs S. Depressive episodes and dysphoria resulting from conjugal bereavement in a prospective community sample. *Am J Psychiatry* 1990;**147**:608–11.

28 Murphy E. Social origins of depression in old age. *Br J Psychiatry* 1982;**141**:135–42.

29 Goldberg E, Van Natta P, Comstock GW. Depressive symptoms, social networks and social support of elderly women. *Am J Epidemiol* 1985;**121**:448–56.

30 Palinkas LA, Wingard DL, Barrett-Connor E. The biocultural context of social networks and depression among the elderly. *Soc Sci Med* 1990;**30**:441–7.

31 Murphy E. The prognosis of depression in old age. *Br J Psychiatry* 1983;**142**:111–9.

32 Baldwin RC, Jolley DG. The prognosis of depression in old age. *Br J Psychiatry* 1986;**149**:571–83.

33 Cole M. The course of elderly depressed out-patients. *Can J Psychiatry* 1985;**30**:217–20.

34 Kennedy G, Kelman H, Thomas C. Persistence and remission of depressive symptoms in late life. *Am J Psychiatry* 1990;**148**:174–8.

35 Old Age Depression Interest Group. How long should the elderly take antidepressants? A double-blind placebo-controlled study of continuation/prophylaxis therapy with dothiepin. *Br J Psychiatry* 1993;**162**:175–82.

36 Benbow SB. The role of electroconvulsive therapy in the treatment of depressive illness in old age. *Br J Psychiatry* 1989;**155**:147–52.

37 Gallagher DE, Thompson LW. Treatment of major depressive disorder in older adult outpatients with brief psychotherapies. *Psychotherapy Theory Res Pract* 1982;**19**:482–9.

38 Thompson LW, Gallagher D, Breckenridge JS. Comparative effectiveness of psychotherapies for depressed elders. *J Consult Clin Psychol* 1987;**55**:385–90.

31 Osteoporosis

STEFANIA MAGGI

Definition and diagnostic criteria

Osteoporosis is a disease characterised by low bone mass, microarchitectural deterioration of bone tissue leading to enhanced bone fragility, and a consequent increase in fracture risk.[1]

Different approaches can be used to define osteoporosis on the basis of bone mineral density (BMD). For a young healthy adult, a value of BMD 2·5 SD or more below the mean at any site (spine, hip, or mid-radius) is generally used for the diagnosis of osteoporosis, while a value of BMD between 1 and 2·5 SD below the young adult reference mean is adopted to define osteopenia.[2]

Several techniques can be used to measure BMD and morphological changes of the bone. The major limitations are related to their precision (ability to obtain the same results in repeated measurements) and accuracy (ability to obtain a result which is close to the true value).

Conventional radiology is quite insensitive, given that it detects bone loss only when the mass has decreased by about 30–50%. Digital methods for evaluating vertebral dimensions are suggested as more objective methods for fracture identification.[3] Although vertebral body height on x ray can be used to diagnose vertebral fracture (anterior height decrease compared with the posterior height), it should always be kept in mind that vertebral dimensions and structure vary in the normal population and could lead to overdiagnosis of spinal osteoporosis. Among the semiquantitative techniques for assessing trabecular morphology the most commonly used is the Singh index,[4] which provides an indication of the degree of trabecular structural loss in the hip, inferred from the remaining trabecular pattern. This technique is useful in epidemiological studies of hip fracture, but much less so in studies of young healthy people.

Single photon absorptiometry (SPA) has been available for about 30 years. It uses a γ ray source coupled with a scintillation detector, which together scan across the area of interest.

SPA has several advantages, such as reasonable cost, low radiation exposure, short scanning time (10–15 minutes), and high accuracy and precision. The major disadvantage is that it has been used extensively to study bone density at the distal radius and other peripheral sites but the correlations between bone mineral content assessed at these sites and the trabecular bone mass at the femoral neck or in the vertebral body is poor. SPA is therefore inadequate for predicting hip and spinal fractures.

Dual photon absorptiometry (DPA) uses two photon energies and permits separation between bone and soft tissue. It can be used to measure sites at high risk of osteoporotic fractures, such as lumbar spine and proximal femur. Some of the major advantages are the small radiation dose and good precision but there are several disadvantages, such as the long scanning time (30 minutes), the high cost, and the need for frequent replacement of the isotope source (gadolinium), which affects the accuracy of repeated measurements.

In more recent years DPA has been replaced in many sites by dual energy x ray absorptiometry (DEXA). Its advantages are low radiation, a reduced scanning time (10–20 minutes), high accuracy and precision, multiple sites of assessment, including spine and hip, and ease of use. A limitation of DEXA is that the anterioposterior image is affected by osteoarthrosis and aortic calcification at lumbar sites, while the lateral position is affected by the increased soft tissue mass and overlap of the projected image by the ribs and pelvis. Although its capital cost is relatively high, the running cost is modest.

Quantitative computed tomography (QCT) allows the measure of volumetric bone mineral density, and trabecular bone can be examined separately from cortical bone, but the high radiation exposure and the high cost do not allow its use as a screening instrument.

Ultrasonography, more recently developed, seems very promising. It does not involve ionising radiation and provides information not only on the density but also on the structure of the bone. The ultrasonographic attenuation discriminates between patients with and without osteoporosis, and attenuation values are significantly lower in patients with hip fracture than in controls.[5]

Several biomarkers of bone turnover are available. The rate of bone formation can be assessed by measuring serum alkaline phosphatase (particularly sensitive and specific is the bone isoenzyme), osteocalcin, and type 1 procollagen propeptides. Markers of bone resorption include hydroxyproline, serum tartrate resistant acid phosphatase, hydroxylysine, and urinary pyridinium cross link (Pyr and dPyr), which are released from the bone matrix during its degradation by the osteoclasts. Pyr and dPyr seem to have several advantages over the other biomarkers because they are relatively specific for bone turnover and are not metabolised in vivo before their urinary excretion.

Risk

The clinical significance of osteoporosis lies in fractures and many authors have suggested that the term osteoporosis should be used to describe fragility fractures, including mainly hip fracture, vertebral fracture, and Colles' fracture of the wrist. The incidence of fractures is commonly calculated using the number of fractures in the numerator, usually obtained from hospital discharge records, and person years at risk as the denominator. Great care must be taken in comparing available data on incidence of fractures because of major biases that can affect their comparability (box 31.1).

Box 31.1—Potential biases in comparative studies on osteoporotic fractures

Differences in:
- Definition of fracture
- Accuracy of coding
- Case ascertainment
- Hospital transfer rates
- Availability of health services
- Selection of study population
- Period of ascertainment
- Sample size

Magnitude of the problem

Osteoporosis represents a major public health problem because of the high mortality and morbidity associated with some of the resultant fractures. The large majority of osteoporotic fractures occur in older women and the number increases with age. The lifetime risk of osteoporotic fracture in women is probably close to 40%, while in men it is about 13%.[6] The reasons for this sex difference are mainly related to the lower bone mass in women at the age of peak bone mass and the bone loss after menopause. Whereas in women the incidence of osteoporotic fractures increases after the age of 45 years, in men there is a substantial increase only after the age of 75 years.

Most of the data available on incidence of osteoporosis worldwide relate to rates of hip fractures because they are easier to identify. It is estimated that about 1·7 million hip fractures occurred in 1990 worldwide and this number could rise to 6·26 million by 2050. Considering the demographic change and the increasing life expectancy in developing countries, it is expected that 71% of all fractures in 2050 will occur in Africa, Asia, South America, and the eastern Mediterranean region.[7]

The incidence of vertebral fractures is difficult to determine because many are asymptomatic and there is no general agreement about the criteria for their diagnosis. Estimated annual incidence in England and Wales ranges from 70 000 to 140 000 people affected.[8] Although they

292

are less important than hip fractures in terms of morbidity and mortality, vertebral fractures are relevant from a public health point of view because they give rise to deformity, pain, and eventually to the need for medical treatment. Estimates from the United States indicate that about one third of all patients are clinically attended and one tenth are hospitalised.[9]

The incidence of fracture of the distal forearm increases rapidly after the menopause. For European women the lifetime risk is about 15%, and it is approximately four times higher than in men.[8] The consequences of these fractures are mainly disability and consequent dependence on others until healing has taken place. Other sequelae, such as algodystrophy (pain; stiffness; swelling; vasomotor disturbance of the hand, due to an abnormal neurovegetative response caused by the fracture), may present in up to 30% of patients.[10]

The total cost of osteoporosis is hard to assess because it includes hospital care, loss of working days, long term care, and drugs. The different health care systems and the different assumptions on which cost estimates are made make any comparative analyses between countries impossible. Annual cost estimates for the United States are about $7–10 billion, in England and Wales about £614 million, and in France about Fr 3·7 billion.[2] These costs are largely due to hip fractures because of the high rates of hospitalisation and nursing home admission and the high disability rate in these patients.

Variation

Time

Most studies have shown a significant increase in age and sex specific rates of osteoporotic fractures since the early 1960s in Hong Kong and in most of Europe and North America. The reasons for this secular trend are unclear. Improvement in case assignment might be in part responsible but changes in lifestyle, such as the increased frequency of cigarette smoking and alcohol consumption, decreased amount of heavy physical labour, and increased use of psychotropic drugs (related to a higher risk of falls) could also account for the trend.[11]

Place

Considerable variation in incidence of osteoporotic fractures has been reported from various parts of the world; most of the data relate to hip fractures. Figure 31.1 presents the hip fracture rates per 100 000 persons in different countries. These data show that the highest rates are found in northern Europe and North America. The lowest rates are found in Africa.[11]

293

It has been suggested that the rates in Hong Kong are approaching those of the North American white population[12] but careful attention should be given to some methodological problems, as listed in box 31.1. In a recent study, for instance, Ho et al[13] have compared hospital discharge data in Hong Kong and in the United States and found that the transfer rate (cases counted twice) was about 7% in the United States, whereas it was close to 30% in Hong Kong. Inclusion of transferred cases minimised differences between the countries and despite the increased rates in the last 30 years in Hong Kong the rates are still significantly lower than those in the United States.

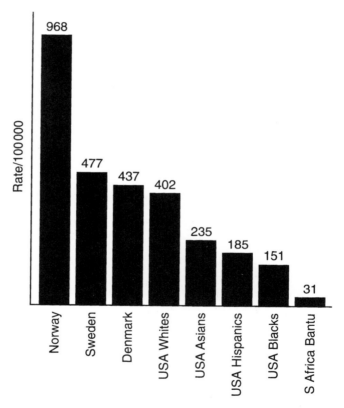

Fig 31.1 Age and sex adjusted incidence rates of hip fracture (adjusted to United States population 1985) in the population over 50 years of age.

The reasons for the international variation in incidence rates are unclear, although differences in diet, physical activity, body build, genetic predisposition, use of drugs, and propensity to fall have been suggested as possible explanations.[11]

294

Person

In all countries in which incidence studies have been undertaken rates of osteoporotic fractures increase with age in both sexes and in all ethnic groups but the increase in rates with age occurs earlier in women than in men, and earlier in white women than in Asian, Hispanic, and black women.[11] The occurrence of an osteoporotic fracture is likely to be the consequence of a combination of constitutional and environmental risk factors, and bone mass has been reported to be the strongest predictor of fractures. Most studies show higher BMD in black people than in white people at each age. Solomon[14] found that white individuals in Johannesburg present a phase of slight but continuous reduction in metacarpal bone density between 30 and 50 years of age, whereas the black population sustain their metacarpal bone density at maximum levels, or actually increase them, at the same age. This could in part explain the lower incidence of osteoporotic fractures in black compared with white populations, although some paradoxes have yet to be clarified. Japanese individuals, for example, have lower BMD than white people but still experience lower rates of hip fracture.[15] There must therefore be other important factors beside bone mineral content, such as those predisposing to falls and those related to neuromuscular reaction, that have to be considered as aetiological agents for fractures.

Determinants of osteoporosis

A number of factors that increase the likelihood of developing osteoporosis have been identified, some of which affect the peak bone mass, others bone loss. Already mentioned in the previous section are the risks related to increasing age, female gender (particularly thin, small framed women), and white racial group. Menopause represents the most important cause of osteoporosis, in addition to the bone loss related to age or to the diseases and conditions listed in box 31.2.[2] Obesity is protective, probably because it is associated with higher oestrogen levels and hence with greater bone mass. The high prevalence of obesity in black women, as well as their higher bone mass compared with white women, might account for some of the racial differences. It is interesting to note that weight loss in adults has been reported to be a significant risk factor for loss of bone mass independent of the effect of current weight.[16] A family history of osteoporosis is important and there is evidence of a genetic role in the determination of peak bone mass. Sowers et al[17] estimated that in premenopausal women genes account for 67%, 47%, and 58% of the variability in bone mineral density in the femoral neck, trochanter, and Ward's triangle, after adjusting for age and body size. Cigarette smoking has been suggested as a potential risk factor for osteoporosis and several reasons could justify this association: female smokers are usually thinner than non-smokers, experience an earlier menopause, and have lower endogenous oestrogen levels.[18]

Box 31.2—Diseases and conditions related to secondary osteoporosis

- *Endocrine diseases*
  Cushing's syndrome
  Hyperparathyroidism
  Hypogonadism
  Thyroid toxicosis
  Hypopituitarism
  Insulin dependent diabetes mellitus
  Anorexia nervosa

- *Nutritional causes*
  Malabsorption/malnutrition
  Chronic liver disease
  Scurvy
  Vitamin D deficiency
  Alcoholism
  Gastrectomy

- *Drugs*
  Chronic corticosteroids administration
  Excess thyroxine replacement
  Chronic heparin administration
  Anticonvulsants

- *Inflammatory disorders*
  Rheumatoid arthritis
  Ankylosing spondylitis

- *Other*
  Myeloma and some cancers
  Osteoporosis of pregnancy
  Immobilisation
  Oophorectomy

A lifetime low intake of calcium results in low peak bone mass and higher bone mass loss in adults. Calcium supplementation and/or vitamin D enhance gain in bone mass and slow bone loss.[19]

Intervention

Prevention

The discussion on determinants of osteoporosis points out that lifestyle factors, such as appropriate level of exercise, improved nutrition, and smoking cessation, might affect the bone mass and are important components of general health measures that should therefore be adopted by the general population. Of the treatments proposed to decrease the rate of bone loss, hormone replacement therapy (HRT) seems to be the most effective, leading to a reduction of 30–50% in the incidence of fractures with an exposure to HRT of 3–10 years. Randomised trials have shown that HRT prevents bone loss at the menopause and thereafter. There is also evidence that bone preserved by HRT is not rapidly lost when the treatment is stopped, as previously believed.[2] The side effects of HRT are well investigated. Oral unopposed oestrogen use is associated with a reduction in the incidence of coronary heart disease and mortality from cardiovascular disease. Combined oestrogen and progestogen seems to attenuate the beneficial effects of oestrogen on cardiovascular disease but data are still inadequate for any firm conclusion. Oestrogen use has been found to be associated with an increased risk of endometrial carcinoma (relative risk 2·4) but the addition of a progestogen seems to prevent this risk.[2] Although controversial, oestrogen use has been reported to be associated with increased risk of breast cancer when taken for a long period (15 years or more) and at high doses.[20] Before they receive HRT, women should be carefully evaluated and a familial or personal history of breast cancer or endometrial carcinoma should be considered as contraindications to such treatment.

Other interventions used in the prevention of osteoporosis and fractures include administration of calcium, calcitonins, bisphosphonates, and vitamin D.

Treatment

Several treatments are approved for use in established osteoporosis; examples are those affecting bone resorption, including hormone replacement therapy, vitamin D and its derivatives alfacalcidol and calcitriol, calcitonin, intermittent bisphosphonates, anabolic steroids, calcium, thiazide diuretics, and those stimulating bone formation, including intermittent parathyroid injections and sodium fluoride. Fluoride is used for vertebral osteoporosis because it increases cancellous bone mass; however, it has been shown to alter bone qualitatively and, in one study, to increase fractures other than spinal fractures.[21]

Health policy

Burden of osteoporosis

Of all bone disorders in the elderly, osteoporosis is the most relevant from the public health point of view because of its high prevalence, the risk of dependency or death, and the large costs incurred by health services in treating fractures.

297

Prevention and treatment

Although it is likely that factors such as adequate nutrition, appropriate rate of exercise, and avoidance of smoking can affect the bone mass, the ability of public health policy to influence these factors is not yet known.

The argument for screening all women to evaluate their BMD is weak; however, screening women at 65 years of age could enhance the effects of interventions. Indeed at this age the incidence of bone loss in women is high and there is a substantial influence on bone mass; while the risk of hip fracture is still low, it will keep increasing and the benefits of intervention have been proved. The cost effectiveness of screening programmes might therefore be favourable. Bone mass measurements meet many of the essential criteria of a screening test because they identify individuals at high risk of developing fractures and are quick, safe, reliable, simple, painless, and relatively inexpensive. In particular, DEXA at the hip is currently the best predictor of hip fractures, the most devastating consequence of osteoporosis.[2]

It would be advisable for perimenopausal women to receive professional information on the risks of osteoporosis and on the risks and benefits of HRT. Several other interventions, such as calcium, calcitonins, bisphosphonates, and various forms of vitamin D, are effective in preventing osteoporotic fractures. Their use is increasing and this fact further underlies the need for targeting individuals at high risk by an effective screening programme, in order to avoid unnecessary treatments.[2]

1 Consensus Development Conference. Prophylaxis and treatment of osteoporosis. *Osteoporosis Int* 1991;**1**:114–7.
2 World Health Organization Study Group. Assessment of fracture risk and its application to screening for postmenopausal osteoporosis. *WHO Tech Rep Ser* 1994:843.
3 Eastell R, Cedel SL, Wahner HW, Riggs BL, Melton J III. Classification of vertebral fractures. *J Bone Miner Res* 1991;**6**:207–15.
4 Singh M, Nagarth AR, Maini PS. Changes in trabecular pattern of the upper end of the femur as an index of osteoporosis. *J Bone Joint Surg [Am]* 1970;**52**:457–67.
5 Heaney RP, Avioli LV, Chestnut CH III, Lappe J, Recher RR, Brandenburger GH. Osteoporotic bone fragility. Detection by ultrasound transmission velocity. *JAMA* 1989;**261**:2986–90.
6 Melton LJ III. How many women have osteoporosis? *J Bone Miner Res* 1992;**9**:1005–10.
7 Cooper C, Campion G, Melton LJ III. Hip fractures in the elderly: a world-wide projection. *Osteoporosis Int* 1992;**2**:285–9.
8 Kanis JA, Pitt FA. Epidemiology of osteoporosis. *Bone* 1992;**13**:S7–15.
9 Jacobsen SJ. Hospitalization with vertebral fracture among the aged: a national population-based study, 1986–1989. *Epidemiology* 1992;**3**:515–8.
10 Atkins RM, Duckworth T, Kanis JA. The features of algodystrophy following Colles' fracture. *J Bone Joint Surg [Br]* 1990;**72**:105–10.
11 Maggi S, Kelsey JL, Litvak J, Heyse S. Epidemiology of hip fracture: a cross-national comparison. *Osteoporosis Int* 1991;**1**:232–41.
12 Lau EMC, Cooper C. Epidemiology and prevention of osteoporosis in urbanized Asian populations. *Osteoporosis Int* 1993;**1**(suppl):S23.
13 Ho S, Bacon E, Harris T, Looker A, Maggi S. Comparison of hip fracture rates from Hong Kong and the US for 1988–89. *Am J Public Health* 1993;**83**:692–4.
14 Solomon L. Bone density in ageing Caucasian and African populations. *Lancet* 1979;**iv**: 1326–7.

15 Yano K, Wasnich RD, Vogel JM, Heilbrun LK. Bone mineral measurements among middle-aged and elderly Japanese residents in Hawaii. *Am J Epidemiol* 1984;**119**:751–5.
16 Bauer DC, Browner WS, Cauley JA. Factors associated with appendicular bone mass in older women. *Ann Intern Med* 1993;**118**:657–60.
17 Sowers MFR, Boehnke M, Jannausch ML, Crutchfield M, Corton G, Burns TL. Familiality and partitioning the variability of femoral bone mineral density in women of child-bearing age. *Calcif Tissue Int* 1992;**50**:110–5.
18 MacMahon B, Trichopulos D, Cole P. Cigarette smoking and urinary estrogen. *N Engl J Med* 1982;**307**:1062–4.
19 Heaney RP. Bone mass, nutrition, and other lifestyle factors. In Consensus Development Conference on osteoporosis. *JAMA* 1993;**95**:5A–29–32S.
20 Steinberg KK. A meta-analysis of the effect of oestrogen replacement therapy and breast cancer. *JAMA* 1991;**265**:1985–90.
21 Kanis JA. What constitutes evidence for drug efficiency in osteoporosis? *Drugs Aging* 1993;**3**:391–9.

32 Proximal femoral fracture

J GRIMLEY EVANS

Magnitude of the problem

There are appproximately 50 000 proximal femoral fractures (PFFs) annually in Britain; about a quarter of victims die within six months of injury, up to two thirds of survivors have persistent leg swelling or pain, and only a minority of survivors attain the level of their preinjury functioning.[1][2]

Definitions

PFFs are divided anatomically into intracapsular and extracapsular for purposes of treatment. Both increase steeply in incidence with age in later life but the ratio of cervical to trochanteric fractures falls from approximately 3:1 at age 60 to 1·3:1 at age 80 in women. In men the change is less dramatic, from 1·9:1 to 1·2:1 over the same age range. On average, therefore, patients with trochanteric fracture will be older and frailer than patients with cervical fracture. Otherwise the epidemiology of the two types of fracture seems similar and it is customary to discuss them as a single entity.

Sources of data

Virtually all patients with PFF are referred to hospital and generate health service data, but there are important problems in the use of routine data for the epidemiological study of PFF. Mortality data are highly unreliable as death certificates of patients who die after PFF often fail to mention the injury. Hospital admission data can be more accurate but also may have errors in coding. Studies are only reliable if restricted to all and only those cases of PFF arising within a specified period in a population defined by geographical area of residence.

The three groups of causes

Three groups of factors involved in the genesis of PFF are weakness of bone, falls, and factors determining whether a fall results in sufficient energy being transmitted to the proximal femur to break it (box 32.1).

Box 32.1—Factors in the pathogenesis of proximal femoral fracture

- Bone weakness
    Osteoporosis
    Osteomalacia
    Bone dystrophy
    Malignant disease
    Paget's disease

- Falls
    Occurrence
        Environmental hazards
        Drugs
        Sensory impairments
        Motor impairments
        Vestibular or hindbrain disorder
        Cognitive impairment
        Impairment of consciousness (for example, hypotension, epilepsy)
    Nature
        Direction (sideways, forwards, backwards)
        Energy (height, body weight)

- Absence of protective factors in falling
    Lack of subcutaneous fat
    Hard floors
    Non-protective clothing
    Muscle weakness
    Slow or inadequate protective responses
        Failure to perceive the incipient fall
            Sensory impairment
            Cognitive impairment
            Drugs
        Failure to respond appropriately
            Neurological defects
            Cognitive impairment
            Stiff or immobile joints
            Drugs
            Cold

Bone weakness

Pathological causes of bone weakness in PFF are rare. In the Newcastle population based studies[1] the proportion of patients with pathological fractures due to metastatic deposits or Paget's disease was 4% (95% confidence limits 1·5 to 7%). There is evidence of abnormalities other

301

than osteoporosis in some patients with PFF. Microfractures (possibly a consequence of osteoporosis or low bone turnover rates), mineralisation defects, and abnormal bone crystal size have been described in a proportion of cases. Surveys in the United Kingdom have found lower mean levels of serum vitamin D metabolites in patients with PFF than in controls and up to a third of cases have been reported to have histological changes of osteomalacia. Compston *et al*[3] have recently found evidence of osteomalacia in only one of 49 patients from Cardiff with PFF and suggest that the high rates described earlier were due to non-specific histological criteria.

PFF is clearly linked to osteoporosis[4] but is more closely related to bone mineral density measured at the hip than elsewhere in the body. In case–control studies the relationship of PFF to osteoporosis is more obvious at younger than older ages. This is because in later life the majority of women have bone mineral density below the level associated with strength sufficient to resist the kinetic energy of a "normal" fall and controls will be as osteoporotic as the cases. None the less, the prevalence of osteoporosis in the population, manifested in the proportion of the population falling below the fracture threshold, will still be a major determinant of the incidence of PFF.[5] Other things being equal, the epidemiology of PFF in a population will follow the prevalence of osteoporosis and its risk factors. Conversely, the three component model (bone strength, falls, nature of fall) of box 32.1 emphasises that variation in the incidence of PFF cannot necessarily be interpreted as reflecting the prevalence of osteoporosis (see chapter 31).

Falls

The great majority of PFFs in later life are incurred in a simple fall from the standing position. Some patients with PFF appear not to have broken the femur in a fall but rather to have fallen because of a spontaneous fracture, perhaps due to the accumulation of fatigue fractures of trabeculae. This is probably rare; of the 75% of patients able to give a clear history in the Newcastle studies[1] only 3% (95% confidence limits 0·5 to 5·5%) might have fallen because of a spontaneous fracture.

Several factors linked to the causes and mechanisms of falls emerge as risk factors for PFF. Body sway is linked to the risk of certain types of fall in later life and is a predictive factor of fractures.[6] Quadriceps strength is also negatively associated with PFF incidence, probably as a consequence of its effect in reducing the likelihood of a fall.[6]

It is thought that the majority of PFFs are due to direct impact on the greater trochanter and this is supported by a case–control study comparing patients with PFF with controls who had fallen without sustaining a fracture.[7] The patients with PFF were significantly more likely to have fallen sideways and the kinetic energy of the fall, calculated from body

302

weight and height of fall computed for the subject's centre of gravity, was significantly associated with PFF. Taller subjects are therefore at greater risk of PFF.

Protective factors

As described elsewhere in this volume (see Chapter 39) the incidence of falls increases steeply with later age. This increase in risk of falls is matched by a steep increase in the incidence of PFF, but the incidence of distal forearm fracture does not increase consistently at ages above 65.[5] This suggests that as one grows older one is more liable to fall, but less able to mobilise one's protective responses in time to put out an arm to break a fall (and a wrist) but protect the proximal femur. "Passive" protective factors that prevent a fall from resulting in a fracture include cushioning effects from soft carpets and protective clothing, and perhaps most importantly from subcutaneous fat.[7]

Interactions of risk factors

A general problem with the interpretation of the epidemiology of PFF is that not only are there three groups of factors involved in the genesis of fractures but some factors appear in more than one group and may even acquire thereby opposite associations with femoral fracture; for example, obesity protects against PFF by preventing osteoporosis and its effect in increasing the kinetic energy of a fall seems to be generally outweighed by the cushioning effect of subcutaneous fat.

General risk factors

Age and sex

Up to the age of 55, PFF is usually due to severe trauma, such as road traffic accidents; rates are generally low but are higher in men. At later ages in Western populations incidence rates increase exponentially at approximately the same rate in both sexes, doubling every seven years, but because the increase begins earlier in women their rates are twice as high as those in men. Annual incidence rates of PFF in England rise from 1–2 per 1000 in women and 0·5–1 per 1000 in men at age 65, to around 25 per 1000 and 10 per 1000 respectively by the age of 85. These rates are broadly similar to those given in recent reports from elsewhere in Europe.

Rates are thought to be higher in women because of their greater prevalence of osteoporosis and their greater propensity to falls. Although all Western populations that have been studied show higher incidence of PFF in women than in men in old age, in some earlier studies in other national groups—for example, in Singaporeans and black South Africans—the sex ratio was closer to unity or reversed.[8]

Race

In the United States the incidence of PFF is lower in the black population than in the white population. Rates are lower in Maoris than in Europeans in New Zealand.[8] Rates in white Americans are higher than in Japanese Americans who, despite adopting a more Western lifestyle, have rates similar to those observed in Japan.[9]

The black–white difference is largely attributable to a higher prevalence of osteoporosis in white people. It has also been suggested that the angle at which the femoral neck leaves the shaft differs between black and white people and affects the likelihood of fracture.

Levels of physical activity may be relevant to racial variation in PFF incidence in some settings. Some Asian women have a high risk of osteoporosis, attributable at least in part to dietary factors, and PFF is an important and increasing problem among urban Asians.

Secular trends

An increase in age specific incidence rates of PFF over the last 40 years has been reported from a number of countries, including Hong Kong, the United States, Spain, and Scandinavia.[8] In the United Kingdom, where the increase has been most rigorously documented, it may have ceased in the last decade. Figure 32.1 presents data on hospital admissions for PFF from the Hospital Inpatient Enquiry (HIPE) and the Oxford Record Linkage Study (ORLS).[10] Detailed analysis of the HIPE data suggest a steady increase in risk of PFF in successive cohorts of people born between 1883 and 1912. In addition, the HIPE data show a strong period effect over the years 1974–1979 that is much less apparent in the ORLS data and is possibly due to increasing accuracy of diagnostic coding. In neither set of data is there clear evidence that incidence was rising after 1980.

It is likely that no single factor has been entirely responsible for the secular increase in PFF. Several explanations have been suggested, including an increasing prevalence of osteoporosis due to a decrease in physical activity, exposure to ultraviolet light, the smoking epidemic, reduction in obesity, and poor diet. Archaeological evidence suggests that there may indeed have been a reduction in mean femoral bone density in the British population over the last 200 years[11] but there is no direct evidence on recent trends in the prevalence of either osteoporosis or falls.

One factor to be considered is body height, which is known to have increased in successive birth cohorts from the end of the nineteenth century in Britain, and, as noted above, is associated with increased risk of PFF. The kinetic energy transmitted to the femur in a fall will be equal to the potential energy of the person before the fall. This will be the product of the person's weight and the height of his or her

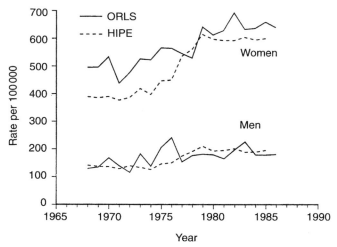

Fig 32.1   Hospital admission rates from the Oxford Record Linkage Study (ORLS) and Hospital Inpatient Enquiry (HIPE) data standardised to 1981 populations by 5-year age groups from 65 to 85 and over.[10] *In order to avoid coding errors the data are restricted to immediate admissions and relate to fractures coded to proximal femur and femur not otherwise specified (codes N820 and N822).*

centre of gravity above the ground. Assuming that the centre of gravity is at the midpoint of the body and that body weight increases in proportion to the square of height, as assumed in the computation of the body mass (Quetelet's) index, an increase in mean height of women by one inch (2·5 cm) would lead, other things being equal, to an increase in the energy generated in a fall of only 4–5%. Since the increase in height in the British population over the relevant period was at a rate of the order of one inch per 25 years, this effect would be too small to account entirely for the cohort differences in our data. The kinetic energy effect would, however, be amplified to an uncertain degree by the corresponding increase in the length of the femoral neck enhancing its fragility.[12]

Region

Identification of regional differences from published data is complicated by the interference of secular and racial effects. There do appear to be unexplained differences with rates in Norway in the early 1980s being higher than in white Californians, for example.[8] Hospital admission data in the United States suggest a north–south gradient with higher rates in the south east.[13] No explanation is apparent. There is no evidence of a north–south gradient in the United Kingdom at present.

305

Season

In the United Kingdom and North America the incidence of PFF is higher in the winter than the summer months. This is not attributable to falls outdoors in snow or ice and several explanations have been suggested.

Increased activity—Part of the effect may be due not to seasons but to increased levels of activity in unfamiliar surroundings. In Newcastle upon Tyne, England, the winter peak differed between fractures due to falls indoors and those due to falls in public places. Fractures due to falls in shops, streets, or public transport peaked in December and January, perhaps owing to the hazards of Christmas shopping and January sales. Where the fracture followed a fall indoors the highest incidence was in late spring.[5]

Nutrition—The late spring peak for fractures after falls indoors in Newcastle upon Tyne coincides with the period when blood levels of vitamin D, particularly in housebound people, tend to be low. Low levels of vitamin D activity in the winter may affect neuromuscular function, so increasing risk of falls, as well as reducing bone strength by increased parathyroid hormone secretion.

Temperature—In a study from Nottingham, England it appeared that seasonal variation in PFF was more prominent among thin people than fat and there was a close relationship between daily low temperatures and numbers of patients with PFF referred to hospital.[14] The authors suggested that the seasonal effect was due to thin undernourished old people becoming mildly hypothermic, with the consequent neuromuscular incoordination increasing the risk of falling.

The general importance of both temperature and seasonal exposure to sunlight is called into question by the observation that the magnitude of the seasonal variation in PFF incidence does not differ with latitude between the north and the south of the United States.[15] It seems most likely that the seasonal variation in PFF is a composite effect of several different causes, but its elucidation clearly has possible preventive implications.

Fluoride

Early epidemiological studies suggested that the presence of fluoride in drinking water might reduce the prevalence of osteoporosis. Experimental work in rats suggests that the relationship between bone strength and fluoride is bell shaped, with intakes above or below an optimal level resulting in bone weakness. The consensus arising from a number of studies indicates that water fluoride levels up to 1 ppm have no consistent effect one way or the other on PFF rates. At higher levels of fluoride there may be an increased risk of PFF.[16]

Sedative drugs

There is consistent evidence linking PFF to the consumption of sedative and antidepressant drugs, particularly those with a long half life.[17] The effect is presumably mediated at least in part through the genesis of falls and impairment of protective responses to falling.

Thiazide diuretics

A number of reports have suggested that thiazides protect against osteoporosis and fractures,[18] although not all studies have confirmed this. An association with risk of PFF mediated by a beneficial effect on bone strength will be confounded by an association with increased risk of falls as a result of thiazide use by patients with illnesses predisposing to falling.

Caffeine

American studies have found a relationship between PFF and caffeine intake, mostly in the form of coffee,[19] but not all studies have confirmed this. Any effect of caffeine is probably mediated through osteoporosis; it is likely to be small and confounded by smoking.

Alcohol

Several studies have found a relationship between alcohol intake and risk of PFF at ages under 65. The effect is presumably the result of an increase in the risk of trauma and an association with osteoporosis. At ages over 65, perhaps because very high intakes of alcohol are less common, there is no consistent relationship.[20]

Oestrogens

A number of case–control studies have shown a protective effect of postmenopausal hormone replacement therapy (HRT) on the incidence of PFF.[4] The finding is compatible with the known effects of oestrogens in preventing postmenopausal osteoporosis and increasing muscle strength. All case–control studies of HRT are subject to selection bias in that women who opted for HRT tended to follow a number of other health promoting lifestyles. A randomised controlled trial is needed to measure the effect of HRT on the incidence of PFF, particularly as the benefit has not yet been shown to outlast the duration of the therapy. No consistent relationship has been found between risk of PFF and age of menarche or menopause.

Smoking

Case–control studies of younger patients with PFF show an association with cigarette smoking, probably mediated through osteoporosis and lower body weight. Smoking has an antioestrogenic effect and may block the beneficial effect of postmenopausal oestrogen therapy.[21]

Physical activity

Past physical activity and moderate levels of recent activity appear to protect against PFF in case–control studies.[4] The mechanism is likely to be complex, acting through a beneficial effect on bone strength and a relationship with muscle strength and agility affecting the frequency and nature of falls. Physical activity in childhood may be important in the prevention of osteoporosis in later life.[22]

Dietary calcium

Studies in Western populations have not shown any consistent relationship between dietary calcium and PFF, although positive findings have been reported.[4] Among elderly women of Hong Kong there does appear to be an inverse association between risk of PFF and dietary calcium but their calcium intakes are very low by Western standards. The effect is probably mediated through osteoporosis.[23] It seems probable that individuals differ genetically in their ability to adapt to low calcium diets, and the ability to detect an effect of calcium intake in epidemiological or interventional studies will depend on the range of intakes in the population studied and the number of susceptible subjects included in the study sample. If it is calcium intake during childhood and early adolescence that has the most effect, case–control studies involving elderly PFF patients may not be a sensitive method of study.

Cognitive and neurological disorders

It has been known for many years that the incidence of PFF among residents in mental hospitals is higher than average. The mechanism is assumed to be mostly an increased frequency of falls, partly due to sedative drugs, but vitamin D deficiency due to lack of sunlight and consumption of enzyme inducing drugs (typically anticonvulsants) have also been suggested as causes. Case–control studies also link PFF to cognitive impairment and neurological conditions, especially parkinsonism and stroke. The mechanism is presumably through increased risk of falls. Stroke patients fracture their hemiplegic leg more often than expected by chance; this is probably due to a tendency to fall that side, together with impaired protective responses, but may also reflect disuse osteoporosis in the weak leg.

Conclusion

Age associated loss of bone mineral is universal and so partly an intrinsic (genetically determined) process, but the amount of bone laid down in childhood and its rate of loss are affected by extrinsic (environment and lifestyle) factors. Some important determinants of the frequency of trauma and its impact on the proximal femur are also extrinsic. There are therefore good prospects for partial prevention of PFF but the relevant controlled trials to assess cost effectiveness need to be performed. Apart from other interventions aimed specifically at treatment and prevention of osteoporosis, notably HRT, exercise programmes to reduce the frequency of falls and improve protective responses in falling, avoidance of sedative drugs, and dietary supplementation with calcium and vitamin D all merit study at a community level. The design of floors and floor coverings and the use of hip protectors need attention in institutional settings for older people.

1 Grimley Evans J, Prudham D, Wandless I. A prospective study of proximal femoral fracture: incidence and outcome. *Public Health* 1979;**93**:235–41.
2 Marottoli RA, Berkman LF, Cooney LM. Decline in physical function following hip fracture. *J Am Geriatr Soc* 1992;**40**:861–6.
3 Compston JE, Vedi S, Croucher PI. Low prevalence of osteomalacia in elderly patients with hip fractures. *Age Ageing* 1991;**20**:132–4.
4 Law MR, Wald NJ, Meade TW. Strategies for prevention of osteoporosis and hip fracture. *BMJ* 1991;**303**:453–9.
5 Grimley Evans J. The epidemiology of osteoporosis. *Rev Clin Gerontol* 1993;**3**:13–29.
6 Nguyen T, Sambrook P, Kelly P, *et al.* Prediction of osteoporotic fracture by postural instability and bone density. *BMJ* 1993;**307**:1111–5.
7 Greenspan SL, Myers ER, Maitland LA, Resnick NM, Hayes WC. Fall severity and bone mineral density as risk factors for hip fracture in ambulatory elderly. *JAMA* 1994;**271**: 128–33.
8 Maggi S, Kelsey JL, Litvak J, Heyse SP. Incidence of hip fractures in the elderly: a cross-national analysis. *Osteoporosis Int* 1991;**1**:232–41.
9 Ross PD, Norimatsu H, Davis JW, *et al.* A comparison of hip fracture incidence among native Japanese, Japanese Americans, and American Caucasians. *Am J Epidemiol* 1991; **133**:801–9.
10 Grimley Evans J, Seagrove V, Goldacre MJ. The increase in incidence of fractures of the proximal femur: evidence from the Oxford Record Linkage Study. In preparation.
11 Lees B, Molleson T, Arnett TR, Stevenson JC. Differences in proximal femur bone density over two centuries. *Lancet* 1993;**341**:673–5.
12 Reid IR, Chin K, Evans MC, Jones JG. Relation between increase in length of hip axis in older women between 1950s and 1990s and increase in age specific rates of hip fracture. *BMJ* 1994;**309**:508–9.
13 Jacobsen SJ, Goldberg J, Miles TP, Brody JA, Stiers W, Rimm AA. Regional variation in the incidence of hip fracture. *JAMA* 1990;**264**:500–2.
14 Bastow MD, Rawlings J, Allison SP. Undernutrition, hypothermia, and injury in elderly women with fractured femur: an injury response to altered metabolism? *Lancet* 1983;**i**: 143–6.
15 Jacobsen SJ, Goldberg J, Miles TP, Brody JA, Stiers W, Rimm AA. Seasonal variation in the incidence of hip fracture among white persons aged 65 years and older in the United States, 1984–1987. *Am J Epidemiol* 1991;**133**:996–1004.
16 Gordon SL, Corbin SB. Summary of workshop on drinking water fluoride influence on hip fracture and bone health (National Institutes of Health, 10 April 1991). *Osteoporosis Int* 1992;**2**:109–17.
17 Ray WA, Griffin MR, Malcolm E. Cyclic antidepressants and the risk of hip fracture. *Arch Intern Med* 1991;**151**:754–6.

18 LaCroix AZ, Wienpahl J, White LR, *et al*. Thiazide diuretic agents and the incidence of hip fracture. *N Engl J Med* 1990;**322**:286–90.
19 Kiel DP, Felson DT, Hannan MT, Andersen JL, Wilson PWF. Caffeine and the risk of hip fracture: the Framingham study. *Am J Epidemiol* 1990;**132**:675–84.
20 Felson DT, Kiel DP, Anderson JJ, *et al*. Alcohol consumption and hip fractures: the Framingham study. *Am J Epidemiol* 1988;**128**:1102–10.
21 Kiel DP, Baron JA, Anderson JJ, Hannan MT, Felson DT. Smoking eliminates the protective effect of oral estrogens on the risk for hip fracture among women. *Ann Intern Med* 1992;**116**:716–21.
22 VandenBergh MFQ, DeMan SA, Witteman JCM, Hofman A, Trouerbach Th, Grobbee DE. Physical activity, calcium intake, and bone mineral content in children in The Netherlands. *J Epidemiol Community Health* 1995;**49**:299–304.
23 Lau E, Donnan S, Barker DJP, Cooper C. Physical activity and calcium intake in fracture of the proximal femur in Hong Kong. *BMJ* 1988;**297**:441–3.

33 Arthritis

ELIZABETH M BADLEY, LINDA ROTHMAN

Definitions and diagnostic criteria

This chapter will focus on osteoarthritis (OA), which is a major cause of morbidity and disability in the elderly and the most frequently occurring type of arthritis in the population. OA has a population prevalence of 10% or higher (see below), compared with a prevalence of around 1% for rheumatoid arthritis (RA).[1] RA is an autoimmune disorder that causes inflammation of the joints and can also affect other organ systems of the body. It is an important cause of disability in the population; however, even though a smaller proportion of people with OA than RA experience disability, because of its much higher overall prevalence OA is the most frequent cause of disabling arthritis. Data from both American and British population studies show that there are more than seven people with OA and severe disability (for example, dependence in activities of daily living) for one with RA.[2 3]

OA is a degenerative disorder that is characterised by destruction of articular cartilage followed by changes in subchondral bone.[1] It primarily affects the knees, hips, and small joints of the hands and spine. Progressive pain is the chief complaint, together with joint stiffness, resulting in loss of physical function, interruption of sleep, psychological stress, and change in quality of life.[4] Radiographic features associated with the disease include joint space narrowing and osteophytes (bony spurs) at the margins of the joints.[1]

Diagnosis of OA is difficult for a variety of reasons. There is no clear disease marker and there is great heterogeneity in the nature of the disease.[4] Although there is agreement that consideration of pathological, radiological, and clinical components are necessary in the diagnosis of OA, there is no consistent correlation between these different manifestations of the disease. It has been estimated that fewer than 50% of all those with radiographically identifiable OA have symptoms.[1] It is not yet known why so many people with radiographic evidence of OA have no symptoms or disability.

The most recent diagnostic criteria for OA have been developed by the American College of Rheumatology.[1] As the disease presents differently in each of the joints, criteria have been developed for the knee, hip, and hand separately. The criteria are based on combinations of clinical, radiographic, and laboratory evidence. They have been found to provide approximately 90% sensitivity and 90% specificity.[1]

Risk

Mortality from arthritis is low; the major impact in the population is in terms of morbidity and disability. The burden of arthritis in the population has been underestimated as a result of its low mortality rates and its insidious onset. Problems in defining disease onset and lack of longitudinal data make the measurement of the incidence of OA, and musculoskeletal disorders in general, very difficult.[1] As a result, very little data exist that measure the incidence of OA. Prevalence data indicate that OA increases with age, which is the most powerful risk factor for the disease.[2 5-7] Other risk factors for OA are described in following sections.

Magnitude of the problem

Estimates of the prevalence of OA can vary depending on which diagnostic method is used, namely through radiographic or symptomatic evidence, self report, or disability. Generally estimates for arthritis are highest when using radiographic diagnosis, somewhat lower for symptomatic disease, and lowest for disease resulting in functional limitations.[5]

The prevalence of OA in the population aged 65 years and older ranges from 33% for symptomatic disease[6] to more than 80% for OA defined by radiographic changes.[1 7] Data on the prevalence of OA of the knee from the Framingham population survey show an overall prevalence of 10% for symptomatic OA and 33% for radiographic OA for people aged 63 years and older. There was a linear increase with age in the prevalence of radiographic OA of the knee, which was found in over half of women aged 80 years and older.[8] Generally, the prevalence of both symptomatic disease and radiographic changes increases markedly with increased age.[7 9]

Arthritis is the leading chronic condition and the most frequent cause of long term disability in the population aged 65 years and older.[10 11] The prevalence of arthritis associated disability in the senior population is over 10%.[2 3 5] OA leads to extensive use of health care resources and is a leading cause of economic loss to those affected.[11 12 13] It is the most common condition for which knee and hip replacement procedures are performed and the most common disease affecting hand function in the elderly.

Variation

Time

No data are available with regards to secular trends in incidence or prevalence of arthritis. With the ageing of the population in Western societies, however, it has been estimated that the number of adults disabled by arthritis will almost double in many Western countries by the year 2020.[14]

Although climate does not appear to be a factor in the pathogenesis of the disease, some work has been done on seasonal variation in the number of medical consultations for symptoms related to OA. The number of medical consultations for OA has been found to peak in spring and autumn, when climatic influences are the most variable.[15] Climatic factors, which have been found in some studies to be related to pain in OA, include temperature, precipitation, barometric pressure, and wind speed.[16]

Place

Geographic differences in prevalence have been reported, although they are often difficult to interpret because of differences in sampling procedure and diagnostic consistency.[9] Greater variation has been found in the distribution of hip OA, with low rates reported among black populations from Jamaica, South Africa, Nigeria, and Liberia. Low rates have also been found in Asian Indians and Hong Kong Chinese. Higher rates of hip OA were generally evident in Europe. Hand osteoarthritis was, however, as common in Chinese as in Europeans. It has been suggested that racial differences in hip OA may be indicative of a greater variety of causes of OA in the hip than in other joints.

Person

The individual risk factors for OA can be divided into two categories: (a) factors related to a generalised susceptibility to the condition; and (b) mechanical factors resulting in abnormal biomechanical loading of joints.[17] Risk factors for OA included in the first category are increased age, obesity, heredity, and female sex.[9 17] Factors that are negatively associated with OA are the presence of osteoporosis (especially at the hip joint) and cigarette smoking. In some population based studies cigarette smoking has been found to have a protective influence on the development of OA.

Mechanical factors that are associated with OA include trauma at the joint, joint incongruency, and occupational or leisure physical activities involving repetitive use of particular joint groups.[9 17]

Determinants of osteoarthritis

Individual factors, such as age, obesity, heredity, sex, and abnormal biomechanical loading of joints, are strong determinants of OA in individuals and in the population in general. Low socioeconomic status has also been associated with increased rates of arthritis.[6] Determinants of secular and geographic variability in the rates of OA have not been adequately explained.

Intervention

Primary prevention

There has been little work done in the area of primary prevention, which may be due to the lack of longitudinal data. There is a potential for primary prevention with a focus on diet and physical activity to reduce the effects of obesity and to maintain the integrity of the musculoskeletal system to prevent joint injury. Preventive measures should be directed toward the reduction of occupational hazards related to repetitive movements and joint trauma as well as toward injury prevention in sport.

Secondary prevention

Currently there is no specific therapy available that has been found to be efficacious in preventing or slowing the progression of OA. Much of the medical management of OA is devoted to symptomatic relief of the disease by reducing pain, and preserving and improving physical function. Drug therapy is used primarily for the symptomatic relief of pain. The use of drugs in the management of OA is controversial.[18] Surgical interventions, such as arthroplasty, osteotomy, and joint fusion, are also important, in particular in the treatment of severe OA.[118] Total joint replacement is an efficacious and cost effective procedure for individuals with advanced hip and knee disease.

Exercise as a potential treatment of OA has been neglected in the literature. Limited work has been carried out to look at the effects of exercise. Some evidence suggests that cartilage repair occurs when biomechanical factors are altered and that individuals with OA are able to tolerate weight bearing exercises.[19] The long term effects of exercise on the musculoskeletal system have not, however, been studied in a controlled manner. It is generally thought that therapeutic exercise, as well as general fitness and exercise programmes, may be positive interventions for the prevention and treatment of this disease. More work needs to be done in this area.

Acute treatment

OA is generally slowly progressive in nature and may take years to evolve. Over time, symptoms can come and go with some periods of flare when symptoms are especially severe. As there is no acute phase of OA, acute treatment is generally not appropriate for this condition.

Rehabilitation

Physiotherapy and occupational therapy are important in the management of OA, although there has been little research to date investigating efficacy of therapy interventions.[18] Therapy strategies include exercises that aim to maintain muscular strength and joint range of motion, joint protection techniques to reduce pain and improve joint alignment, energy conservation to prevent muscle fatigue, and supportive devices, such as insoles and splints, to protect weakened joints. The provision of assistive devices, such as mobility devices and home adaptations, are also important to facilitate independence.

Hydrotherapy has been used by physical, occupational, and recreational therapists to improve an individual's physical abilities, such as strength, range of motion, and endurance, using water as a therapeutic medium. Despite numerous anecdotal reports that cite the benefits of hydrotherapy, there are few studies that have critically evaluated its efficacy in the management of arthritis. There is a need for a controlled study of the use of hydrotherapy for people with OA.

Recent developments in the understanding of OA are redirecting the emphasis of management of the disease toward non-medical interventions and multidisciplinary strategies. Education provided to patients to assist them to adapt and cope with their disability is felt to be essential in the management of OA. Educational and community support interventions have been found to have a positive impact on many aspects of health status, including knowledge, pain, compliance with medication, emotional and social well being, and disability.[18 20] Programmes that include and emphasise problem solving, self efficacy, and endurance exercise may prove more effective than traditional programmes that emphasise pathophysiology, range of movement, and joint protection.

Health policy

OA presents as a major burden to individuals, their families, and the population as a whole. As indicated above it is a major cause of ill health and disability in the population and people with OA have been reported to use health care services at an extremely high rate. Despite the high prevalence and consistently high contribution of OA to long term disability, the population impact of this disorder is insufficiently appreciated in comparison to conditions such as heart disease and cancer, which are associated with high mortality.

OA has often been incorrectly dismissed as a normal component of ageing by both physicians and patients. The moderate disabling potential of OA together with its slowly progressive nature may also obscure the large overall population impact, which does not lend the same sense of urgency as that given to rare diseases with a higher disablement rate.[11] As a result the public and the professional perception of OA is that it is not an important or compelling health problem.

There is currently little available that has been found to affect the disease progression of OA. There are, however, many options with regards to

315

symptomatic relief, which can help to improve individuals' quality of life. Policies directed at the treatment of OA should emphasise the importance of developing strategies to increase physician awareness of management options, and to further develop services in the community for people with osteoarthritis. Primary prevention of OA is also an important option for future directions in its management. Evidence indicates that efforts to reduce the impact of OA and arthritis in general could substantially improve the health of the population and greatly reduce the cost of health services.

1 Schumacher HR, Klippel JH, Koopman WJ, editors. *Primer on the rheumatic diseases.* 10th ed. Atlanta: Arthritis Foundation, 1993.

2 LaPlante MP. *Data on disability from the National Health Interview Survey 1983–1985. An InfoUse report.* Washington: US National Institute on Disability and Rehabilitation Research, 1988.

3 Badley EM, Tennant A. Impact of disablement due to rheumatic disorders in a British population: estimates of severity and prevalence from the Calderdale rheumatic disablement survey. *Ann Rheum Dis* 1993;**52**:6–13.

4 Dieppe P. Osteoarthritis: clinical features and diagnostic problems. In: Klippel JH, Dieppe PA, editors. *Rheumatology.* London: Mosby–Year Book Europe, 1994;7:4.1–16.

5 Reynolds DL, Chambers LW, Badley EM, *et al.* Physical disability among Canadians reporting musculoskeletal diseases. *J Rheumatol* 1992;**19**:1020–30.

6 Cunningham LA, Kelsey JL. Epidemiology of musculoskeletal impairments and associated disability. *Am J Public Health* 1984;**74**:574–9.

7 Lawrence RC, Hochberg MC, Kelsey JL, *et al.* Estimates of the prevalence of selected arthritic and musculoskeletal diseases in the United States. *J Rheumatol* 1989;**16**:427–41.

8 Felson DT. The epidemiology of knee osteoarthritis: results from the Framingham osteoarthritis study. *Semin Arthritis Rheum* 1990;**20**:42–50.

9 Felson DT. Epidemiology of hip and knee osteoarthritis. *Epidemiol Rev* 1988;**10**:1–27.

10 Badley EM, Rasooly E, Webster GK. Relative importance of musculoskeletal disorders as a cause of chronic health problems, disability, and health care utilization: findings from the 1990 Ontario health survey. *J Rheumatol* 1994;**21**:505–12.

11 Verbrugge LM. Physical and social disability in adults. In: Hibbard H, Nutting P, Grady ML, editors. *AHCPR conference proceedings. Primary care research: theory and methods.* Washington: US Department of Health and Human Services, Public Health Service, Agency for Health Care Policy and Research, 1991.

12 Kramer JS, Yelin EH, Epstein WV. Social and economic impacts of four musculoskeletal conditions: a study using national community-based data. *Arthritis Rheum* 1983;**26**:901–7.

13 Pincus T, Mitchell JM, Burkhauser RV. Substantial work disability and earnings losses in individuals less than age 65 with osteoarthritis: comparisons with rheumatoid arthritis. *J Clin Epidemiol* 1989;**42**:449–57.

14 Badley EM. Population projections and the effect on rheumatology. *Ann Rheum Dis* 1991;**50**:3–6.

15 Harris CM. Further observations on seasonal variation. 1. Osteoarthritis. *J R Coll Gen Pract* 1986;**36**:316–8.

16 Laborde JM, Dando WA, Powers MJ. Influence of weather on osteoarthritics. *Soc Sci Med* 1986;**23**:549–54.

17 Cooper C. Osteoarthritis: epidemiology. In: Klippel JH, Dieppe PA, editors. *Rheumatology.* London: Mosby–Year Book Europe, 1994;7:3.1–4.

18 Dieppe P. Osteoarthritis: management. In: Klippel JH, Dieppe PA, editors. *Rheumatology.* London: Mosby–Year Book Europe, 1994;7:8.1–8.

19 McKeag DB. The relationship of osteoarthritis and exercise. *Clin Sports Med* 1992;**11**:471–87.

20 Buckelew SP, Parker JC. Coping with arthritis pain: a review of the literature. *Arthritis Care Res* 1989;**2**:136–45.

34 Breast cancer

ASTRID FLETCHER

International and temporal trends

Worldwide, breast cancer is the most common cancer in women, comprising 18% of all cancers.[1] The relative importance of breast cancer shows some geographical variation; for example, in those countries (including the United Kingdom) where there has been a marked increase in smoking prevalence in women, lung cancer incidence has increased exponentially and overtaken breast cancer as the most common cause of cancer incidence and mortality in women. The highest rates for breast cancer are found in European and North American countries and the lowest in Asia. Even within European countries there are marked differences in the rates. The United Kingdom has the highest mortality from breast cancer both in Europe and worldwide, while the Mediterranean countries experience approximately a third of the rate (fig 34.1).[2]

Breast cancer incidence rates rise with age but the rate of increase is attenuated around and after the age of 50. It is considered that the slowed rate of increase around the menopause reflects the aetiological importance of hormonal factors. At ages 65–69 years the rate is almost double that of women aged 40–49 years and in elderly women breast cancer contributes about 20% of female deaths.

In all countries for which data are available, breast cancer incidence rates have been increasing in all age groups (with the exception of China). At least a part of this increase could be due to increased identification through screening programmes. It might also reflect temporal changes in breast cancer risk factors, such as early age at menarche and nulliparity. Age at menarche has decreased considerably in most countries, probably reflecting nutritional factors, while social trends have led to decreases in fertility.

It is interesting to speculate that the changes in hormonal patterns in women that unfavourably influence breast cancer rates may have produced considerable benefits on coronary heart disease (CHD) rates. Striking temporal differences in the patterns of CHD mortality for men and women are observed in all countries for which data are available.[3] In women, apart from in eastern Europe, all countries have shown a marked decline in the rate, including countries where the pattern for male CHD mortality has been in the opposite direction. Even in eastern European countries the trends for women are noticeably different from those for men. Hormonal

317

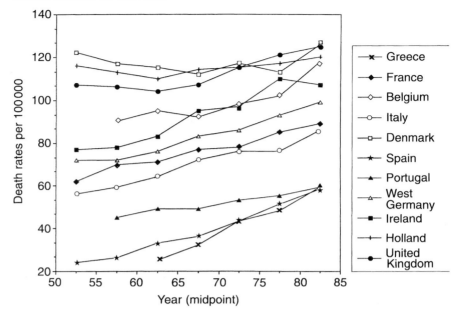

Fig 34.1   Death rates from breast cancer in women aged 65–74 years in some European countries.

factors are generally considered to be the major protective factor explaining the differences in absolute CHD risk between men and women, which persists even at equivalent levels of risk factors. A plausible explanation for the consistent fall in CHD mortality in women across different countries is a change in factors influencing the female hormonal status. Earlier age at menarche and reduced parity are temporal trends that may favourably influence possible protective endogenous hormones.

Increases in breast cancer mortality paralleling the rise in incidence have been observed in countries with low incidence rates but have also been observed in the oldest age group in many European countries with high incidence rates (fig 34.1). In other countries, such as the United States, the rate of increase of incident breast cancer has not been matched by the rate of increase in breast cancer mortality. The increase in identification of early cancers with a more favourable prognosis, as a result of increased surveillance and screening, may in part explain the gap. Case fatality rates, which are a measure of the difference between incidence and mortality, vary considerably between countries, with some countries, including the United Kingdom, having case fatality rates exceeding 40%. At present these striking differences are not fully understood.

Within countries there is considerable variation by sociodemographic factors. Breast cancer is more common in single women and in women of higher socioeconomic status, with these groups having almost 50% excess of this cancer compared with married or widowed women or women from the lowest socioeconomic groups.

Determinants of breast cancer

Hormonal factors

The influence of hormonal factors is suggested from studies showing the excess risk associated with nulliparity, late age at first birth, early menarche, and late menopause but the physiological basis remains poorly understood.

Oral contraceptives are known to increase breast cancer risk in young women but the risk does not extend to postmenopausal women. Of considerable relevance to the elderly is the debate over postmenopausal oestrogen and breast cancer risk. Increasing use of hormone replacement therapy has been postulated as at least a part of the explanation for the sharp increase in breast cancer incidence in postmenopausal women observed in the United States.[4] There have been several meta-analyses of studies of postmenopausal women taking oestrogen, with two of the meta-analyses reporting no increase in risk and two a small association. It is possible that excess risk associated with oestrogen use exists only for women who are already at excess risk by virtue of factors such as family history of breast cancer, nulliparity, and increased age at first pregnancy[5] or with duration of use of 10 years or more.[6] In the other meta-analysis that reported a positive association the increased risk of breast cancer was observed with use of oestrogen given after a natural menopause.[7] The great majority of studies have taken place in the United States, where unopposed oestrogen use was more common. In contrast, European studies have included women taking combined oestrogen and progestin preparations. The studies have had mixed results, showing both an increased risk with the combination therapy and no additional adverse effect of the progestin component.[6]

Dietary factors

A correlation is observed across countries between a high fat diet and breast cancer rates but the evidence for a relationship within populations is weaker and less consistent.[8]

Obesity is a strong and independent risk factor for postmenopausal breast cancer, whereas the effects of excess alcohol consumption continue to be controversial. It is possible that a weekly consumption of more than 21 units of alcohol (1 unit = 8 g alcohol) is associated with an increase in risk[9] but even moderate alcohol consumption may increase risk. In the nurses' health study, consumption of 3–9 drinks weekly was associated with a 30% excess breast cancer risk, and for more than nine drinks a week there was a 60% increase in risk.[10]

Intervention

Screening for breast cancer

The effectiveness of mammographic screening for breast cancer has been demonstrated by randomised controlled trials showing an overall 30% reduction in mortality from the disease.[11 12] The upper age limits of the trials ranged from 64 to 74. The largest reduction in breast cancer mortality in the trials was observed in women aged 50–69 (29%). Only the Swedish two county study included women up to the age of 74 years and showed a relative risk for ages 70–74 of 0·77 (95% CI 0·5 to 1·3) after an average eight years of follow up, which was reduced to 0·98 (0·6 to 1·5) after 12 years of follow up.[12] The wide confidence interval and inconsistency with the earlier results published by the two county study leave considerable uncertainty about the case for screening elderly women, at least in the age range 70–74 years. For women aged 65–69 years there is consistent evidence of benefit from screening, with 30% reduction in breast cancer mortality (95% CI 50 to 90%).

Reduction in mortality from breast cancer is not the only end point of screening programmes, although undoubtedly it is the paramount objective. Identification of early cases may also result in treatment options that are more favourable to the patient's quality of life; for example, in the Edinburgh trial conservation therapy rather than mastectomy was more frequent in screened women, reflecting smaller tumour size.[13]

Regular screening by physician examination of the breasts is sometimes advocated for elderly women. The poor sensitivity of palpation and inspection, especially in large breasted postmenopausal women, suggests that this is a poor screening method when used without mammography.

Self examination of the breast

The effect of breast self examination on the prognosis of breast cancer is highly controversial.[11] Although a number of studies have reported favourable effects, with the result from a meta-analysis showing a 40% reduction in tumour size in women with self report of self examination,[14] and other studies showing an increase in survival, there are considerable methodological biases in such studies. Randomised controlled trials in the United Kingdom, Russia, and China are still underway but to date results from these offer little evidence of benefit from breast self examination. In the 10 year follow up of the British study no reduction in mortality was observed in the districts where women were instructed in self examination, but the uptake for self examination instruction was low. Five year results from the Russian trial indicated no difference in cancer detection rate or tumour size and class but more self referrals in the self examination group to hospital clinics. Given the poor sensitivity of self examination (26% compared with 90% for mammography), together with the high number of false positives, it seems unlikely that self examination can be promoted because most cancers will be missed and there will be a large number of unnecessary referrals for further tests.[11] There is also evidence that women are reluctant to practise breast self examination because of the fear of detecting a lump. It is probably better to advise women about changes in the breast that may be indicative of cancer so that they are encouraged to report early. This is particularly important in older women because for a range of cancers, including breast cancer, studies have shown that elderly people tend to present at a later stage than younger and middle aged people. This factor alone accounts for the apparent poorer survival of elderly people with cancer rather than age alone.[15] The reasons for delay in presenting with symptoms are complex and include, in addition to age, lower educational levels and psychological factors. Initiatives aimed at improving early presentation in elderly people are required.

Management of elderly people with cancer may also be suboptimal; for example, in the United States it has been shown that elderly patients with breast cancer receive less active treatment,[16] although there is no consistent evidence to support the widely held view that breast cancers presenting in late life are less aggressive.

Health policy

Strategies for breast cancer prevention

It is difficult to identify strategies to reduce the burden of breast cancer in elderly women because many of the established risk factors for breast cancer, such as reproductive and menstrual history, are not amenable to modification in later life. The opportunities for risk factor modification in the elderly are also limited by uncertainty about the likely latency period of breast cancer and the effect of duration of exposures on risk.

Reduction in postmenopausal obesity would seem to be a sensible strategy for elderly women because it is unlikely to do harm and will have additional benefits on cardiovascular risk factors.

Advice on drinking is more controversial and needs to take account of the association between alcohol and cardiovascular diseases. Moderate alcohol intake, 1–2 drinks daily, protects against CHD and ischaemic stroke but increases the risk of subarachnoid haemorrhage.[3] In an American population of predominantly middle aged people the overall risk associated with different amounts of alcohol consumption was optimal for women at intakes of less than 1–2 drinks a day but more than once a month.[17] Men consuming more than six drinks a day had a relative risk of 1·3 compared with those who never drank, while women drinking this amount had an excess risk of 2·2 compared with non-drinkers, in part reflecting the added risk for women drinkers of breast and other cancers. Similar data that would guide recommendations on alcohol intake in elderly people are not available and might differ, because CHD is a more common cause of morbidity and mortality in elderly women than is breast cancer. It is unlikely that recommendations to maximise CHD protection by increased drinking would be acceptable as the social and psychological consequences might be profound.

Similarly advice on hormone replacement therapy must take account of the possible adverse effects on breast cancer against the possible benefits on cardiovascular diseases and osteoporosis. For postmenopausal women there is substantial evidence that oestrogen replacement therapy is associated with a lower risk of CHD, with an overall estimate of a 44% reduction in CHD.[3] In nearly all these studies unopposed conjugated oestrogen without progestin was given. Oestrogens have beneficial effects on a range of cardiovascular risk factors, most noticeably they increase high density lipoprotein cholesterol and lower low density lipoprotein cholesterol, and may improve blood flow. Adverse effects of unopposed oestrogens on endometrial cancer risk make it unlikely that unopposed oestrogen will be prescribed other than for women without uteri. The risks and benefits of modern combination therapies, such as oestrogen–progestin, require to be fully examined in a randomised trial evaluating their long term effects on cardiovascular disease, osteoporotic fractures, and breast cancer. Current trials examining these and other interventions are underway in other countries and are in preparation in the United Kingdom. The women's health initiative study in the United States will examine the effects of a low fat diet, hormone replacement therapy, and a calcium/vitamin D component on the risk of CHD, breast cancer, colon cancer, and hip fracture. Other breast cancer prevention trials underway in the United States and the United Kingdom include the therapeutic agent tamoxifen.

Screening policy

Population screening for breast cancer has been established in many western European and North American countries. In the United Kingdom screening started in 1988. Women aged 50–64 years are being screened with a single view mammography, initially at a three year interval, although this will be kept under review. Women over the age of 65 years are not included in the British screening programme on the basis of expected poor response rates, although screening is available on demand. Some recent data suggest that response rates may be higher than anticipated[18] and, although lower than at younger ages, the higher incidence of breast cancer in older women is likely to produce a higher yield of preventable deaths, at least in the age range 65–74 years.

In contrast, the National Board of Health and Welfare of Sweden includes women up to the age of 74 in its screening programme recommendations. In the Netherlands, the National Council of Public Health recommends screens every two years in the age group 50–69. In the United States a large number of professional and government bodies recommend annual mammograms in women 50 years or older.[19]

At present there is little optimism for preventing breast cancer in elderly women by modification of risk factors but randomised trials of nutritional and other interventions are underway. Any preventive recommendations for elderly people must take account of risks from other diseases and weigh the relative benefits of preventing one disease against the possible undesirable effects on others. With respect to screening programmes, there seems inadequate justification for excluding the 65–69 age group from breast cancer screening but the case for including women over 70 is less certain. Alternative study designs to randomised trials, such as case–control studies, could be used to explore the possible benefits for this age group. Moreover, for elderly women it is important to consider how we can improve their relatively poor survival, reflecting both delay in presentation and less than optimal treatment.

1 Ursin G, Bernstein L, Pike MC. Breast cancer. In: Doll R, Fraumeni JF, Muir CS, editors. *Trends in cancer incidence and mortality.* Cold Spring Harbor: Imperial Cancer Research Fund and Cold Spring Harbor Laboratory Press, 1994:241–64.
2 World Health Organization. *World health statistics 1988.* Geneva: WHO.
3 Fletcher AE. Epidemiology of cardiovascular disease in women. *Vasc Med Rev* 1995;6: 7–21.
4 Barret Connor E. Postmenopausal estrogen and the risk of breast cancer. *Ann Epidemiol* 1994;4:177–80.
5 Steinberg KK, Thacker SB, Smith SJ, *et al.* A meta analysis of the effect of estrogen replacement therapy on the risk of breast cancer. *JAMA* 1991;265:1985–9.
6 Hunt K, Vessey M, McPherson K, Coleman M. Long-term surveillance of mortality and cancer incidence in women receiving hormone replacement therapy. *Br J Obstet Gynaecol* 1987;94:620–35.
7 Sillero-Arenas M, Delgado Rodriguez M, Rodrigues-Canteras R, Bueno-Cavanillas A, Galvez-Vargas R. Menopausal hormone replacement therapy and cancer. A meta analysis. *Obstet Gynecol* 1992;79:286–94.
8 Hunter DJ, Willett WC, Diet, body size and breast cancer. *Epidemiol Rev* 1993;15:110–32.
9 Longnecker MP, Beilin JA, Orza MJ, Chalmers TC. A meta analysis of alcohol consumption in relation to breast cancer. *JAMA* 1988;260:252–6.
10 Colditz GA. A prospective assessment of moderate alcohol intake and major chronic diseases. *Ann Epidemiol* 1990;1:167–77.
11 Austoker J. Screening and self examination for breast cancer. *BMJ* 1994;309:168–74.
12 Nystrom L, Rutqvist LE, Wall S, *et al.* Breast cancer screening with mammography: overview of Swedish randomised trials. *Lancet* 1993;341:973–8.
13 Roberts MM, Alexander FE, Anderson TJ, *et al.* Edinburgh trial of screening for breast cancer: mortality at seven years. *Lancet* 1989;335:241–6.
14 Hill D, White V, Jolley D, Mapperson K. Self examination of the breast: is it beneficial? Meta analysis of studies investigating breast self examination and extent of disease in patients with breast cancer. *BMJ* 1988;297:271–5.
15 Holmes F, Hearne E III. Cancer stage-to-age relationship: implications for cancer screening in the elderly. *J Am Geriatr Soc* 1981;29:55–7.
16 Greenfield S, Blanco D, Elashoff R, Ganz P. Patterns of care related to age of breast cancer patients. *JAMA* 1987;257:2766–70.
17 Klatsky AL, Armstrong MA, Friedman GD. Alcohol and mortality. *Ann Intern Med* 1992; 117:646–54.
18 Hobbs P, Kay C, Friedman EHI, *et al.* Response by women aged 65–79 to invitation for screening for breast cancer by mammography: a pilot study. *BMJ* 1990;301:1314–6.
19 Fletcher A. Controversies in screening for breast and cervix cancer. In: George J, Ebrahim S, editors. *Health care for older women.* Oxford: Oxford University Press, 1992:

35 Prostatic cancer

KLIM McPHERSON

Definitions and diagnostic criteria

Prostatic cancer is a common cause of death in elderly men. In England and Wales in 1992 8700 men died of prostatic cancer, of whom only 200 were aged under 60. In contrast to the other common gender specific cancer for women, breast cancer, the incidence and mortality are concentrated among the elderly (table 35.1). At age 50, women suffer 20 times the mortality rate from breast cancer than men from prostate cancer, but mortality rates at age 85 or more from prostate cancer become twice as high as those from breast cancer among elderly women. As the longevity of the male population increases so the burden of morbidity and mortality from prostate cancer will, in the absence of adequate preventive measures, become increasingly important.

Table 35.1   Cancer death rates (per million): England and Wales 1992

Age (years)	Prostate	Lung (male)	Lung (female)	Breast (female)
15–24		1		1
25–35		4	3	36
35–44		67	41	203
45–54	21	380	197	557
55–64	239	1547	709	949
65–74	1206	4398	1669	1295
75–84	3919	6667	1924	1963
85 +	7627	7306	1368	3097

The disease has a wide variation in clinical progression and manifestation: in some patients the disease metastasises rapidly and causes death within a year of diagnosis, whereas in others with localised disease a prostatectomy may cure the patient. About two thirds of patients appear clinically to have localised disease. The ability to distinguish histologically between in situ and invasive cancer in the prostate is limited. The disease can present with symptoms similar to obstructive benign hypertrophy or metastatic disease with bone pain. Early cancer is symptomless and can only be diagnosed by a combination of digital rectal examination, serum prostate specific antigen (PSA) determinations, transrectal ultrasonography, and biopsy.

324

The natural course of the disease among the 20% of elderly men with undetected (or detected) foci of prostate cancer is very inadequately understood.

Magnitude of the problem

In the European Union it is estimated that, by age 75, 33% of men will have latent cancer, 4% will have been diagnosed, and 1% will have died from the disease.[1] In a recent study[2] in the United States the incidence of prostate cancer was reported to have increased by 6·4% a year in the years between 1983 and 1989. This increase was attributed in part to increased detection of early stage disease because no increase was observed in metastatic cancer. An increase of 30% a year in the rate of radical prostatectomy among men aged 60–80 was also observed during the same period. In this period no increase in mortality was observed and moreover no correlation was observed between incidence rates for an area and their corresponding mortality rates.

Hence prostate cancer represents a very common cancer among elderly men, a common problem, and a common cause of death. Yet effective and efficient interventions to reduce the burden of this disease have yet to be developed, tested, and implemented. Management of localised prostate cancer is controversial and highly variable with both time and place.[3] Provision of screening facilities are scandalously haphazard and, if provided, based on inadequate evidence of benefit.

Variation: time and place

Trends in incidence in the United States have already been mentioned and the greatest problem with the interpretation of these figures is the changing methods of detection in attempts to diagnose the disease at a curable stage. This obviously leads to designation of prostate cancer among men who may have no disease, no life threatening disease, or possibly some men who otherwise would not have been diagnosed (or suffered) at all during their lives. Notwithstanding this consideration a doubling of incidence between the 1940s and the 1970s has been reported in the Connecticut cancer registry.[4] Since the 1960s prostate cancer incidence rates have increased in nearly all regions with continuous incidence registries.[5] An 11-fold increase has been observed in Japan during the past 30 years,[6] which appears to be, at least in part, consistent with changing rates of cancer detection at autopsy.[7]

In terms of variations by country table 35.2 gives a selection of the reported age standardised annual incidence rates per 100 000 males in the middle to late 1970s. Thus the disease is more common among black males than white males (+60%) and nearly a hundred times as common among black males from North America than Chinese males. Obviously part of this difference will be attributable to more aggressive screening and detection strategies. It does seem that international studies tend to find a similar prevalence of latent cancer at autopsy between populations who show a systematic variation in recorded incidence of up to 10-fold.[8]

Table 35.2   Reported age standardised annual incidence rates per 100 000 males in the middle to late 1970s

Place	Population	Incidence
Atlanta	Black	96
Bay area	Black	92
New Orleans	Black	72
Seattle	All	59
Connecticut	All	43
England and Wales	All	30
Nigeria	All	13
Poland	All	6
India	All	6
Hong Kong	All	5
Japan	All	3
Shanghai	All	1

The lifetime risk of prostate cancer can be seen in table 35.3, in which the cumulative risk of the disease is compared with breast cancer in women in four geographic areas.

Table 35.3   Cumulative risk (%) of breast cancer in women and prostate cancer in men up to age 74 years

Place	Breast	Prostate
California	4·0	3·1
Alameda County (black)	9·5	11·7
Birmingham UK	7·2	2·6
Japan	2·9	0·8

Determinants

The risk factors for this disease have largely to do with sexual history, diet, and family history. It is a hormonal cancer because there is evidence that hormonal milieu affects both the aetiology and the progression of the disease. Research has found strong associations with numbers of premarital sexual partners and a history of venereal disease—particularly a history of syphilis. Trends in the mortality rates for prostate cancer also appear to correlate with trends in gonorrhoea.[9] The argument is that exposure to the infection before the antibiotic era might have an effect resulting in cancer detected some 45 years later.

As far as diet is concerned the findings appear to indicate an effect associated with increased fat consumption, possibly eggs, cheese, and meat.

The effect is around a fourfold increase in risk between the highest quintile of fat consumption compared with the lowest. A diet rich in green or yellow vegetables may be associated with a decrease in risk by modification of the circulating sex hormones.[10] It should be remembered that studies indicating this kind of effect probably attenuate the real effect because of measurement error of true dietary habits at the appropriate period in a person's life. Cadmium exposure also increases the risk of prostate cancer, possibly by as much as sixfold.[11]

A first degree relative with prostate cancer gives rise to around a fivefold increase in risk, as apparently does a history of the disease among second degree relatives.[12] Vasectomy has been found to be associated with an increased risk,[13] as has, not surprisingly, a history of benign hypertrophy of the prostate.[14]

Intervention

Routine clinical practice on diagnosis usually involves some form of androgen withdrawal, which is associated with a 60–80% response rate; however, most patients, even those who respond, will ultimately present with recurrent disease that is resistant to hormonal interventions. It is probably the case, as for other common solid cancers, that the majority of patients when diagnosed are already in the advanced, ultimately incurable stages of disease. As with these other cancers, such a state of affairs leads inexorably to increasingly invasive therapies designed to effect a cure. The evidence for the ultimate efficacy of such procedures often relies on arguments of biological plausibility and hope rather than on evidence.

The hypothetical advantages of the increasing use of radical prostatectomy noted above should, however, be set against the known side effects; these are a mortality rate of about 1–2%, cardiopulmonary complications in 4–8% of men aged 65–69, impotence in 34%, urethral strictures in 6%, and incontinence in 5%.[15] Of course, some will question these figures in their own series, which may or may not be well validated. In all such discussion enthusiasts inevitably use the data most convenient to their belief, which may of course involve implicit (or explicit) claims of superior techniques in circumstances where there may be a substantial learning curve.

Comparison of effectiveness by the many clinical trials in progress is beginning to provide sensible insights for choosing optimal treatments: choices between "watchful waiting", radical prostatectomy, and radiotherapy that are commensurate with disease stage. Of course, the dilemma is exacerbated by knowing that staging is unreliable, and hence that these treatments may not be at all specific. The use of neoadjuvant luteinising hormone releasing hormone treatment is being tested in a large clinical trial in the United States.[16] The preliminary results are promising, suggesting an important improvement in local control rates.

327

This is all further complicated by the several purposes of treatment, which of course have as their objective palliation as well as cure. Thus patients with a relatively short life expectancy need not be subjected to invasive therapies with significant postoperative morbidity, such as decreased libido, impotence, and hot flushes.[17] At the very least the options ought to be discussed, taking account of the latest clinical trial (and other) information, so that patients may decide between options that have very different and predictable incidental consequences and are no panacea for dealing with the disease.

Health policy

The essence of useful health policy for this enormous burden among elderly men must depend on reliable information on effectiveness set against reliable information on costs. The results of clinical trials will provide some important further insight into the determinants of the clinical course of the disease. It is, however, clear that a very effective combination of treatments for any significant well defined subgroup of patients is not available now. Thus the considerable dilemmas facing urologists and geriatricians will remain acute for the foreseeable future, indeed they will grow in intensity as the burden increases. In these circumstances the pressures to indulge in mass or opportunistic screening programmes using PSA, digital rectal examination, transrectal ultrasonography, or some other modality are extremely strong. This, as we shall see, will do nothing to alleviate these problems—in the short term at least.

Screening interventions must be relatively harmless, as well as specific and sensitive, and give rise to more effective treatment opportunities than are available to patients who present with symptoms in the normal course of their lives. In circumstances where latent cancer is well described but poorly understood, finding and treating localised disease therefore has to be especially well justified. At the moment it seems that more men die with prostate cancer than from it and thus the widespread adoption of prostate cancer screening facilities could in principle simply cause more men to die "from" it than "with" it, if the aggregate diagnostic advantages failed to affect significantly the natural course.

It is clear that PSA determination is currently potentially the most useful screening modality. The specificity of the test is, however, incompletely known, partly because the pertinent disease entity itself is poorly defined. Latent, and hence possibly benign, prostate cancer is not reliably distinguishable from the invasive form of the disease in localised lesions. (At autopsy some distinction is possible but even this clearly cannot be validated).[8] Specific and effective screening modalities must usefully detect only the latter. Since it is found that a major determinant of serum PSA level among cancer patients is cancer volume, this test will anyway be less specific for small tumours than for larger ones. Even in the best studies

PSA levels of more than 4 µg/l in screened men are associated with 70% of them having no cancer on biopsy. Of those men with levels above 10 µg/l, 40% appear to be clear on biopsy.

Moreover, since around 20% (or more) of men of the relevant age will have foci of prostate cancer at autopsy, the finding that only 4% of a PSA screened population will have prostate cancer detected hardly supports enormous optimism.[18] The other modalities are even less specific,[19] as far as is known, and gratuitous digital rectal examinations are obviously problematic.

Starting with considerable problems with the ability of the best test reliably to detect early disease that is amenable to and requires treatment, it is therefore even more essential to offer treatments that demonstrably provide a significant contribution to cure. No proper randomised clinical trial has yet been undertaken to discover whether radical prostatectomy or irradiation in early disease is effective.[20] There is no clear evidence that these treatments improve survival in patients with apparently localised disease. A recent observational comparison of series of patients given watchful waiting, radical prostatectomy, and irradiation found a 10 year prostate cancer survival rate of 83, 93 and 74% respectively.[21] Such observations are subject to problems of selection by astute clinicians with some insights into prognosis, but even acknowledging that, the treatments are not unequivocally providing a significant contribution to cure.

The basic policy questions thus have to do with optimising the productivity of appropriate health research. As things are, screening is not justified. Indeed even the randomised evaluation of a screening programme is hardly, if at all, justified[22] because of the real possibility that harm could well be greater than any plausible benefit. Hence the research agenda should now be concentrating on the development of more highly specific tests for identifying presymptomatic localised life threatening disease. The study of the natural history of the disease should be improved but the development of therapies without side effects but with targeted potency remains a dream. In these circumstances the active involvement of the patient in the evidence, and possibly the uncertainties, to enable sensible decision making is crucial. The responsibilities of clinicians to ensure and to demonstrate that more harm than good does not result from many well intentioned interventions has rarely been greater.

1 Schroder FH. Prostate cancer: to screen or not to screen? *BMJ* 1993;**306**:407–8.
2 Lu-Yao GL, Greenberg ER. Changes in prostate cancer incidence and treatment in USA. *Lancet* 1994;**343**:251–4.
3 Lu-Yao GL, McLerran D, Wasson J, Wennberg JE. An assessment of radical prostatectomy. Time trends, geographic variation and outcomes. *JAMA* 1993;**269**:2633–6.
4 Roush GC, Holford TR, Schymura MJ, White C. *Cancer risks and incidence trends: the Connecticut perspective.* Washington: Hemisphere Publishing, 1987.
5 Zaridge DG, Boyle P, Smans M. International trends in prostatic cancer. *Int J Cancer* 1984;**33**:223–30.

6 Hirayama T. Epidemiology of prostate cancer with special reference to the role of diet. Epidemiology and cancer registries. *Natl Cancer Inst Monogr* 1979;**53**:149–53.

7 Araki H, Misina T, Miyakoda K, *et al*. An epidemiological survey of prostatic cancer from the Annual of the Pathological Autopsy Cases in Japan. *Tohoku J Exp Med* 1980;**130**: 159–64.

8 Yatani R, Chigusa I, Akazaki K, Stemmermann GM, Welsh RA, Correa P. Geographic pathology of latent prostatic carcinoma. *Int J Cancer* 1982;**29**:611–6.

9 Heshmat MY, Kovi J, Herson J, *et al*. Epidemiologic association between gonorrhoea and prostatic carcinoma. *Urology* 1975;**6**:457–60.

10 Hill PB, Wynder EL. Effect of vegetarian diet and dexamethasone on plasma prolactin, testosterone and dehyroepiandrosterone in men and women. *Cancer Lett* 1979;**7**:273–83.

11 Kolonel L, Winkelstein W Jr. Cadmium and prostate cancer. *Lancet* 1967;**ii**:566–7.

12 Krain LS. Some epidemiologic variables in prostatic carcinoma in California. *Prev Med* 1974;**3**:154–9.

13 Guess HA. Is vasectomy a risk factor for prostate cancer? *Eur J Cancer* 1993;**29**:1055–9 [abstract no 7].

14 Meikle AW, Smith JA. Epidemiology of prostate cancer. *Urol Clin North Am* 1990;**17**: 709–18.

15 Bilgrami S, Greenberg BR. Why so many operations for localised prostate cancer? *Lancet* 1994;**344**:700–1.

16 Shearer RJ, Davies JH, Gelister JSK, Bearnaley DP. Hormonal cytoreduction and radiotherapy for carcinoma of the prostate. *Br J Urol* 1992;**69**:521–4.

17 Fleming C, Wasson J, Albertsen P, Barry M, Wennberg JE. A decision analysis of alternative treatment strategies for clinically localized prostate cancer. *JAMA* 1993;**269**:2650–8.

18 Neal DE, Hamdy FC. Screening for prostate cancer. *Lancet* 1994;**343**:1438.

19 Kramer BS, Brown ML, Prorok PC, Potosky AI, Gohagan JK. Prostate cancer screening: what we know and what we need to know. *Ann Intern Med* 1993;**119**:9144–23.

20 Flemming C, Wasson JH, Albertson PC, Barry MJ, Wennberg JE. A decision analysis of alternative treatment strategies for clinically localised prostate cancer. *JAMA* 1993;**269**: 2650–8.

21 Adolfsson J, Steineck G, Whitmore WF. Recent results of management of palpable clinically localised prostate cancer. *Cancer* 1993;**72**:310–1.

22 Adami H-O, Baron JA, Rothman KJ. The ethics of a prostate cancer screening trial. *Lancet* 1994;**343**:958–60.

36 Visual impairment

DARWIN C MINASSIAN

Definition and diagnostic criteria

The World Health Organization Prevention of Blindness Programme (WHO/PBL) has defined five categories of visual impairment, which are included in the International Statistical Classification of Diseases, and Related Health Problems, tenth revision (ICD-10). The WHO/PBL definition of blindness is a visual acuity of less than 3/60 (or <0·05) using the Snellen notation, with best possible spectacle correction (visual impairment categories 3–5 in ICD-10). This is equivalent to the inability to count fingers at a distance of three metres. Low vision is defined as a visual acuity of poorer than 6/18 but not blind, and visual acuity of 6/18 or better is labelled as "adequate vsion", again with best possible correction. In defining the level of visual impairment for a person the visual acuity of the best eye is used. Further details and guidelines on methods of assessment of visual impairment are described in a WHO Offset Publication.[1]

Having a standard definition of blindness and low vision has allowed sensible comparison of prevalence data from different countries or regions, as has having a standard method of sampling, data collection, and analysis in eye surveys. Most surveys of blindness and eye disease carried out over the past decade in developing countries have used the standard WHO/PBL eye examination record and coding instructions and have followed the WHO general guidelines on sampling design.[1] The data from these, and other population based surveys that have used the WHO definition of blindness, have formed the main bulk of the "blindness databank" used by the WHO/PBL to compare the burden of blindness in different regions of the world and to estimate the global prevalence of blindness and low vision.[2]

The legal definition of blindness and impaired vision for registration or certification purposes in some countries does not follow the WHO criteria. In the United Kingdom there is no legal definition of partial sight and the National Assistance Act 1948 says that a person can be certified as blind if they are "so blind that they cannot do any work for which eyesight is essential." According to the BD8(1990) guidelines issued by the Department of Health to ophthalmologists, to certify a person as blind or partially sighted depends not only on the level of visual acuity, but also on how contracted the visual fields are, how recently the person's eyesight has

331

failed, and how old the person was when the eyesight failed. Such blindness registration data have limited use in epidemiological studies. Incomplete registration adds to the problem. In the United States visual acuity of poorer than 6/12 is considered as impaired vision and persons with visual acuity of 6/60 or less are classified as blind.

Magnitude of the problem

There are about 38 million blind in the world and a further 110 million have low vision.[2] These are the most recent (1995) estimates based on the WHO/PBL blindness databank, using the WHO definition of blindness and low vision to compute the global prevalence for 1990.[3]

The only published direct epidemiological measure of incidence of blindness comes from a population based cohort study in central India, reporting the incidence of blindness from cataract to be 470 new cases per 100 000 per year.[4] The incidence in persons aged 65 or older is 5810 new cases per 100 000, some 30 times higher than that in the 35–39 year age group (fig 36.1). An epidemiological model is being developed to simulate the dynamics of world blindness, to project global and regional estimates of the magnitude of visual disability, under various demographic scenarios.

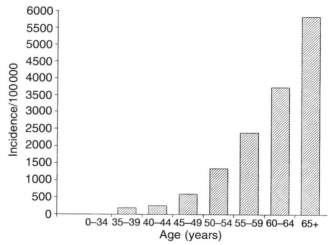

Fig 36.1   Annual age specific incidence of cataract blindness in Central India. Data from a population based longitudinal study.

Visual impairment is strongly related to age, occurring mainly in the elderly. Figure 36.2 shows a typical example of age specific prevalence of visual impairment derived from a population based survey. The expected growth of the elderly population in the coming decades presents a major challenge to ophthalmic services throughout the world. In the United Kingdom, for example, the proportion of the NHS budget allocated to eye services (or to any particular eye service, such as cataract surgery) is best

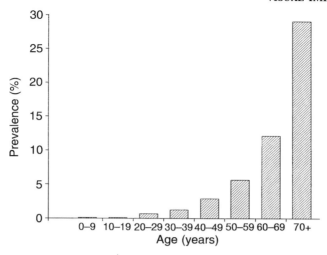

Fig 36.2   Age specific prevalence of visual impairment (blindness and low vision) in the Gambia (1986). Data from a national sampling survey.

considered unknown, in preference to adopting a baseless figure. Reliable estimates will require painstaking research.

The global distribution of visual impairment is far from uniform, the main burden being in developing countries of Asia and Africa, particularly in remote rural populations.

The main disorders leading to binocular visual impairment in adults and the elderly are cataract, age related macular degeneration, chronic open angle glaucoma, and diabetic retinopathy, together with onchocerciasis (river blindness), which is limited to parts of Africa and Latin America, and severe trachoma, which mainly affects poor rural populations and slum dwellers in developing countries.

Cataract is by far the most common blinding disorder worldwide. Table 36.1 summarises the findings from some recent (1980 onwards) population based prevalence surveys that have used a standard or well described method to ascertain the principle cause of blindness.[5-14] These indicate that more than half of the blindness in most developing countries is due to cataract and its sequel. In developed countries that have advanced medical services much of the cataract is treated surgically before the onset of severe visual disability. Sight restoring cataract surgery constitutes the biggest workload in ophthalmic units throughout the world. More than one million cataract operations are performed each year in the United States.[15] In the United Kingdom there were about 105 100 cataract operations in 1990, amounting to an average of about 200 cataract operations under each consultant ophthalmic surgeon.[16] In India about 1·2 million cataract surgeries are performed annually; however, an epidemiological model of the population dynamics of cataract incidence and management predicts that more than three million operations are

Table 36.1 Main disorders causing binocular blindness and visual impairment

Country		Cataract	Glaucoma	Trachoma	Other corneal	Phthisis	Onchocerciasis	Macular degeneration	Retinopathy	Refractive	Other	Sampled population
Gambia[5]	Blindness	55·0	2·0	17·0	11·0	9·0					6·0	Whole country
	Low vision	67·0	1·0	9·0	6·0					11·0	6·0	Whole country
Congo[6]	Blindness	81·0	9·0						5·0		5·0	Whole country
	Low vision	80·0	3·4		1·4			5·5		3·4	6·3	Whole country
Togo[7]	Blindness	39·0	3·5	14·5	4·0		29·0	3·5		7·0		Kara region
	Low vision	70·0	4·0			3·5	2·0	5·5		9·0	5·5	Kara region
Benin[8]	Blindness	54·0	15·0		11·0	4·0		9·0			16·0	Whole country
	Low vision	64·0	3·4		4·0					9·6	10·0	Whole country
Morocco[9]	Blindness	54·6	14·3	3·9	6·5	5·2		3·9	2·6	1·3	7·7	Whole country
	Low vision	47·8	3·4	1·3	0·4	1·7		2·2	1·7	36·2	5·3	Whole country
Turkey[10]	Blindness	50·0	12·0	3·0	12·0	6·0		2·0			17·0	South east
	Low vision	52·0		4·0	2·5					26·0	13·5	South east
Saudi Arabia[11]	Blindness	68·4	5·3			10·5			5·3	5·3	5·3	Bisha region
	Low vision	20·6	1·0	1·9	1·9				1·9	67·9	4·8	Bisha region
Nepal[12]	Blindness	72·1							3·3	14·0		Whole country
	Low vision		3·2	2·4	5·0							Whole country
Vanuatu[13]	Blindness	84·6						7·7			7·7	All islands
United Kingdom[14]	Impaired vision	63·0	7·0					20·0			10·0	Inner London

Cause (%)

Data from recent population based surveys.

needed each year in order to bring the cataract blindness problem in the country under control. The projection takes into account the higher mortality associated with cataract, assumes successful outcome of surgery in 90%, and is based on prevailing demographic trends.

The relative importance of the other main blinding disorders are also shown in table 36.1. Cataract, macular degeneration, and glaucoma collectively account for more than 60% of the world's blindness and are all primarily diseases of the elderly. In addition, diabetic retinopathy is responsible for about 5% of the global blindness and 10% of the blindness in people over age 65 in the United States.[15] Trachoma causes blindness as a consequence of repeated episodes of infection that begin in early childhood and go on to sustain prolonged chronic inflammation over many years, eventually leading to blindness in late life. Trachoma can, however, occasionally lead to acute corneal damage that causes blindness in young adults or even in children. The estimates for the proportion of the world's blindness that is caused by trachoma vary from about 8 to 25%, the most recent being 15·5%.[2] As for most of the global estimates mentioned, precise figures are not available. Eye complications of leprosy are largely avoidable[17]; they may be responsible for about 1% of the blindness in the world.

Variation

Time

It is widely believed that the global prevalence of blindness and low vision is increasing. The previous WHO estimate in 1987 was 31 million blind worldwide, compared with the current estimate of 38 million blind; however, direct comparison of the two estimates is problematic because the methods used for estimation differed.[2] It might be reasonable to assume increasing numbers of visually impaired persons in line with population growth, the "ageing trend", and the general failure of basic ophthalmic services to cope adequately with the population needs in much of the world. There are as yet no known effective measures for reducing the incidence of at least three of the main blinding disorders that affect the elderly—cataract, macular disease, and glaucoma; we can expect an increasing burden on ophthalmic services for management of these problems and of the resulting visual disability.

Place

The prevalence of blindness in different regions of the world is shown in table 36.2. Less than half (48%) of the world's population live in developing countries of Africa and Asia (excluding China), whereas about 70% of the world's blind are to be found in these continents, in spite of their younger population.

335

Table 36.2 Blindness prevalence in different regions of the world

Region	Population in 1990		Estimated number blind		% Prevalence of blindness
	Millions	%	Millions	% of all blind	
Sub-Saharan Africa	510	10	7·1	19	1·4
India	850	16	8·9	23	1·0
Middle-East and Other Asia	1186	23	9·4	25	0·8
China	1134	22	6·7	18	0·6
Latin America and the Caribbean	444	8	2·3	6	0·5
Europe, North America, Australia, New Zealand, Japan	1144	22	3·5	9	0·3
WORLD	5267	100	37·9	100	0·7

Data from Thylefors et al.[2]

The clustering of the world's blind and visually disabled in developing countries of Africa and Asia is primarily caused by two interrelated phenomena. Firstly, the relatively poor access to eye care services—in particular that of elderly people to sight restoring cataract surgery and subsequent management; and, secondly, the higher incidence of blindness and low vision, which is largely due to higher incidence of cataract, particularly in Asia.

There is ample evidence in support of the poor access phenomenon in terms of the number of people served per ophthalmologist, the number of untreated curable visually disabled persons discovered during population based surveys, and the estimated need for basic ophthalmic services in relation to the actual services available.[5-12 18] The shortfall in eye care services also contributes to the high incidence of visual disability, as early treatment of some disorders is expected to prevent subsequent loss of vision. Evidence for the higher incidence of some of the major blinding disorders in developing countries is more scarce but is found through comparison of age specific or age standardised prevalence in developed and developing nations. An example is the prevalence of cataract in the Punjab compared with that in Framingham, USA, whereby the prevalence of cataract in persons aged 52–64 was 4·5% in Framingham and 29·4% in the Punjab.[19] More obvious differences occur in incidence of severe blinding trachoma and in incidence of onchocerciasis, which are virtually absent from the developed North.

Determinants of the main vision impairing disorders

Ageing is the best known and most powerful determinant of blindness and visual disability, as the main blinding disorders are strongly age related. Cataract, macular degeneration, and glaucoma, which collectively account for more than 60% of the world's blindness, are all primarily diseases of the elderly. In addition, the major bulk of the blindness from diabetic retinopathy, trachoma, onchocerciasis, and leprosy occur in the elderly.

Cataract

Three main risk factors—sunlight, severe dehydration, and malnutrition—have been proposed for cataract. A well designed detailed recent study found an association between exposure to ultraviolet B sunlight radiation and cortical cataract but no association was found with nuclear or vision impairing cataract.[20] The epidemiological and other evidence concerning lifelong exposure to high levels of ultraviolet radiation from sunlight and risk of cataract has been critically reviewed.[21 22] The evidence in support of the dehydration hypothesis suggests that repeated episodes of severe dehydrational crises from cholera-like diarrhoeal disease or heat stroke may be a major risk factor accounting for nearly 40% of cataracts in some populations[23]; however, these findings have yet to be repeated in other locations and in more convincing longitudinal studies and randomised intervention trials. The data concerning the nutritional factors have also been recently reviewed.[21] There is some evidence that low total protein consumption is associated with higher risk of cataract and that food rich in antioxidant vitamins may be protective. Other proposed risk factors include diabetes, smoking,[24] and glucose 6-phosphate dehydrogenase deficiency.[25] More obvious causes of cataract such as physical trauma to the eye, intraocular inflammation, prolonged use of steroids, and exposure to industrial sources of radiation (microwave, infrared, and ultraviolet rays), account for only a tiny proportion of the cataract blindness problem.

Age related macular degeneration

The prevalence of this potentially blinding disorder in the United States is projected to increase from 4·5 million (1990) to 7·5 million by the year 2020.[15] It is largely untreatable (apart from very few patients who benefit from early detection and laser photocoagulation therapy) and, as no major risk factors or protective factors have yet been identified, it remains unavoidable. Cardiovascular disease, postmenopausal exogenous oestrogen use, higher levels of serum cholesterol, and smoking have been proposed as possible risk factors.[26] The epidemiology and clinical features are outlined in a review.[27]

Chronic open angle glaucoma

Glaucoma is often quoted as the second most common cause of visual impairment in the elderly in developed countries, second only to macular degeneration. Early detection and treatment of glaucoma, including regular follow up and monitoring of the intraocular pressure and the visual fields, are generally expected to reduce the risk of progressive damage to the optic nerve and of visual disability. No primary prevention is feasible, as no important root causes have yet been identified. There is evidence that the disease is more severe and has an earlier onset in the Afro–Caribbean ethnic groups and that untreated systolic hypertension and smoking may be risk factors.[28] Other suspect risk factors include positive family history and diabetes.

Diabetic retinopathy

In addition to poor control of diabetes, other factors that might enhance the risk of diabetic retinopathy include younger age of onset, dependence on insulin, and education. Proliferative retinopathy is more likely to develop in women with younger onset diabetes who have had less education than in those with more education. Apparently education is not a factor in older onset diabetics.[29]

Trachoma

Poverty and related factors, including poor housing, overcrowding, poor sanitation and hygiene (personal, family, and community), and poor utilisation and access to water, are generally accepted risk factors that may enhance the transmission of trachoma within communities and, perhaps more importantly, within families. High pressure of transmission leads to repeated episodes of infection and prolonged chronic inflammation of the external eye over many years, causing scarring and deformity of the eyelid, opacity of the cornea, and eventual impairment of vision. The importance of face washing behaviour as a protective factor to reduce transmission has been documented in a number of studies. The epidemiology and clinical aspects of trachoma have been reviewed by Taylor.[30]

Intervention

A recent publication gives the WHO perspective of the problem of world blindness and possible solutions: the role of primary eye care, manpower development, and establishment of national programmes for prevention of blindness throughout the world.[3]

Cataract surgery

The burden of blindness and visual disability in the developing nations of the world could be halved by a single intervention—the provision of an equitable cataract surgery and aftercare service. The challenge is to make the service reliable, accessible, and acceptable to the bulk of the rural populations and to the disadvantaged in urban areas. This and other measures to reduce blindness are discussed in several publications.[3 18 31] In developed regions that have advanced medical services the main challenges include improvements in the cataract management systems, in relation to the population need as assessed through sound epidemiological methods, to reduce waiting time, to hasten visual rehabilitation, and to reduce costs, and the proper evaluation of new high cost technologies before their incorporation into routine use. The search for effective anticataract drugs or nutrients continues and randomised trials of antioxidant vitamins are awaited.

Cataract is treatable by surgical removal of the lens with or without implantation of an artificial intraocular lens. The modern intraocular lens implants tend to give more satisfactory postoperative visual function, compared with aphakic spectacle correction, and are now routinely used in almost all ophthalmic units in developed countries that have advanced medical services. In most developing country situations, however, implantation of intraocular lenses is not used routinely because of the relatively high technological requirements and related costs, the relative slowness of the surgical procedure, the need for follow up to treat possible

339

complications (opacity of the lens capsular bag left behind), and the additional training necessary to achieve the required level of surgical expertise. There is currently much debate concerning mass adoption of the high tech "Western" cataract surgical techniques in developing countries. The possible advantages have to be weighed against the potentially disastrous opportunity costs. Randomised clinical trials are currently in progress in Nepal, India, and Bangladesh, comparing standard intracapsular cataract extraction and spectacle prescription with cataract surgery that involves implantation of an intraocular lens in the anterior chamber of the eye in front of the iris. This type of implantation requires relatively less time and additional training and is therefore a more practicable option in most developing countries; however, it is considered less than ideal by many Western ophthalmic surgeons who prefer implantation of the intraocular lens in the intact capsular bag of the lens in the posterior chamber of the eye behind the iris, a more natural place for the lens.

The outcome of cataract surgery has been the subject of recent research. A follow up study in a voluntary hospital and associated eye camps in central India found that in 92% the outcome was successful and the patients had adequate vision (6/18 or better) one year after surgery.[32] A recent study in the United States reported that up to 96% of the patients had improved visual acuity at four months after surgery and 85% had improved satisfaction with their vision.[33] In the United Kingdom the national survey of cataract surgery found that 80% of all patients had visual acuity of 6/12 or better three months after surgery.[34] Serious perioperative and postoperative complications are generally rare, the annual cumulative incidence for endophthalmitis being 0·08%.[35]

Glaucoma

The incidence of visual loss from glaucoma can be reduced by early diagnosis, surgical treatment, and ongoing follow up. Effective continuous screening systems aimed at the over 50s, to identify early cases of glaucoma, might be a key component of the intervention. Such systems are yet to be developed for most of the world's population and to be evaluated by randomised screening trials.

Diabetes

Similarly, effective screening to detect early cases of diabetic retinopathy needs to be developed and tested. Even in the United Kingdom, with its relatively advanced health care system, much of the irreversible damage to the eye occurs in diabetic patients who have not had timely ophthalmic assessments by competent clinicians. There is no consensus as to who should examine the eyes of diabetics to detect early cases of diabetic retinopathy. The main candidates seem to be ophthalmologists, general

340

practitioners, or diabetologists. The technology of intelligent computer imaging systems that could identify early diabetic retinopathy is at present in its infancy.

Trachoma

The importance of trachoma as a cause of blindness in many countries has diminished substantially since the 1960s, seemingly because of effective trachoma control programmes and the general improvements in housing and related development. The remaining pockets in need of maintained intervention are mostly in the remote and poor areas that have little or no economic potential. Inflammatory trachoma may be prevented by improved hygiene and sanitation. The active inflammation can be treated with tetracycline eye ointment, which is highly effective in treating infected individuals but not so in treating communities. Single dose oral antibiotic therapy is now available and, if successful, may revolutionise trachoma control programmes. Damaged eyelids with inturned eyelashes can be treated surgically. About 100 years ago trachoma was prevalent in poor overcrowded city areas of much of Europe, including London. Its disappearance was probably the result of the dramatic improvement in socioeconomic conditions rather than any mass treatment by antibiotics. While waiting for general development to eliminate trachoma gradually in the least developed areas, it seems that practicable interventions to provide access to and better utilisation of water and to improve personal hygiene, particularly in children, may substantially reduce the risk of severe potentially blinding trachoma.[30]

Onchocerciasis

Onchocerciasis can be prevented by larviciding to control the vector. Within the onchocerciasis control programme area in west Africa, substantial regression of the disease has resulted from many years of vector control.[36] Infected patients can now be safely treated with ivermectin, a potent microfilaricide. A single dose is effective for 6–12 months. Work is in progress to develop systems for cost effective distribution of ivermectin in large populations at risk. The main challenges in onchocerciasis control are outlined by Thylefors.[3]

Thus more than half of the adult blindness in the world is "avoidable blindness",[37] that is, it could be prevented or relieved within the limits of the resources that could reasonably be used. Foster[18] suggests that "four of the five million adults going blind each year would not do so if appropriate eye care was made available, at an affordable cost, to all people."

341

1 World Health Organization. Methods of assessment of avoidable blindness. *WHO Offset Publ* 1980;54.

2 Thylefors B, Negrel AD, Pararajasegaram R, Dadzie KY. Global data on blindness. *Bull World Health Organ* 1995;**73(1)**:115–21.

3 Thylefors B. The World Health Organization's programme for the prevention of blindness. *Int Ophthalmol* 1990;**14**:211–9.

4 Minassian DC, Mehra V. 3·8 Million blinded by cataract each year: projections from the first epidemiological study of incidence of cataract blindness in India. *Br J Ophthalmol* 1990;**74**:341–3.

5 Faal H, Minassian DC, Sowa S, Foster A. National survey of blindness and low vision in the Gambia—results. *Br J Ophthalmol* 1989;**73**:82–7.

6 Negrel AD, Massembo-Yako B, Botaka E, Minassian DC, Coddyzitsamele R. Prévalence et causes de la cécité au Congo. *Bull World Health Organ* 1990;**68**:237–43.

7 Schemann J-F, Minassian D, Negrel D. Prévalence et causes de cécité dans la region de kara au Togo. *Cah Sante* 1993;**3**:24–30.

8 World Health Organization. Prevalence and causes of blindness and low vision, Benin. *WHO Weekly Epidemiol Rec* 1991;**66**:337–40.

9 World Health Organization. Prevalence and causes of blindness and low vision, Morocco. *WHO Weekly Epidemiol Rec* 1994;**69**:129–36.

10 Sayek F. Ophthalmology in Turkey. *Arch Ophthalmol* 1990;**108**:894–5.

11 Al Faram MF, Al-Rajhi AA, Al-Omar OM, Al-Ghamdi SA, Jabak M. Prevalence and causes of visual impairment and blindness in South Western region of Saudi Arabia. *Int Ophthalmol* 1993;**17**:161–5.

12 Brilliant LB, Pokhrel RP, Grasset NC, *et al.* Epidemiology of blindness in Nepal. *Bull World Health Organ* 1985;**63**:375–86.

13 Newland HS, Harris MF, Walland M, *et al.* Epidemiology of blindness and visual impairment in Vanuatu. *Bull World Health Organ* 1992;**70**:369–72.

14 Wormald RPL, Wright LA, Courtney P, Beaumont B, Haines AP. Visual problems in the elderly population and implications for services. *BMJ* 1992;**304**:1226–9.

15 Pizzarello LD. The dimensions of the problem of eye disease among the elderly. *Ophthalmology* 1987;**94**:1191–5.

16 Courtney P. The national cataract surgery survey: I. Method and descriptive features. *Eye* 1992;**6**:487–92.

17 Ffytch T. Blindness in leprosy: a forgotten complication. *Aust N Z J Ophthalmol* 1989; **17**:257–60.

18 Foster A. World blindness, increasing but avoidable! *Semin Ophthalmol* 1993;**8**:166–70.

19 Chatterjee A, Milton RC, Thyle S. Prevalence and aetiology of cataract in Punjab. *Br J Ophthalmol* 1982;**66**:35–42.

20 Taylor HR, West SK, Rosenthal FR, *et al.* Effect of ultraviolet radiation on cataract formation. *N Engl J Med* 1988;**319**:1429–33.

21 Evans J, Minassian DC. Epidemiology of age-related cataract. *Community Eye Health* 1992;**9**:2–6.

22 Dolin PJ. Assessment of the epidemiological evidence that exposure to solar ultraviolet radiation causes cataract. *Br J Ophthalmol* 1994;**78**:478–82.

23 Minassian DC, Mehra V, Verrey J-D. Dehydrational crises: a major risk factor in blinding cataract. *Br J Ophthalmol* 1989;**73**:100–105.

24 Harding JJ. *Cataract: biochemistry, epidemiology, and pharmacology.* London: Chapman and Hall, 1991.

25 Orzalesi N, Sorcinelli R, Guiso G. Increased incidence of cataract in male subjects deficient in glucose-6-phosphate dehydrogenase. *Arch Ophthalmol* 1981;**99**:69–70.

26 Eye Disease Case–Control Study Group. Risk factors for neovascular age-related macular degeneration. *Arch Ophthalmol* 1992;**110**:1701–8.

27 Boldt HC, Bressler SB, Fine SL, Bressler NM. Age-related macular degeneration. *Curr Opin Ophthalmol* 1990;**1**:247–57.

28 Wilson MR, Hertzmark E, Walker AM, Childs-Shaw K, Epstein DL. A case-control study of risk factors in open angle glaucoma. *Arch Ophthalmol* 1987;**105**:1006–71.

29 Klein R, Klein BEK, Jenson SC, Moss SE. The relation of socioeconomic factors to the incidence of proliferative diabetic retinopathy and loss of vision. *Ophthalmology* 1994;**101**: 68–75.

30 Taylor HR. Trachoma. *Int Ophthalmol* 1990;**14**:201–4.

31 Adamsons I, Taylor HR. Major causes of world blindness: their treatment and prevention. *Curr Opin Ophthalmol* 1990;**1**:635–42.

32 Reidy A, Mehra V, Minassian DC, Mahashabde S. Outcome of cataract surgery in Central India: a longitudinal follow-up study. *Br J Ophthalmol* 1991;**75**:102–105.

33 Steinberg EP, Tielsh JM, Shien OD, *et al.* National study of cataract surgery outcomes. Variation in 4-month postoperative outcomes as reflected in multiple outcome measures. *Ophthalmology* 1994;**100**:1131–41.

34 Desai P. The national cataract surgery survey: II. Clinical outcomes. *Eye* 1993;**7**:489–94.

35 Jarvitt JC, Street DA, Tielsch JM, *et al.* National outcome of cataract extraction. Retinal detachment and endophthalmitis after outpatient cataract surgery. *Ophthalmology* 1994;**101**:100–6.

36 Dadzie KY, Remme J, Rolland A, *et al.* The effect of 7–8 years of vector control on the evolution of ocular onchocerciasis in West African savannah. *Trop Med Parasitol* 1986;**37**:263–70.

37 Jones BR. In: International Agency for Prevention of Blindness. J Wilson, editor. *World blindness and its prevention.* Oxford: Oxford University Press, 1980:36–43.

343

37 Hearing impairment

KATIA GILHOME HERBST

Types of hearing impairment

The term "conductive loss" is usually applied to hearing loss that arises from obstruction or disease of the outer and middle ear. The causes of conductive loss are listed in box 37.1. Conductive losses can often be treated medically or surgically and lend themselves to remediation by a hearing aid.

Box 37.1—Causes of conductive hearing loss

- Any obstruction of the external ear canal by wax or debris
- Perforation of the tympanic membrane—after infection or injury
- Otosclerosis—causing fixation of the ossicular chain in the middle ear so that bones do not move freely
- Arthritis in the ossicular chain
- Head injuries—which might dislocate one bone from the next in the ossicular chain
- Otitis media

The term "sensorineural loss" (or inner ear, perceptive, or nerve deafness) refers to hearing loss that originates in the sensory cells and neurones of

---

Box 37.2—Causes of sensorineural deafness

- Diseases affecting the organ of Corti in the inner ear—for example, Ménière's disease, mumps and measles
- Diseases of the acoustic nerve—such as acoustic neuroma
- Rare diseases of the brain itself
- Iatrogenic damage—by such drugs as streptomycin, quinine, and nicotine
- Noise induced injury to the hair cells of the cochlea
- High blood pressure
- Effects of ageing on the auditory system

---

the cochlea and central (brainstem and cortical) dysfunction—the inner ear. The causes of sensorineural loss are listed in box 37.2. Sensorineural losses are irreversible and by their very nature are rarely if ever relieved by a hearing aid.

"Old age" deafness—presbyacusis

The most common cause of sensorineural loss is conventionally considered to be damage to hair cells in the cochlea as a result of the ageing process; the progressive loss of hearing produced is called presbyacusis. The characteristics of presbyacusis are listed in box 37.3.

Box 37.3—Characteristics of presbyacusis

- Sensorineural losses—with some conductive overlay
- Bilateral losses
- Losses for the high frequencies in particular—a progressive deterioration with age
- Recruitment—the abrupt transition from hearing little or nothing to hearing sounds very loudly

---

Onset and rate of functional decline vary among individuals. As some causes of such sensorineural losses are preventable and as there is a strong association between such losses and low socioeconomic group, particularly in places where noisy industry is common, there is some evidence to suggest that it might not, however, be entirely unavoidable.

Prevalence

Hearing impairment in the elderly has been investigated by researchers since the early 1940s in their quest to assess the needs of elderly people that would have to be met by the new welfare state. The presence of the disorder was always established by self report alone. In this way it was estimated that about 30% of all those of retirement age had some form of hearing loss.[1]

Such estimates were challenged by two community studies of elderly people that used audiometric techniques to establish the presence of hearing loss. One was undertaken in London by Gilhome Herbst and her colleagues in the late 1970s.[1] The other was carried out in Scotland.[2] These studies, both using audiometry, found that some 60%—not 30%—of those aged 70 years or over had some significant hearing loss. These findings were confirmed more recently by other researchers who also used audiometric techniques to establish the presence of hearing loss among people aged 70 years and over in the Welsh Valleys.[3]

The results of the Edinburgh study[2] have been adjusted to be compatible with those of the London investigation (table 37.1). "Deafness" was defined in all three studies as an average loss over the speech frequencies at 1, 2, and 4 kHz of 35 dB or more in the better ear—a loss of 35 dB being generally regarded as reflecting a level of impairment sufficient to necessitate the use of a hearing aid.

Table 37.1 Prevalence of hearing impairment (defined as a mean loss of 35 dB or more in the better hearing ear—35 dB BEA) in different older populations

	Inner London	Edinburgh	Welsh village
Hearing impairment in total sample population aged 70+ years (%)	60	68	77·5
Hearing impairment in total sample population aged 80+ years (%)	82	94	93

By comparing the results of those studies that use audiometry to assess the presence of acquired deafness with those that do not, the extent to which it is not noticed or is denied (or at least not accepted or volunteered) by the sufferer is exposed.

Between 1980 and 1986 the Institute of Hearing Research in Nottingham, England embarked upon the first large scale national study of the prevalence of deafness that did not rely solely on self report—the national study of hearing. Its findings are based upon data from 2708 people (aged between 18 and 80 years) who underwent audiological investigation after initial contact by postal questionnaire.[4]

Using as an index of impairment an average loss of 25 dB or more over the speech frequencies at 0·5, 1, 2 and 4 kHz in the better ear (the better ear average or BEA), the study found that 16·1% of the adult population in the United Kingdom had some hearing loss.[4] An earlier national survey, which did not use audiometric techniques, had suggested that 3% of the adult population were hearing impaired.

The national study reported that the majority of hearing impairments (some 87%) are of a sensorineural type rather than conductive. As severity of loss increases, so the likelihood of there being a conductive overlay also increases. As severity increases, so prevalence decreases. The study confirmed that the prevalence of hearing impairment is significantly age related, as is severity of impairment (table 37.2).

The study did not include persons over the age of 80 years, in whom it is known that hearing impairment is most prevalent; however, it provides the best available estimates in the United Kingdom for bilateral severe and profound hearing impairments. It suggests that hearing impairment is one of the most widespread of all physical disabilities. This is amply confirmed by the survey of the prevalence of disability among adults conducted by the Office of Population Censuses and Surveys, England, which found that hearing disabilities are the most common, after locomotor disabilities, in

346

Table 37.2   National estimates of acquired deafness showing the prevalence in each age cohort at a better ear average (BEA) of 25 dB hearing loss (HL) or more as a function of age and median BEA, pooled for women and men[4]

Age (years)	Prevalence (%)	Median BEA (dB HL)
20–24	3·0	3·8
25–29	0·8	4·5
30–34	2·7	6·0
35–39	2·3	6·3
40–44	4·8	8·0
45–49	19·7	9·3
50–54	18·5	12·3
55–59	19·0	13·0
60–64	29·7	15·0
65–69	44·2	22·5
70–74	45·4	23·3
75–79	76·6	36·0

Great Britain—even when not using audiometric techniques to assess their presence.[5]

Most deafness of whatever severity is acquired. Even when looking at severe impairments producing a BEA of 95 dB it is probable that 15 000 people in the United Kingdom of all ages are prelingually (before acquiring language) deaf—out of a total number of 100 000.[4]

Other problems associated with acquired deafness

Ménière's disease and tinnitus sometimes accompany acquired hearing loss.

Ménière's disease is a distressing combination of sensorineural deafness with tinnitus and vertigo that attacks the sufferer intermittently, causing acute giddiness and vomiting. These symptoms of dizziness and nausea are due to disturbances of the mechanism of balance and may be of vascular origin. It is thought that Ménière's disease may have a psychogenic component or be triggered in those so predisposed by excessive stress.

Tinnitus is the term used to describe a subjective head noise of internal origin, which in consequence is not heard by others. Such noises are to be distinguished from auditory hallucinations, which are more complex, such as music or voices; nor should they be mistaken for autophony—hearing one's own breathing and other internal bodily functions.

It is well established that the presence of tinnitus is correlated with acquired hearing loss.[4] The findings of the UK national survey of hearing suggest that one in three adults report some experience of tinnitus but only 10% of the population report noises in the head which last for 5 minutes or more.[6] The proportion of people reporting intrusive tinnitus increases with severity of hearing impairment such that 15% of those with average losses of 85 dB in the better ear are afflicted in this way. Indeed, of all those who seek medical advice concerning any hearing impairment, about one third do so on account of tinnitus. Thus the onset of tinnitus may draw a person's attention to a previously unrecognised or unacknowledged hearing difficulty.[6]

Very few types of tinnitus can be cured or treated. Since it is considered unwise to undertake surgery of the middle or internal ear where the primary complaint is tinnitus, the problem is generally managed by counselling and by desensitising the sufferer from the sound of the tinnitus with a preferred noise ("masking"), usually with a small device like a hearing aid.[7] Counselling has had to be used as a rehabilitative device, much as it would or could have been used for those with more standard hearing problems had the hearing aid not usurped the status of counselling by virtue of the ease and cheapness with which it can be dispensed.

Rehabilitation

As long ago as the 1950s psychologists showed that if people internalise and hold society's negative attitudes to a certain condition or state in life, which they know and accept to be theirs (for example, their deafness or their skin colour), they are more likely to be maladjusted than if they do not.

Researchers now agree that in general those with acquired hearing loss tend to attempt to "pass" or deny their hearing loss and that this is a natural healthy response—a protecting mechanism against society's negative attitudes to their disorder.[7–9] The corollary of such behaviour is that there is felt to be something intrinsically shameful or unpleasant about deafness that is worthy of being hidden.

This capacity to deny or reject the presence of an acquired hearing impairment needs to be taken seriously for three main reasons.

Firstly, because it is likely that those who deny it in themselves and strive to conceal it will succeed in so doing and may not recognise in others the problem that they themselves have. This may exacerbate feelings of aloneness—or loneliness—namely, the feeling of being the only one with a dreadful disability to cope with.

The second reason why denying their deafness is important is because those who are unwilling to accept that they have a problem are unlikely to come forward for deafness specific rehabilitation services. At the moment "rehabilitation" is likely to mean the issue of a hearing aid. Thomas and Gilhome Herbst found that 40% of their sample of people of employment age knew that they had had a hearing loss for 20 or more years before coming forward to seek an aid.[10] Humphrey and her colleagues found that, in a sample of hearing impaired people over the age of 70 years who would admit to experiencing a hearing loss, 45% knew that they had had such a loss since before reaching retirement age.[11]

Between 21 and 25% of those older people who would benefit from wearing an aid actually possess one. The reasons for this are varied but are likely to be a combination of lack of understanding and dislike of the disorder by both clinicians and sufferers.[11]

The third reason why denial of deafness is important is its role or function within the rehabilitative process. The conventional principles of rehabilitation demand acceptance of the problem before therapeutic intervention can either take place or be effective. Perhaps this is why rehabilitation of those with acquired hearing loss is still relatively speaking in its infancy. Lip reading classes, counselling, and individual attention by a specialist to help with the social problems encountered by those with acquired hearing loss have never been universally available. Interventions other than the hearing aid are rare; yet given the very complex responses of those with acquired hearing loss the simple issue of an aid will seldom be sufficient to achieve satisfactory rehabilitation.

Social and psychological effects of acquired hearing loss

The social effects of hearing impairment, though diverse, stem from two sources: the disability—namely, the functional restriction caused by the impairment; and the handicap—namely, the unpleasant results of society's attitude. Combined, the major social and psychological effects of acquired hearing loss are a greater tendency to experience loneliness and isolation than do normally hearing people and a greater tendency to experience feelings of low self esteem, shame, and frustration.[10] The extent to which the sociosomatic imbalances associated with acquired hearing loss may produce or contribute to more serious psychological disturbance must now be considered.

Depression—Community studies in the United Kingdom have consistently reported a relationship between deafness and depression in old age. Indeed, in the summary of their review of mental health and acquired hearing impairment, Jones and White report that the only area in which there seems to be some consistent agreement among researchers is in the association between acquired hearing loss and depression—for both younger and older adults.[12] Similar findings have also been reported by a range of researchers in a variety of locations—by Carabellese *et al*, Italy[13] and Ihara in Japan[14]; however, researchers in the United States were unable to document an association between hearing loss and depression after adjusting for potential confounders, such as age and visual acuity.[15] Such work concerning the implication of poor sight coupled with poor hearing in old age needs to be developed.

Paranoia—The debate about the association of acquired hearing loss and paranoia has been raging for the past 30 years or so. Researchers have sampled hearing impaired people and attempted to discover whether they are more or less likely to suffer from paranoid illnesses than are the normally hearing. Researchers have also sampled mentally ill people and attempted to assess whether the paranoid are more or less likely to be deaf than are the not paranoid. All studies so far undertaken are beset with methodological problems and do not stand up to close scrutiny. The reviews of Thomas in 1984,[16] Meadow-Orlans in 1985,[17] and Jones and White in 1990[12] are consistent in their observations that any association between acquired hearing loss and paranoid illness needs further work before it can be confirmed or refuted.

Organic brain syndrome—The prevalence for moderate to severe cognitive impairment in those aged 80 years and over has been assessed at about 20%. Whether there is any association between hearing impairment and organic brain syndrome in older age is unclear because both conditions are so prevalent in advanced old age. This is disputed, however, by Peters and her colleagues, who found cognitive decline more rapid in the demented hearing impaired after follow up of 6–16 months (even when age was controlled for) and concluded that there is an interaction between acquired sensorineural loss in later life and Alzheimer's disease.[18]

At least a third of the deafness found in the elderly is probably of onset in middle age. It is possible that there is some causal link between deafness and dementia derived from a complicated interweave of cause and effect of time of onset, type of deafness, and type of dementia. As a strong component of organic brain syndrome is poor memory recall, it is not possible to determine accurately duration of deafness amongst the demented without recourse to longitudinal studies.

The disease–disease interaction theory is now proposed by researchers studying the observed consistent pattern of degeneration in the auditory system of sufferers from Alzheimer's disease.[19 20]

With regard to the effects on cognitive function of acquired hearing loss in older age, a slightly clearer picture is now unfolding. In a review of the literature on the subject, Gennis and colleagues came to the view that hearing ability is related to cognitive status in those with organic brain syndromes but that there is little to suggest that in normal elderly people hearing impairment leads to cognitive decline.[21] The precise nature of the interplay between hearing impairment, dementia, and cognitive functioning is unclear—leaving room for further research.

Management

Improvements in general health and prescribing techniques, further legislation designed to reduce occupational or noise induced hearing loss, and the absence of war in some countries may have some effect in controlling the prevalence of hearing impairment in the future. The size of the older population is, however, steadily increasing and will continue to do so well into the twenty first century; the number of people with age related hearing impairment will still pose a substantial and largely unrecognised public health problem.

Only a third of those older people who might benefit from rehabilitation currently have a hearing aid. At the same time the hearing aid service is overloaded. In some parts of the United Kingdom patients are waiting for more than a year to be fitted with an aid.[22] The government is taking steps to improve the service. In 1990 it set up 12 pilot projects using a direct referral system. This provides for a general practitioner to refer patients with simple age related sensorineural deafness direct to a hearing aid clinic, bypassing the ear, nose, and throat (ENT) hospital consultant. The aim of the scheme is to speed up referral time, reduce costs, and release the ENT consultant for more complex cases. First reports of the experiment confirm that waiting time is halved; that there are no cost savings; and that the direct referral system entails a small increased risk to the patient.[23] For this system to be universally adopted, general practitioners and hearing aid technicians will have to be better trained than they are at present.

It is appropriate that the hearing aid service for older people is improved and should reach all who need it. For many, however, the aid will be of limited value in view of the predominantly sensorineural nature of their impairment. In the United Kingdom there are only 75 hearing therapists, whose job it is to provide counsel and social support to the millions of hearing impaired people of all ages in this country.

Personal services on the scale and of the type that are undoubtedly required (namely, counselling, case work, domiciliary visiting, and destigmatisation of deafness) are labour intensive, hard to administer, and expensive. What is more, such needs are, as with most welfare imperatives, extraordinarily difficult to pin down in terms of specific service content. The result has been the channelling of the needs of older deaf people towards services that are relatively easy to provide rather than the development of services that might help overcome the very marked social and psychological problems they face. Rehabilitation of older deaf people has become equated with the issue of the hearing aid—regardless of the value to the sufferer to be derived from it.

1 Gilhome Herbst KR, Humphrey CM. Prevalence of hearing impairment and mental state in the elderly living at home. *J R Coll Gen Pract* 1981;**31**:155–60.
2 Milne JS. A longitudinal study of hearing loss in older people. *Br J Audiol* 1977;**11**:7–11.
3 Gilhome Herbst KR, Meredith R, Stephens SDG. Implications of hearing impairment for elderly people in London and in Wales. *Acta Otolaryngol (Stockh)* 1991;**476**(suppl): 209–14.
4 Davis A. The prevalence of deafness. In: Ballantyne J, Martin MC, Martin A, editors. *Deafness*. London: Uhurr Ltd, 1993.
5 Martin J, Meltzer H, Elliot D. *The prevalence of disability among adults*. London: HMSO, 1988. (OPCS surveys of disability in Great Britain, report 1.)
6 Coles R, Davis A, Smith P. Tinnitus; its epidemiology and management. In: Jensen JH, editor. *Presbyacusis and other age related aspects*. 14th Danavox symposium, 1990. Copenhagen: Danavox Jubilee Foundation, 1990:377–402.

7 Weinberger M, Radelet M. Differential adaptive capacity to hearing impairment. *J Rehab* 1983;**4**:64–9.
8 Hetu R, Riverin L, Getty L, Lalande NM, St-Cyr C. The reluctance to acknowledge hearing difficulties among hearing impaired workers. *Br J Audiol* 1990;**24**:265–76.
9 Hallberg LR-M, Carlsson SG. Hearing impairment, coping and perceived hearing handicap in middle-aged subjects with acquired hearing loss. *Br J Audiol* 1991;**25**:323–30.
10 Thomas AJ, Gilhome Herbst KR. Social and psychological implications of acquired deafness for adults of employment age. *Br J Audiol* 1980;**14**:76–85.
11 Humphrey CM, Gilhome Herbst KR, Faruqi S. Some characteristics of the hearing impaired elderly who do not present themselves for rehabilitation. *Br J Audiol* 1981;**15**: 25–30.
12 Jones EM, White AJ. Mental health and acquired hearing impairment: a review. *Br J Audiology* 1990;**24**:3–9.
13 Carabellese C, Appollonio I, Rozzini R, *et al.* Sensory impairment and quality of life in a community elderly population. *J Am Geriatr Soc* 1993;**41**:401–7.
14 Ihara K. Depressive states and their correlates in elderly people living in a rural community. *Nippon Koshu Eisei Zasshi* 1993;**40**(2):85–94.
15 Mulrow CD, Aguilar C, Endicott J, Velez R, Tuley MR, Charlip WS. Association between hearing impairment and the quality of life of elderly individuals. *J Am Geriatr Soc* 1990; **38**:45–50.
16 Thomas AJ. *Acquired hearing loss: psychological and psychosocial implications.* London: Academic Press, 1984.
17 Meadow-Orlans K. Social and psychological effects of hearing loss in adulthood: a literature review. In: Orlans H, editor. *Adjustment to adult hearing loss.* London: Taylor and Francis, 1985:35–57.
18 Peters CA, Potter JF, Scholar SG. Hearing impairment as a predictor of cognitive decline in dementia. *J Am Geriatr Soc* 1988;**36**:981–6.
19 Oyer HJ, Solberg LC. Audiological rehabilitation of older people: visual and vibro-tactile considerations. *Br J Audiol* 1989;**23**:33–7.
20 Sinha UK, Hollen KM, Rodriguez R, Miller CA. Auditory system degeneration in Alzheimer's disease. *Neurology* 1993;**43**:779–85.
21 Gennis V, Garry PJ, Haaland KY, Yeo RA, Goodwin JS. Hearing and cognition in the elderly. New findings and a review of the literature. *Arch Intern Med* 1991;**151**:2259–64.
22 Royal National Institute for the Deaf. *A survey of National Health Service hearing aid services.* London: RNID, 1984.
23 Reeves D, Mason L, Prosser H, Kiernan C. *Direct referral systems for hearing aid provision.* London: HMSO, 1994.

38 Incontinence

CATH McGROTHER, MIKE CLARKE

Definitions and diagnostic criteria

Urinary incontinence is not a homogeneous condition. Most classifications of incontinence distinguish extrinsic disorder—for example, immobility—from intrinsic disorder, including overt neurological disorder and lower urinary tract dysfunction. The International Continence Society recognises categories of the latter based on the functionality of the detrusor muscle, the urethral closure mechanism, and bladder sensation, which are helpful in the clinical management of the condition.[1] Four main clinical categories of lower urinary tract dysfunction are recognised on the basis of cystometric investigation: (a) *detrusor instability*, in which the bladder contracts despite the patient attempting to inhibit micturition; (b) *genuine stress incontinence* reflecting a demonstrably incompetent urethral closure mechanism in the absence of a detrusor contraction; (c) *voiding difficulties* encompassing underactive detrusor function, overactive urethral closure mechanism, and mechanical obstruction due to prostate or urethral stricture; and (d) *hypersensivity* including primary sensory urgency and interstitial cystitis. In addition, *infection* may be superimposed, particularly when the bladder fails to empty completely, and may or may not give rise to symptoms. *Senile urethrovaginitis* is also commonly recognised in older women and may exacerbate other symptoms. Considerable controversy persists over distinctions between these clinical categories.[2]

The majority of cases are related to underlying detrusor instability and genuine stress incontinence in women or prostatic obstruction in men.[3][4] These distinct conditions need to be considered separately as they are likely to have different incidence and remission rates and different prognostic indicators. In a majority of cases the underlying condition can be inferred from the prominence of symptoms, for example, urge incontinence in relation to detrusor instability, stress incontinence in relation to genuine stress incontinence, and hesitancy in relation to prostatism. In practice, however, distinctions are complicated by a confusing overlap of symptomatology between accepted categories, and combinations of dysfunction are not uncommon. Diagnostic confirmation relies on urodynamic investigation, which is particularly important for the more complex symptom presentation and for those who fail to respond to first line treatment.

Urinary incontinence is often defined as "any leakage of urine occurring more than once a month." Although this may be easily understood for the purposes of population surveys, this level of disorder is too mild to constitute a significant need.[5] Leakage of urine that renders a person "wet" or "damp" rather than "dry" has more relevance for service provision,[6] although more trivial incontinence may constitute an early phase of the disorder relevant to studies of incidence, natural history, and prevention.

People present with a range of symptoms of urinary dysfunction, including urgency, frequency, nocturia, hesitancy, pain, and others within which incontinence may be a minor feature, depending on the underlying condition.[3] In terms of describing the clinical picture or defining need for the more specialist services, leakage of urine may be too narrow a description. A definition expressed in terms of "having difficulty in controlling urine" is suggested as the more appropriate indication for this broader group of conditions and the related level of need.

There has been far less research into faecal incontinence in the community and it is not clear how to describe the problem in terms that estimate the extent of need. Definitions based on "leakage of faeces" are known to identify a high proportion of trivial disorders, including staining relating to haemorrhoids.[7] Two main categories of significant faecal incontinence are generally recognised: neurogenic incontinence and faecal incontinence secondary to impaction.

Incidence

There are no reliable estimates of the incidence of urinary incontinence or dysfunction in older age. Provisional estimates suggest that any incontinence may occur in 2·7% of middle aged women per annum[8]; in the elderly the more stringent definition of difficulty in control may affect a minimum of 1% per annum.[6] There have been no studies of the incidence of faecal incontinence in old age.

Magnitude of the problem

Estimates of the prevalence of urinary incontinence vary widely depending on the definition used (Table 38.1). In Great Britain it is estimated that up to 4% or one million adults over 40 are affected with socially disabling urinary incontinence and around 10% of older adults may have a significant problem. The prevalence of significant urinary dysfunction is somewhat higher, mainly as a result of a substantial number of men with voiding difficulties and minimal or no incontinence. Prevalences are considerably higher in residential care compared with the community, with between a quarter and a third of elderly residents in some areas having difficulty in controlling their urine.[9]

354

Significant faecal or double incontinence has been estimated to affect around 4/1000 adults in the community, with rates of 11/1000 and 13/1000 in men and women aged 65 or more respectively.[3] Fewer than a quarter of cases have been shown to be receiving services. Similar degrees of faecal incontinence affect between a fifth and a third of elderly people in residential homes, depending on the setting.

Urinary incontinence in the elderly is associated with significant reduction in five year survival compared with that for continent elderly people[10]; however, the excess mortality is greatest for those with associated physical and mental handicaps.

The overall cost of incontinence is difficult to ascertain. Recently the Association of Continence Advisors estimated NHS expenditure on continence aids alone at £68 000 000 per annum and suggested that there was scope for reducing some costs by better management.[11] The true overall cost is likely to be higher as a consequence of hidden and indirect costs; for example, approximately 20% of elderly people in the community pay for their own continence aids.[12] Incontinence can incur other social costs—for example, among informal carers of the elderly inability to tolerate incontinence and sleep disturbance due to problems with micturition were cited as contributing factors in the breakdown of community care in a substantial proportion of cases.[13]

Variation and determinants

The prevalence of urinary incontinence increases with age (table 38.1). In women the prevalence increases substantially after the childbearing years but declines slightly after the menopause before increasing again in old age. In men incontinence is less prevalent and rises progressively with age.[5] Urinary dysfunction as a whole is, however, equally common in men and women in old age, affecting 12% of a total population aged 75 or more.[6] The prevalence of the different categories of dysfunction on the basis of symptoms for men and women is shown in table 38.2.[3]

The only prospective study to have explored aetiological factors focused on the effects of childbirth and showed that in the decade after giving birth a fifth of women developed persistent stress incontinence.[14] The strongest associations were with high birth weight, prolonged second stage of labour, use of forceps, and vaginal delivery. Maternal age was the dominant predictor of late starting and persistent stress incontinence. Members of social classes I and II and non-Asian women were at increased risk, independent of maternal age. These results suggest that stress incontinence is a condition of heterogeneous aetiology in which social, obstetric, and age factors play a substantial part. Associations identified from prospective studies of selective healthy women could be misleading.[8]

Cross-sectional studies show a number of strong relationships with stroke,[15] cognitive impairment, including possibly depression, and mobility/

Table 38.1   Prevalence of urinary incontinence

Age (years)	Prevalence (%)			
	More than minimal*		Any regular leakage	
	Women	Men	Women	Men
35–44	5·6	1·0	10·2	1·5
45–54	6·5	1·0	11·8	1·6
55–64	6·6	1·9	11.9	2·9
65–74	4·6	1·7	8·8	6·1
75–84	8·3	2·3	16·0	8·1
85 +	8·4	4·3	16·2	15·4

* Estimated from interview of a sample.[5]

Table 38.2   Prevalence of subtypes of urinary dysfunction predicted on the basis of symptoms in an elderly population living at home

Category of dysfunction	Prevalence (%)		
	Women	Men	All
Unstable bladder	3·7	1·9	3·1
Unstable + genuine stress incontinence	1·5		1·0
Unstable + obstruction		0·8	0·3
Genuine stress incontinence/	1·9	—	1·7
urethral incompetence	—	1·4	—
Obstruction/voiding difficulties		3·6	1·2
Other dysfunction	0·7	0·3	0·5
All urinary dysfunction	7·7	8·0	7·8

dexterity problems.[10] The strongest relationships occur with dementia and stroke, which may point towards common underlying causes of atherosclerosis and hypertension, implicating a number of lifestyle factors. Interestingly, cigarette smoking shows a strong relationship and obesity is also related to incontinence.[16] Certain aspects of diet, including the consumption of coffee, tea, alcohol, fizzy drinks, and citrus fruits, are also commonly recognised clinically.

Intervention

Primary prevention

The possible relationship of incontinence with obstetric factors and cardiovascular risk factors as well as psychological morbidity and ageing raises the potential for primary prevention; however, considerably more research is needed, especially a prospective study of the various types of urinary dysfunction, before guidance on primary prevention can be formulated with confidence.

Secondary prevention

There is considerable stigma attached to the presence of urinary incontinence or dysfunction, which inhibits communication and early detection of the condition. In addition, services are rarely oriented to early intervention, tending perhaps to offer reassurance or even disdain for apparently trivial problems. The decline in prevalence of incontinence after menopause points to a self limiting problem in some cases. In the absence of systematic information on the natural history of the subtypes of urinary dysfunction it is perhaps not surprising that clinicians find it difficult to interpret the significance of early symptoms and to respond appropriately.

Treatment

Detrusor instability accounts for just over 40% of urinary incontinence in older adults.[34] Preliminary treatment is based on retraining the bladder by developing a new habit of micturition, which alone may improve or cure 40–50% of patients at least in the short term.[17] Anticholinergic drugs, particularly imipramine and oxybutynin, are usually used as a secondary measure to help suppress unstable bladder contractions, with possible benefit for a further 20% or so of patients.[18 19] Oestrogen also affects detrusor muscle contractions and preliminary studies suggest it may have a supportive role in the management of detrusor instability.

Genuine stress incontinence accounts for around 40% of urinary incontinence in older women.[34] Management is based on strengthening the pelvic floor musculature and surrounding tissues by exercises using physiotherapy. Substantial benefits have been reported in three quarters of patients but studies need to be controlled for possible placebo or attention effects.[20] Weighted vaginal cones constitute an alternative approach that includes an element of biofeedback. Preliminary studies suggest cure rates comparable with pelvic floor exercises, at lower cost, but the results are inconclusive because of the small numbers of patients studied.[21] Here too there is a suggestion that oestrogen may help in strengthening pelvic tissues in women with signs of deficiency. Surgery is also beneficial but it is regarded as best reserved for those who fail to respond to less invasive treatments, which include weight reduction.

Unfortunately many patients never come to the attention of the primary care team and reports suggest that 90% of elderly patients in need receive no specialist treatment.[12]

Information on the response of faecal incontinence to conservative management is very limited. In a study of frequent faecal incontinence among elderly people in residential care half were diagnosed as having neurogenic incontinence and half had faecal incontinence secondary to impaction.[22] Both problems occurred mainly in association with dementia, whereas incontinence associated with diarrhoea was rare. Fewer than 4%

of patients had received medical attention. Management involving laxatives or constipating medication and enemas, designed to regulate bowel action, proved successful in 60% of patients.

Long term support

Overall, little attention has been given to the long term support needs of elderly people with incontinence. There has been little follow up of specialist treatment but there is some indication that initial improvement may not be sustained in a fair proportion of cases.[23] Patients who fail to receive specialist services or to respond must rely on incontinence pads, pants, and other aids.

In one area, of 8% of the elderly living in the community who were incontinent only a third received NHS incontinence pads or aids and fewer than half of these managed to prevent external wetting of clothes.[12] The main problems with incontinence aids services identified were failure to communicate the problem to and between the primary care team, lack of proper assessment procedures, shortages in the supply of pads, difficulty in accessing the distribution centre, the poor quality of pads provided, and the lack of any systematic follow up.

Health policy

Health policy is in confusion at present, with uncertainty about the relative merits of treatments, including their long term efficacy, and the organisation of services, particularly the role of specialist nursing.[24] There is also awareness of the lack of information to guide the development of preventive measures and the rational use of surgery. It is, however, commonly perceived that development should be in the direction of early active phases of low and then higher level interventions, in which incontinence aids are used in support rather than as the centrepiece of treatment.

Traditionally care has centred on the primary care team with very limited special training but with access to specialist referral. Attempts have been made by general practitioners to supplement primary care, with encouraging results. O'Brien and colleagues recently evaluated primary care non-specialist nurse continence classes and showed 68% of patients were improved or cured compared with 5% in the general practitioner control group.[25] Other service developments include specially trained district nurses supported by a continence adviser, which in some areas has achieved improvement for 50% of patients seen.[26] Alternatively, a continence nurse may practise as part of a specialist medical team, which typically report improvement rates of over 70%.[27] These results suggest considerable scope for improvement but there are a number of problems in comparing these models of service because of differences in selection factors affecting the type and severity of condition, the age of patients seen, and the lack of standard criteria and resource information.

In conclusion it is apparent that incontinence constitutes a common and substantial problem for older people and services, yet only a small proportion of people affected come to the attention of services. Recent developments in treatments and services appear to offer potential relief for a majority of older people and more effective use of resources; however, further evaluation is needed as a guide to the rational development of services.[28] Knowledge of the epidemiology of the dysfunctions underlying incontinence in older people is at present insufficient to support the development of effective preventive measures. For example, it has been suggested that a high fibre diet may be inappropriate for many elderly people.[29]

1 Abrams P, Blainas JG, Stanton SL, Anderson J. Standardisation of terminology. *Neurourol Urodyn* 1988;7(5):403–27.
2 Peattie AB. The management of sensory urgency. In: Drife JO, Hilton P, Standon SL, editors. *Micturition*. London: Springer, 1990:315–25.
3 McGrother CW, Castleden CM, Duffin H, Clarke M. A profile of disordered micturation in the elderly at home. *Age Ageing* 1987;16:105–10.
4 Feneley RCL, Shepherd AM, Powell PH, Blannin J. Urinary incontinence: prevalence and needs. *Br J Urol* 1979;51:493–6.
5 Thomas TM, Phymal KR, Blannin J, Meade JW. Prevalence of urinary incontinence. *BMJ* 1980;281:1243–5.
6 McGrother CW, Castleden CM, Duffin H, Clark M. Provision of services for incontinent elderly people at home. *J Epidemiol Community Health* 1986;40:134–8.
7 Thomas JM, Egan M, Walgrove A, Meade TW. The prevalence of faecal and double incontinence. *Community Med* 1984;6:216–20.
8 Burgio KL, Matthew KA, Engel BJ. Prevalence, incidence and correlates of urinary incontinence in healthy, middle-aged women. *J Urol* 1991;146:1255–9.
9 Peet SM, Castleden CM, McGrother CW, *et al.* The prevalence of urinary and faecal incontinence in hospital, residential and nursing homes for older people. *BMJ* 1995 (in press).
10 McGrother CW, Jagger C, Clarke M, Castleden CM. Handicaps associated with incontinence: implication for management. *J Epidemiol Community Health* 1990;44:246–8.
11 Sanderson JM. *Agenda for action on continence services*. London: Department of Health, 1991 (unpublished report).
12 McGrother CW, Castleden CM, Duffin H, Clarke M. Do the elderly need better incontinence services? *Community Med* 1987;9:62–7.
13 Sanford JRA. Tolerance of debility in elderly dependants by supporters at home: its significance for hospital practice. *BMJ* 1975;3:471–3.
14 McArthur C, Lewis M, Knox G. *Health after childbirth*. London: HMSO, 1991.
15 Brocklehurst K, Andrews K, Richards B, Laycock PJ. Incidence and correlates of incontinence in stroke patients. *J Am Geriatr Soc* 1985;33:540–2.
16 Bump RC, McClish DK. Cigarette smoking and urinary incontinence in women. *Am J Obstet Gynecol* 1992;167:1213–8.
17 Pengelly AW, Booth CM. A prospective trial of bladder training as treatment for detrusor instability. *Br J Urol* 1980;52:463–6.
18 Castleden CM, Duffin H, Gulato RS. Double-blind study of imipramine and placebo for incontinence due to bladder instability. *Age Ageing* 1986;15:299–303.
19 Thüroff JW, Bunke B, Ebner A, *et al.* Randomised double-blind multicenter trial on treatment of frequency, urgency and incontinence related to detrusor hyperactivity; oxybutynin versus propentheline versus placebo. *J Urol* 1991;45:813–7.
20 Wells JT, Brink C, Diokno A, Wolfe R, Gillis GL. Pelvic muscle exercises for stress urinary incontinence in elderly women. *J Am Geriatr Soc* 1991;39:785–91.
21 Haken J, Bennes C, Cardozo L, Cutner A. A randomised trial of vaginal cones and pelvic floor exercises in the management of genuine stress incontinence. *Neurourol Urodyn* 1991; 10:393–4.

22 Tobin GW, Brocklehurst JC. Faecal incontinence in residential homes for the elderly: prevalence, aetiology and management. *Age Ageing* 1986;**15**:41–6.
23 Snape J, Castleden CM, Duffin HM, Ekelund P. Long-term follow-up of habit retraining for bladder instability in elderly patients. *Age Ageing* 1989;**18**:192–4.
24 Rhodes P, Parker G. *The role of continence nurse advisers in England and Wales.* York: Social Policy Research Unit, University of York, 1993.
25 O'Brien J, Austin M, Sethi P, O'Boyle P. Urinary incontinence prevalence, need for treatment and effectiveness of intervention by nurse. *BMT* 1991;**303**:1308–12.
26 Hall C, Castleden CM, Grove GJ. Fifty-six continence advisers, one peripatetic teacher. *BMJ* 1988;**297**:1181–2.
27 Castleden CM, Duffin HM, Asher MJ, Yeomanson CW. Factors influencing outcome in elderly patients with urinary incontinence and detrusor instability. *Age Ageing* 1985;**14**:303–7.
28 Royal College of Physicians. *Incontinence: causes, management and provision of services.* London: Royal College of Physicians, 1995.
29 Barrett JA. *Faecal incontinence and related problems in the older adult.* London: Edward Arnold, 1993.

39 Falls

JOHN CAMPBELL

Definitions and diagnostic criteria

Different types of falls have different risk factors and careful determination of the circumstances of the fall is required both in clinical evaluation and for classification in epidemiological research. In studies of the incidence of falls, the falls are usually required to be unintentional and to result in contact with the ground—rather than just falling back into a seat.

Fit active elderly people who fall because they participate in vigorous and risky activities differ from frail elderly people who fall because of their instability. Risk factors and preventive measures for the two groups are different. The different types of fall may be separated by:

- Determining the external contribution to the fall and assessing whether it would have been sufficient to cause a fit, younger person to fall[1]
- Only investigating those who have had two or more falls[2]
- Classifying the amount of the movement at the time of the fall.[3]

There have been both retrospective and prospective studies of falls but retrospective studies underestimate the incidence of falls by 13–32% depending on the time period of recall.[4] Risk factors for falls resulting in injury do differ from risk factors for non-injurious falls[5] and falls resulting in injury may be investigated by, for example, drawing a sample from those who present to hospital.[6]

Magnitude of the problem

The fall rate per year by age and sex for a total population of older people living in both the community and in institutions is given in table 39.1. The rate increased with age but in the study reported there was no difference in fall rate between men and women.[7]

The majority of falls cause either no injury or bruising and abrasions only. Fractures have been shown to result from about 5% of falls.[8] A prolonged lie after a fall of an hour or more also occurs after about 5% of falls.

In a prospective Finnish study of the general population the incidence of injurious falls leading to either hospitalisation or death was highest in the older age groups. The incidence per 1000 person years was 3·7 for

361

Table 39.1   Falls per 100 person years by sex and age group[7]

Age (years)	Falls per 100 person years		
	Women	Men	Total
70–74	47·9	46·7	47·4
75–79	68·9	60·2	65·3
80–84	91·1	99·1	94·1
85–89	106·6	125·0	111·8
90 +	198·6	40·0	152·2

those 60–69 years, 7·0 for those 70–79 years and 27·0 for those 80 years and over.[6]

Of 149 504 patients aged 65 years and older discharged from hospitals in Washington state in 1989, 7873 (5·3%) were hospitalised for injuries from falls. The majority of persons admitted for falls were women, and patients tended to be older than those hospitalised for other reasons. Those who fell were also more likely to be discharged to a nursing facility.[9]

There are less obvious but equally serious consequences of falls. People who have fallen experience fear of falling again. Loss of confidence may result in restricted activity and be a significant factor in the person moving to a less independent, more supervised environment, such as a residential home.[10]

Variation

Time

Most falls occur during the hours of maximum activity in the day and only about 20% of falls occur at night.[7] In the winter months and on colder days there is an increase in both the rate of falls in women[11] and in fractures.[12] This increase in fall rate occurs in falls occurring inside as well as outside. Cold days may cause mild hypothermia and slowed responses. If an old person is cold and uncomfortable she may be less cautious when moving, hurrying back to the warmth. In addition, in cold winter weather some elderly women become less active and spend more time in bed, becoming weaker and at increased risk of falling. In winter, daylight hours are fewer and often duller increasing the risk of tripping on home hazards. It is difficult to know why men do not also have an increase in fall rate in winter and in the cold. A possible explanation is that men are more likely to fall outside while involved in activities such as gardening and they participate less in these activities during the winter months.

Place

About 65% of women and 44% of men fall inside their usual residence and about 25% of men and 11% of women fall in their home garden. Falls occur in the most frequently used rooms—bedrooms, kitchen, and dining room. In residential homes most falls occur in the resident's bedroom (64%) or passageways (18·7%).[7]

Person

Although the fall rate is similar for men and women, a greater proportion of women than men will experience a fall in which there is no or only minimal external contribution. The factors that have been shown to contribute to the sex difference in fall rate are the greater age of women than men in most samples, greater use of psychotropic drugs by women, greater inability to rise from a chair, going outside less frequently, and greater likelihood of living alone. Even after allowing for these physical and social factors, women compared with men still have about a one and a half times increased risk of falling.[13]

Secular trends

There are secular changes in the rate of complications from falls. The age adjusted incidence of femoral neck fracture has increased but, in contrast, between 1960 and 1990, deaths from falls among white Americans 75 years and over have decreased by more than 50%.[14 15] We do not have sufficient information to know whether this represents a secular change in fall rate or in the likelihood of complications.

Geographical variation

Comparison between countries of the rate of falls is difficult because of differences in study methodology. Rates for most countries are similar but two retrospective studies from Japan have reported a lower incidence of falls.[16 17] The possible effects of different environments, levels of activity, and life expectancy have not been explored. Although there are racial differences in hip fracture rate both within and between countries, racial differences in fall rate have not been investigated.

Determinants and intervention

The majority of internal falls result from multiple contributing and interrelating factors. Multivariate analysis is therefore necessary in the determination of the significance of potential risk factors. The identification of factors associated with falls has enabled rationally based intervention programmes to be developed. Early intervention trials showed no clear

Table 39.2 Fall determinants and interventions

Type of intervention	Target factor (Relative risk if calculated)	Possible treatment/rehabilitation
Physical activity	Balance and gait: number of abnormalities 0–2 RRA 1·0, 3–5 RRA 1·4 (0·7–2·8), 6–7 RRA, 1·9 (1·0–3·7)[8] lower extremity disability RRA 3·8 (2·2–6·7)[8] diversity of physical activity (≥2 activities in past week) RRA 0·6 (0·4–0·9)[22] weekly walk for exercise RR 0·7 (0·5–1·0)[8]	Gait training Balance training Muscle strengthening Transfer training General activity (for example, dance, t'ai chi)
Medication review	Sedative use RRA 28·3 (3·4–239·4)[8] Psychotropic drugs (women) RRA 1·6 (1·0–2·8)[1] Total number of drugs (women): no drugs RRA 1·0, 1–3 drugs RRA 2·6 (1·2–5·5), ≥4 drugs RRA 4·5 (1·9–10·6)[1]	Review, decrease if possible. Clinical psychologist support for establishing sleep patterns without hypnotics
Alcohol use	Excessive alcohol use: Alcohol intake (g/month) 0 RRI 1·0, ≤99 RRI 0·94 (0·73–1·22) 100–499 RRI 1·43 (1·13–1·82) 500–999 RRI 2·32 (1·71–3·17) ≥1000 RRI 3·05 (2·05–4·55)[6] combination with sedatives may increase this risk	Advice on safe drinking pattern: review, combination with other drugs
Home environment Home safety	Home hazards: ≥1 bedroom hazard RR 3·5 (0·9–13·0)[8] ≥2 living room hazard RR 0·7 (0·5–1·0)[8] As can be seen, home hazards have not been found to be a consistent risk factor[7]	Ensure obstacle free, adequate lighting and contrast, heating, absence of glare, low pile carpet, no loose mats or slippery surfaces, provide night light, hand rails, grip bars, light switches at top and bottom of stairs. Outside: repair cracks in pavement, holes in lawn, remove rocks, wet leaves
Home support	Household tasks beyond ability: Home alone >16 hours/day RRR 1·6 (1·2–2·2)[2] Needs help with ≥1 activity of daily living RRR 2·1 (1·7–3·0)[2]	Social visiting, home help, meals on wheels. Protect against excessive tiredness. Help with tasks beyond capability (rubbish bins, light bulb changing)

Clinical assessment		
Depression, neurological disease, acute illness, hypotension, musculoskeletal disorders, history of falls	Remedial physical and mental conditions: depression RR 1·7 (1·2–2·3)[8] cognitive impairment RRA 5·0 (1·8–13·7)[8] episode of serious illness RR 1·5 (1·1–2·1)[8] history of arthritis RRR 1·9 (1·4–2·6)[2] Parkinson's disease RRR 2·8 (2·1–3·9)[2] stroke (women) RRA 13·6 (2·6–71·3)[1] postural hypotension History of falls: fall in previous two years RR 2·5 (1·9–3·4)[8] ≥1 fall related injury in the past 12 months RRR 2·6 (1·6–4·4)[2]	Treat; advise; refer to other health specialist
Eye examination	Impaired contrast sensitivity, dark adaptation and perception, colour, discrimination, visual acuity, peripheral fields of vision: near-vision loss ≥20% RR 1·7 (1·2–2·3)[8]	Cataract extraction, review spectacles, increase lighting in home environment
Hearing assessment	Impaired hearing: hearing loss at least moderate RR 2·1[23]	Remove cerumen; hearing aid; reduce background noise
Podiatric assessment	Foot problems RRA 1·8 (1·0–3·1)[8]	Trim nails, treat calluses, bunions, deformities
Clothing	Unsafe footwear[24]	Safe footwear (correct size, firm non-skid non-friction sole, low heels, no loose slippers)
Assistive device	Inappropriate walking aids: use of cane or walker RR 1·8 (1·3–2·4)[8]	Appropriate walking aid
	Inappropriate restraint device: restraint use RRI 10·2 (2·8–36·9)[25]	Minimise restraint devices
Cognitive/behavioural/ social programme	Social isolation, loss of confidence: leaves residence once a week or less often RRR 2·5 (1·3–3·8)[2] low social network score RRR 1·6 (1·1–2·4)[2]	Restore confidence, provide social contact, teach avoidance of risk taking behaviour to person or caregiver

RRA, adjusted odds ratio for falls (95% CI) from multiple logistic regression analysis; RR, unadjusted relative risk estimate for falls (95% CI) if given; RRI, odds ratio for fall related injury (95% CI) adjusted for multiple factors; RRR, unadjusted relative risk estimate for two or more falls compared with one or no falls (95% CI).

benefit[18] but major studies are now in progress.[19] The first successful home based intervention study to reduce falls has been reported.[20]

The analysis of results from randomised controlled trials requires definition of a suitable end point, such as the time from randomisation to first fall, or the time of randomisation to injurious fall, or all fall events. There may be difficulty with the effect of those who fall very frequently if total number of falls is used in analysis. One method of dealing with this is to remove such a person from further analysis after a certain number of falls in a specified time period. The person is treated in the analysis in the same way as someone who has withdrawn or died during the study period. Another approach is to compare the number of fallers in the intervention and control groups. Because of the episodic recurrent nature of falls, there are difficulties in analysis using either number of falls or number of fallers as end points.[21]

A summary of potential interventions based on reported determinants of falls is given in table 39.2.

Health policy

Falls are the most prevalent cause of injury in older people. Fall related mortality is high in older adults (18/100 000 per year v 2·7/100 000 per year in young people) and is especially high in those aged 85 years and over (131·2/100 000 per year).[19] Fall related morbidity is also high in older people, who are more likely to injure themselves in a fall, take longer to recover, and may well require relocation after the fall.

Prevention

Fall prevention by either individual or public health programmes can be expensive. A pilot programme in a rural community in Ohio, incorporating the use of the medical community, senior citizens centre, the local college, fire department, local radio stations, and newspapers, had an estimated cost for one year of $52 538.[26]

The Frailty and Injuries: Cooperative Studies of Intervention Techniques (FICSIT) investigators[19] are the only groups reported to be addressing in detail the possible economic costs and benefits of fall intervention programmes.

The study of Rubenstein et al,[18] which showed no significant decrease in the fall rate in the intervention group, did show on follow up that the treated group had significantly fewer hospital admissions and fewer hospital bed days. A falls rehabilitation programme may improve health in a number of different ways and produce secondary benefits; for example, a physical activity programme may have the secondary benefits of increased social contact, improved bone strength, and improved sleep. Evaluation of a fall prevention programme should ideally be broadly based so all potential benefits are measured but this will undoubtedly increase the cost and complexity of the research project. The results of the first major community fall prevention studies are becoming available and these should indicate more clearly the most effective measures and their likely benefits and costs.[20]

1 Campbell AJ, Borrie MJ, Spears GF. Risk factors for falls in a community-based prospective study of people 70 years and older. *J Gerontol Med Sci* 1989;**44**:M112–7.

2 Nevitt MC, Cummings SR, Kidd S, Black D. Risk factors for recurrent nonsyncopal falls. A prospective study. *JAMA* 1989;**261**:2663–8.

3 Isaacs B. Are falls a manifestation of brain failure? *Age Ageing* 1978;**7**(suppl):97–105.

4 Cummings SR, Nevitt MC, Kidd S. Forgetting falls: the limited accuracy of recall of falls in the elderly. *J Am Geriatr Soc* 1988;**36**:613–6.

5 Nevitt MC, Cummings SR, Hudes ES. Risk factors for injurious falls: a prospective study. *J Gerontol Med Sci* 1991;**46**:M164–70.

6 Malmivaara A, Heliövaara M, Knekt P, Reunanen A, Aromaa A. Risk factors for injurious falls leading to hospitalization or death in a cohort of 19 500 adults. *Am J Epidemiol* 1993; **138**:384–94.

7 Campbell AJ, Borrie MJ, Spears GF, Jackson SL, Brown JS, Fitzgerald JL. Circumstances and consequences of falls experienced by a community population 70 years and over during a prospective study. *Age Ageing* 1990;**19**:136–41.

8 Tinetti ME, Speechley M, Ginter SF. Risk factors for falls among elderly persons living in the community. *N Engl J Med* 1988;**319**:1701–9.

9 Alexander BH, Rivara FP, Wolf ME. The cost and frequency of hospitalization for fall-related injuries in older adults. *Am J Public Health* 1992;**82**:1020–3.

10 Tinetti ME, Powell L. Fear of falling and low self-efficacy: a cause of dependence in elderly persons. *J Gerontol* 1993;**48**(special issue):35–8.

11 Campbell AJ, Spears GFS, Borrie MJ, Fitzgerald JL. Falls, elderly women and the cold. *Gerontology* 1988;**34**:205–8.

12 Bastow MD, Rawlings J, Allison SP. Undernutrition, hypothermia, and injury in elderly women with fractured femur: an injury response to altered metabolism. *Lancet* 1983;**1**: 143–6.

13 Campbell AJ, Spears GF, Borrie MJ. Examination by logistic regression modelling of the variables which increase the relative risk of elderly women falling compared to elderly men. *J Clin Epidemiol* 1990;**43**:1415–20.

14 Sorock GS. Falls among the elderly: epidemiology and prevention. *Am J Prev Med* 1988; **4**:282–8.

15 Riggs JE. Mortality from accidental falls among the elderly in the United States, 1962–1988: demonstrating the impact of improved trauma management. *J Trauma* 1993;**35**:212–9.

16 Yasumura S, Haga H, Nagai H, *et al.* Incidence of and circumstances related to falls among the elderly in a Japanese community. *Nippon Koshu Eisei Zasshi* 1991;**38**:735–42.

17 Yasumura S, Haga H, Nagai H, Suzuki T, Amano H, Shibata H. Rate of falls and the correlates among elderly people living in an urban community in Japan. *Age Ageing* 1994; **23**:323–7.

18 Rubenstein LZ, Robbins AS, Josephson KR, Schulman BL, Osterweil D. The value of assessing falls in an elderly population. A randomized clinical trial. *Ann Intern Med* 1990; **113**:308–16.

19 Ory MG, Schechtman KB, Miller P, *et al.* Frailty and injuries in later life: the FICSIT trials. *J Geriatr Soc* 1993;**41**:283–96.

20 Tinetti ME, Baker DI, McAugy G, *et al.* A multi-factorial intervention to reduce the risk of falling among elderly people living in the community. *N Engl J Med* 1994;**331**:821–7.

21 Cumming RG, Kelsey JL, Nevitt MC. Methodological issues in the study of frequent and recurrent health problems. *Ann Epidemiol* 1990;**1**:49–56.

22 O'Loughlin JL, Robitaille Y, Boivin J-F, Suissa S. Incidence of and risk factors for falls and injurious falls among the community-dwelling elderly. *Am J Epidemiol* 1993;**137**: 342–54.

23 Tinetti ME, Williams TF, Mayewski R. Fall risk index for elderly patients based on number of chronic disabilities. *Am J Med* 1986;**80**:429–34.

24 Robbins S, Gouw GT, McClaran J. Shoe sole thickness and hardness influence balance in older men. *J Am Geriatr Soc* 1992;**40**:1089–94.
25 Tinetti ME, Liu W-L, Ginter SF. Mechanical restraint use and fall-related injuries among residents of skilled nursing facilities. *Ann Intern Med* 1992;**116**:369–74.
26 Urton MM. A community home inspection approach to preventing falls among the elderly. *Public Health Rep* 1991;**106**:192–5.

40 Accidents

IRENE HIGGINSON

Definitions and diagnostic criteria

Definitions of accidents vary but the most commonly accepted definition is that an accident is "an unintentional injury or suspected injury, no matter how caused," except for (a) deliberate self inflicted injuries or suicide, or (b) injuries resulting from physical attacks by other persons. These definitions are used by reporting systems such as the Home Accidents Deaths Database (HADD), the Home Accidents Surveillance System (HASS), and the Leisure Accidents Surveillance System (LASS).[1]

Information on the epidemiology and prevention of accidents is available from a very wide range of sources and is often poorly collated. In addition to health journals and reports, data and studies are available from motoring organisations, charities (such as Age Concern), professional organisations (such as the Royal Society of Medicine, College of Occupational Therapists), the police, government departments (such as those for Transport, Health, Trade and Industry, or local government), and many others. This range of different sectors brings with it great variations in definitions and study design, which often make it impossible to compare findings.[2]

The development of national reporting systems—such as, in England and Wales, the HADD, HASS, and the LASS, and in the United States the National Accident Sampling System (NASS), the Fatal Accident Reporting System (FARS) database for motor vehicle related crash deaths, and for non-fatal injuries the National Electronic Injury Surveillance System (NEISS)—provide a very useful source of accident data and national annual estimates of accidents.[3] Information on non-fatal injuries is often based on those people who report to a sample of accident and emergency departments or emergency rooms. These departments must be willing to participate; information on rates within the general population is not usually provided, and data is often incomplete when clerical support is not available within the hospital, for example at night. Thus information is most accurate only for deaths or accidents that result in a person reporting to an accident and emergency department, emergency room, or to the police. Studies of selected communities (for example, people in nursing homes) are available, but prevalence rates are affected by the mechanisms for reporting the accident and the community studied.[24]

Within the general category of accidents, deaths in England and Wales (1991) in people aged 65 years and over were broken down as follows: 55% falls, 22% motor vehicle traffic accidents, 17% other, 5% fire and flame accidents, 2% accidental poisonings.[1] The causes of accidents are, however, complex: they are usually a combination of the interaction of the characteristics of the person injured, the environment, and often the object, product, or vehicle (or its driver) involved.

Magnitude of the problem

Accidents in older people are a major cause of morbidity and mortality in many countries of the world. The death rate for accidents among people aged 65 years and over is around 56/100 000 population in Western countries (tables 40.1 and 40.2).[1-3] These rates are much higher than the death rate for accidents in other age groups, such as that for young adults aged 15–24 years (24/100 000) or for children aged under 15 years (6–7/ 100 000). Over 70% of all fatal home accidents in England and Wales were to people aged over 65 years, and in 1991 there were 4626 deaths and about 500 000 people required hospital attention as a result of home and leisure accidents.[1]

Table 40.1   Fatal accident rate in England and Wales 1991

Age (years)	Men (rate per 100 000)	Women (rate per 100 000)	Increase over rate at 65–74 years	
			Men	Women
65–74	32·9	21·9		
75–84	77·4	68·4	2·4	3·1
85 +	205·5	212·4	6·2	9·7

Table 40.2   Non-fatal accident rate*

	Age 65–74 years		Age 75 +		Total
	Men	Women	Men	Women	
Home accident (England and Wales)	48 000	81 000	42 000	151 000	322 000
Leisure or non-home accident (UK)	29 000	69 000	23 000	63 000	184 000

* Based on national estimates of the total number of patients involved in accidents and reporting to accident and emergency departments (1991).

About 90% of burn and fire deaths occur in residential fires.[1 2 4] The residential fire death rate is higher for adults aged 65 years and over than for individuals aged 5–64 years. The rate increases with age. For adults aged 75 years and over the death rate is higher than that for children aged 0–4 years (deaths per 100 000 persons due to residential fires in the United States, 1985: 12 for men and 6·6 for women aged 75 years and over; 5 for men and 3 for women aged 65–74 years; 5 for boys and 4 for girls aged 0–4 years).

Accidents have significant consequences for the health services. Hip fractures are common sequelae of falls and the incidence of hip fractures has doubled since the mid-1970s.[5] The lifetime cost estimate for the 2·1 million older persons injured in the United States in 1985 was $5·1 billion.[5] The direct expenditures for hospital care, nursing home care, drugs, and other medical and rehabilitation services accounted for $2·8 billion, 55% of the total lifetime costs. Indirect cost for morbidity and mortality are estimated at $1·8 billion and $441 million respectively.[4]

Another important impact of accidents is change in lifestyle. Accidents in older adults may mean the difference between independent lives in their own homes and dependent lives that require supportive care or care in a nursing home. In Washington state, USA, 20% of older adults who entered a hospital for a non-fall accident were discharged to nursing homes or intermediate care facility rather than their own homes.[4]

Variation

Time

Trends since the mid-1970s suggest a decline in the death rate and rate of accidents in people aged over 65 years.[1 2] These data should be interpreted cautiously. The main source of time series data is mortality statistics and national reporting systems, which over the years have varied definitions, population samples, and instructions for coders. With an ageing population the number of falls and accidents will increase. In most Western countries large increases in the number of people in the oldest age groups (over 85 years) are predicted for the coming decade.[5] Accidents and fatal accidents are most common in these oldest age groups.

Place

Data on geographic variation between and within countries is difficult to obtain for accidents among elderly people. This is mainly because of variations in reporting systems. Three studies in Leicestershire, which used data from patient interviews, staff questionnaires, medical and nursing notes, and the accident report forms, demonstrated marked differences between patients' and staff's versions of the events and the accident reports.[6] A literature review, carried out as preparation for this chapter using Medline, found no epidemiological studies comparing accident or injury rates between countries. The *Health for All 2000* World Health Organization database provides rates of accidents among all age groups for most European countries.[7] The standardised death rate of motor vehicle traffic accidents per 100 000 population for all countries within Europe was 14·28 (22·28 for men and 6·74 for women); however, the rate varied, with Russia having the highest standardised death rate for motor vehicle traffic accidents—24·78 total, 40·63 for men and 10·49 for women—compared with 7·53 total, 11·08 for men and 4·12 for women in the United Kingdom. The lowest recorded rate was for Kazakhstan—3·18 total, 5·36 for men and 1·08 for women.[7]

Most (95%) elderly people live in their own homes; the remaining 5% live in residential care or institutions.[2] There is little research on the effect of different environments.[2] Most studies have not linked the presence or absence of environmental factors, such as type of housing, independently with accidents, although pavements have been identified as a factor causing falls outside the home.

A review of building safety has indicated the importance of the inherent slipperiness, maintenance, cleanliness and hardness of floors and the lighting of stairs and corridors as important factors in the cause of falls.[8] Hot water temperatures and hot touchable surfaces of domestic equipment are important in the cause of burns and scalds. The Electricity Research and Development Centre (ERDC) examined 207 electric immersion heater installations in retirement homes and found that 71% of the thermostats inspected were set at temperatures above 65°C—a level that could cause substantial scalding.[9]

Person

The fatal and non-fatal accident rates increases by age for both men and women, as shown in tables 40.1 and 40.2.[1 2 10] In the age group 85 years and over the fatal accident rate can be six times higher for men and almost 10 times higher for women when compared to the rate for those aged 65–74 years. Within the over 65 years age group, 85% of fatal falls, 73% of fatal fires, and 63% of fatal chokings occur in people aged 75 years and over.[10] Poisonings and drowning do not show the same age bias.[12]

Medical and health factors—for example, poor grip strength, impaired mobility, physical disability, poor visual function, health problems, such as cardiovascular disease and dementia, reduced muscle strength, gait disorders, and the taking of benzodiazepines and tricyclic antidepressant drugs—have been associated with an increased risk of accident.[1 2 4 5] Living alone has also been shown to be a risk factor.[24]

Determinants and intervention

Many of the predisposing health problems become common in older people (especially those over 75 years) and it is therefore difficult to separate the risk factors.[2 10] Of most value are multiple regression studies, which seek to identify the most important risk factors.[2] Evaluations of some of the suggested interventions are underway.[1 2 4]

Primary prevention

Health education, environment changes, medical and health assessment, and improvement of fitness have all been advocated to prevent accidents. There is little evidence to suggest that general education can prevent them. There is evidence, however, to suggest that much of the information produced is not seen. In a survey of 902 people over 65 years of age most (86%) of the sample had never seen any information and those who had a home help, district nurse, or social worker were usually in the ill-informed groups.[11] It is probable that the family is more likely than external information to influence behaviour, and any information needs to be targeted.[11]

Improvements in building design, the use of appropriate non-slip, clean, even, softer flooring, adequate indoor lighting, and the control of hot water temperatures have all been suggested but rarely evaluated.[2] Similarly smoke alarms have been strongly advocated and promoted, although evaluative studies are not available.[8]

In an attempt to evaluate multiple interventions, Vetter *et al* found that in a randomised control trial the interventions of a health visitor, including assessment and correction of diet, health, environmental hazards, and fitness, did not alter the number of accidents in 350 people aged 70 years or over.[12]

When considering road accidents, urban safety areas have been demonstrated to be of value in reducing accidents (across all ages) in a number of countries.[13] There are many different types of scheme, most of which are aimed at the general population; they include engineering measures, sometimes together with encouraging walking, cycling, or use of public transport. A number of other campaigns have been developed to target elderly drivers. The accident rate per miles travelled increases after the age of 75 years. Numerous factors may be important here: impaired eyesight (for example, related to cataracts that require surgery), delayed reaction time, and unfamiliarity with the road layout; however, private transport is often a major and sometimes the only form of transport available for elderly people. General transport and driver characteristics are important. A journey by car is three times more likely to injure a pedestrian than a journey made by bus,[14] and the removal of subsidies of public transport in London is suggested to have been partly responsible for the increased number of road casualties.[15] Car speed is also strongly related to the severity of injury: of pedestrians struck by a moving car at 20 miles (32 km) per hour 5% are killed, but at 40 miles (64 km) per hour 85% are killed.[16]

Older drivers have different motor vehicle accident patterns, which usually involve errors of omission, compared with younger drivers.[4] Older drivers are more likely to be involved in intersection and turning crashes and in head on collisions in urban areas. They are also more likely to commit right of way and signal violations and to be charged with inattention.

Conversely older drivers are less likely to be involved in single vehicle crashes or to be cited for reckless driving, driving too fast, or drinking and driving.[4]

Driver education courses for adults aged 55 years and over have been developed in an attempt to update driving knowledge and refresh skills.[4] These are offered throughout the United States through driving schools, automobile and safety organisations, and older adult organisations. The effectiveness of these courses in improving driving is hard to assess because of the possible self selection of those drivers who take the course[4]; however, participants of Californian driver improvement courses had significantly lower rates of fatal or injury collisions and traffic convictions in the six months after the course than comparison drivers after adjusting for age, gender, licence class, prior record, and area of residence.[4]

Older adults have the highest pedestrian death rates of any age group. Figures from the United States suggest a death rate of 4·7/100 000 persons in 1989.[4] The rate for those aged 80 and over was twice as high as for persons aged 70–74 years. Pedestrian–motor vehicle collisions are very different from other types of motor vehicle accidents because very few pedestrians escape injury. Data from the US National Highway Traffic Safety Administration showed that only 1·1% of pedestrians struck by a car are not injured. In contrast, 94% of all motor vehicle crashes involve no injury.[4] Older pedestrian deaths are more likely to occur during daylight.[4]

Few studies of environmental factors have been specifically designed or evaluated for their effect on the risk of pedestrian–motor vehicle collisions in older adults. Pedestrian crossings or crosswalks appear to have benefits in some studies but not in others.[4] Allowing a right turn on a red light has consistently been shown to increase the risk of pedestrian injury, particularly among adults aged 65 years and over. Results from the United States on the use of pedestrian signals are controversial, but in England pedestrian crossings that had both markings and pedestrian activated traffic lights had half the risk of pedestrian injury compared with crossings without such lights for the same levels of vehicle and pedestrian volume. In New York a comprehensive programme introducing pedestrian crossings, altering road markings, and tightening speed limit enforcement decreased the incidence of fatal and near fatal pedestrian injuries by 43 and 86% respectively two years after implementation of the interventions.[4]

Secondary prevention

Intervention to minimise injury after an accident or to prevent future accidents include the following.

Alarms—There is evidence to suggest that people did not receive all the help they wanted after an accident. Alarms do not, however, always solve this problem because the person may be unable to reach the alarm when it is required or there may be problems for the individual summoned in gaining access to the home.[2]

Protection—To prevent or minimise the effects of motor vehicle crashes it is suggested that changes in the environment or the products are more likely to result in a reduction of injuries than is a focus on behavioural change.[4] The most effective methods of occupant protection are seat restraints, including lap and shoulder belts, and air bags. Studies have shown that seat belt restraints are 45% effective in preventing motor vehicle crash deaths and 50% effective in preventing moderate to critical motor vehicle crash injuries.[4] Changes to the bumper, hood, and windshield of vehicles can potentially reduce by one third the risk of serious injury to pedestrians who are struck.[4]

Medical evaluation after an accident—This intervention is based on evidence that once an elderly person has had one accident they are more likely to have another.[25] Intervention at this time may therefore prevent future accidents. Most evaluative studies have concentrated on fall and syncope clinics.[25]

Acute treatment

Evaluation of trauma centres has indicated that severe trauma has a better outcome in terms of mortality and continued morbidity in larger centres that specialise in the management of trauma[24]; however, these studies were largely confined to age groups of those under 65 years and similar results may not necessarily be obtained in older or the oldest age groups.[24]

Rehabilitation

Several trials have demonstrated the benefits of rehabilitation for elderly people, particularly after falls or fracture of the neck of femur, in reducing both mortality and disability.[24]

Health policy and conclusions

The majority of accidents are avoidable and present a major burden for health and social services, patients, and families. Elderly people are the most common group in society to suffer accidents, therefore the prevention of accidents among elderly people should be a high priority.

Definitions

Appropriate monitoring and research into accidents among older people is severely hampered by a lack of standard definitions and poor epidemiological data, especially regarding the severity of injury. Information on accidents is usually extremely disparate, making reviews difficult. Multidisciplinary approaches, particularly those that include representatives from transport or building design, are rarely adopted. To overcome this it is suggested that all funding bodies, including government departments, charities, and research foundations, need to ensure that grants for projects or research are given to well designed projects that use standard definitions and measures, involve other appropriate professionals, and provide clear details of the interventions followed. One way of improving the problems of disparate information would be to develop a central point for the collection of work on accidents among elderly people or on accidents in general. Such central points are available for other age groups, such as children (for example, the Child Accident Prevention Trust).

Prevention

Environmental improvements, improvements in lighting, control of water temperatures, traffic calming,[17] and driver retraining have all been shown to have some small effect on accident rates, although cost effectiveness studies are not available. On current evidence general education is probably not of benefit. Consideration needs to be given to the availability of transport for elderly people.

Secondary prevention where individuals are protected to lessen injury and where medical evaluation is given following an accident appears to be beneficial.

Treatment

The development of trauma units, which specialise in the management of accidents, have been shown to be cost effective. In addition, elderly people suffering from an accident may have multiple pathology and may therefore require input from a multiprofessional team including specialists in the health care of elderly people and rehabilitation.

1 Department of Health. *Key area handbook: accidents.* London: Department of Health, 1993.
2 Higginson I. *Health of the Nation accident reduction targets. A Research Review: What further research is needed.* London: Department of Health, 1995.
3 Kraus JF, Robertson LS. Injuries and the public health. In Last JM, Wallace RB, editors. *Public health and preventive medicine.* London: Prentice Hall, 1992:1021–34.
4 Wolf ME, Rivara FP. Non-fall injuries in older adults. *Annu Rev Public Health* 1992;**13**:509–28.
5 Morris J. Falls in older people. *J R Soc Med* 1994;**87**:435–6.

6 Sutton JC, Standen PJ, Wallace WA. Patient accidents in hospital: incidence, documentation and significance. *Br J Clin Pract* 1994;**48**(2):63–66.

7 World Health Organization. *Health for all 2000 database.* Copenhagen: WHO, 1994.

8 Cox SJ. Buildings and Safety. Garston (Watford): Buildings Research Establishment, 1994.

9 Steven FR, Murray JP. The prevention of hot tap water burns—a study of electric immersion heater safety. *Burns* 1994;**17**:417–22.

10 Consumer Safety Unit. *Accidents to the elderly.* London: Department of Trade and Industry Consumer Safety Unit, 1986.

11 Askham J, Glucksman E, Owens P, Swift C, Tinger A, Yu G. *Home and leisure accident research—a review of research on falls among elderly people.* London: Department of Trade and Industry, 1990.

12 Vetter NJ, Lewis PA, Ford D. Can health visitors prevent fractures in elderly people? *BMJ* 1992;**304**:888–90.

13 Towner E, Dowswell T, Jarvis S. *Reducing childhood accidents. The effectiveness of health promotion interventions.* London: Health Education Authority, 1993.

14 Transport and Health Study Group. *Health on the move. Policies for health promoting transport.* London: Public Health Alliance, TRRL, 1991.

15 Allsop R, Turner E. Road casualties and public transport fares in London. *Accident Anal Prev* 1986;**18**:147.

16 Kimber R. Appropriate speeds for different conditions. In: Parliamentary Advisory Council for Transport Safety (PACTS), *Speed, accidents and injury: reducing the risks.* London: PACTS, 1990 (conference paper).

17 Janeson STMC. Road safety in urban districts. Final results of accident studies in the Dutch Demonstration Projects of the 1970s. *Traffic Eng Control* 1991 Jun:292–6.

41 Locomotor disability

ROWAN H HARWOOD

Definitions and diagnostic criteria

Disability is a restriction or lack of ability to perform a task or activity in a normal manner. The *International Classification of Impairments, Disabilities, and Handicaps*[1] identifies the tasks relevant to locomotion as ambulation (walking on the flat, walking over uneven ground, climbing stairs, climbing obstacles, and running), confinement (transfers from lying and sitting, standing, and reaching a bed or chair), transport (personal, including getting in and out of vehicles or public transport), and lifting. It follows that there are many different locomotor disabilities.

A closely related but distinct concept is that of mobility handicap, the ability to move effectively in one's surroundings, with or without the assistance of aids or modes of transport. A mobility handicap may or may not be experienced in the presence of a locomotor disability and might result from causes other than locomotor disability. Visual or cognitive impairments may cause mobility handicap in the absence of locomotor disability. Mobility handicap may be decreased for a person with a given disability by use of a mechanical aid or may be increased by an obstructive physical environment. The concept of disability predated the *International Classification of Impairments, Disabilities, and Handicaps* and in practice there is considerable overlap in the use of these terms.

Locomotor function is often found as a component part of activities of daily living inventories (such as the Barthel index) or instrumental activities of daily living scales. Strictly, the diagnosis of a locomotor disability is specific to the task or activity specified. Thus there are disabilities associated with being unable to stand up, to walk 50 metres, or to climb stairs. In some cases there is a natural hierarchy of difficulty that may be used to assemble locomotor items into scales.

Locomotor disability is an indicator of disease. An important medical function is to explain it in terms of diagnoses so that appropriate intervention can be instituted. In the case of immobility the causes are legion but a simple classification may be made in terms of time course. Immobility may be acute (for example, acute stroke, hip fracture, pneumonia), chronic deteriorating (arthritis, Parkinson's disease), chronic stable (amputation or old poliomyelitis), acute on chronic, or recurrent (recurrent episodes of heart failure or infection).

378

Magnitude of the problem

Immobility is a "geriatric giant". It is a common non-specific response to acute illness. With the recovery of illness the return of normal functioning is to be expected. Problems arise where recovery is not complete or where there is loss of physiological cardiorespiratory and musculoskeletal reserve such as occurs with age or prolonged illness. Effective locomotion is a prerequisite for many everyday tasks and locomotor disabilities are responsible for dependency on others for basic and instrumental activities of daily living, social isolation, inactivity, loss of autonomy, and the requirement for sheltered or institutional accommodation.

In cross-sectional surveys prevalence increases sharply with age. Estimates are therefore very sensitive to the age structure of the population concerned, making comparisons difficult because no reports have standardised to a reference population.

The British Office of Population Censuses and Surveys (OPCS) disability survey in 1984 screened 185 688 persons in a random sample of 100 000 households and 3794 persons in 595 communal establishments. The threshold for defining locomotor disability was "cannot walk 400 yards [365 m] without stopping or severe discomfort." Prevalence of self reported disability is given in table 41.1. Overall one in 10 of the British population were disabled on this criterion, including nearly half those over 75.[2]

Table 41.1 Prevalence of locomotor disability in the United Kingdom by age (per thousand population)[2]

Age (years)	In private households	Total (including institutions)
16–59	31	31
60–74	195	198
75 +	464	496

A New Zealand study examined disability in 782 subjects aged over 70 from a single town, including those in residential homes, in an interviewer administered survey. Three locomotor functions were included (getting into and out of bed, walking, and use of transportation), with the severity threshold being "the level of ability which threatened capacity to live independently at home." Age and sex stratified proportions are given in table 41.2. Prevalence of disability increased with age, with the difficulty of the mobility task, and was greater in women.[3]

Incidence had been studied in the American Established Populations for Epidemiological Studies of the Elderly cohorts, comprising 10 294 people over 65 in the community at three different geographical locations.[4] At baseline 7225 (70%) were able to climb stairs and walk 800 metres. Annual interviews were used to ascertain subsequent mobility. Table 41.3 shows

Table 41.2   Prevalence of locomotor disabilities in New Zealand by age and sex (per thousand population)[3]

Age (years)	Bed mobility	Walking	Transportation
Men			
70–74 (*n*=106)	9	19	47
75–79 (*n*=100)	0	50	80
80–84 (*n*=55)	55	145	182
85+ (*n*=22)	45	227	227
Women			
70–74 (*n*=164)	6	30	37
75–79 (*n*=163)	12	110	67
80–84 (*n*=111)	54	189	225
85+ (*n*=61)	49	295	557

Table 41.3   Proportion of initially mobile subjects remaining continuously mobile over four years, and incidence of death or mobility loss per 1000 person years[4]

Age (years)	Men		Women	
	Proportion remaining mobile (%)	Incidence of mobility loss or death	Proportion remaining mobile (%)	Incidence of mobility loss or death
65–74	66	104	64	112
75–84	42	136	42	217
85+	16	458	17	443

the proportions who remained continuously mobile over four years amongst 6981 subjects in whom follow up was maintained.

Overall 36% lost mobility, equivalent to a rate of 112 per 1000 person years; 18% of these had regained mobility by the time of a subsequent interview. Thus the incidence of persisting disability was 88 per 1000 person years.

Variation: time and place

There have been no direct comparative studies of secular trends. Several studies that used standardised definitions have examined geographical variations. One found little variation in the proportions of elderly people unable to walk 400 metres or climb stairs across 11 diverse European communities (all <10%).[5] A similar study of four Western Pacific countries, however, revealed marked variation in the proportion unable to walk 300 metres, from 15% in Malaysia and Korea to 29% in the Philippines and 42% in Fiji, with at least twofold variation in each age and sex specific group.[6] The proportions of initially mobile subjects aged 65–74 in the Established Populations for Epidemiological Studies of the Elderly cohorts remaining fully mobile four years later varied from 50% (New Haven women) to 73% (Iowa women). The variation in those over 85 years old was even greater (7% for New Haven men, 30% for Boston women).[4] The explanation for such variation is more likely one of case definition than true variation in prevalence, although differences in the physical environment and expectations may also play a role.

Perception of locomotor disability will depend much on the standpoint of the observer. Prevalence varies greatly among some important and readily identified groups. In a census of all institutional residents over 65 years old in a single English county, for example, Clarke reported proportions achieving various mobility tasks (table 41.4). The proportion who were fully mobile (unadjusted for age) varied among residents of different types of institution, from 14 to 61%.[7]

Determinants

Immobility commonly results from the combined effects of multiple pathologies and is one of a number of non-specific presentations of acute disease in older patients. Box 41.1 lists some of the diagnoses and impairments that may contribute.

Box 41.1—Causes of chronic immobility

Diagnoses	*Impairments*
Arthritis, especially of hip, knee and back	Pain
Fracture, especially of hip and vertebrae	Weakness
Heart failure	Spasticity
Chronic lung disease	Breathlessness
Stroke	Dizziness
Parkinson's disease	Blindness
Dementia	Cognitive impairment
Spinal cord disease	Ataxia and apraxia
Peripheral vascular disease	Depression, agoraphobia
	Fear (of falls, incontinence, attack)
	Fatigue

Table 41.5 contains estimates of population attributable risk fractions calculated from data published from the Established Populations for Epidemiological Studies of the Elderly cohorts.[4] These estimates represent the proportion of subjects with locomotor disability "accounted for" by a given risk factor, taking into account both the prevalence of the risk factor and the relative risk of disability associated with it. Many of the risk factors are associated with each other, hence the "total" proportion accounted for may be greater than 100%. To minimise this, multivariate adjusted relative

381

Table 41.4 *Proportions with different mobility disabilities in institutions in a single English county*[7]

Mobility	Type of institution					
	Acute hospital ward (%)	Geriatric hospital ward (%)	Long stay psychiatric hospital (%)	Residential home for elderly (%)	Home for mentally handicapped (%)	Nursing home (%)
Bedfast	18	37	4	2	6	12
Walk with aid	57	44	23	43	36	56
Walk except stairs	8	5	11	17	18	9
Fully mobile	16	14	61	38	40	23

Table 41.5 Population attributable risk fractions (PARF) based on the prevalence of and crude odds ratios for loss of mobility in the established populations for epidemiological studies of the elderly cohorts[4]

Variable	Men			Women		
	Prevalence (%)	Adjusted relative risk	PARF (%)	Prevalence (%)	Adjusted relative risk	PARF (%)
Age (years)						
65–74	64	1·0	0	65	1·0	0
75–84	29	2·0	14	31	1·9	3
>85	6	4·0	15	5	3·6	12
Income ($k)						
>10	41	1·0	0	25	1·0	0
5–10	43	1·3	1	42	1·3	1
<5	16	1·5	1	32	1·5	1
Education (years)						
>12	14	1·0	0	15	1·0	0
9–12	39	1·5	16	45	1·1	4
<9	46	1·5	19	40	1·1	4
Diagnoses at baseline						
Heart attack	15	1·3	4	6·0	1·2	1
Stroke	5·0	1·5	2	3·1	1·4	1
Cancer	11	1·0	0	15	1·0	0
Diabetes	12	1·3	3	10	1·4	4
Hypertension	33	1·2	6	46	1·2	8
Hip fracture	2·2	1·0	0	2·6	1·0	0
Angina	8·8	1·2	2	8·0	1·2	2
Dyspnoea	27	1·4	10	24	1·4	9
Arthritis	39	1·1	4	45	1·1	4
Leg pain	38	1·4	13	25	1·4	9
Incident diagnoses						
Heart attack	6·4	2·0	6	3·9	2·2	4
Stroke	4·9	2·7	8	3·6	2·6	5
Cancer	10	1·8	7	6·3	2·0	6
Diabetes	4·3	0·9	0	3·8	1·1	0
Hip fracture	1·4	3·0	3	2·2	3·1	4

risk estimates have been used. However, adjustment for age and other sociodemographic factors may lead to underestimation of the impact of diagnosis as the diagnoses may lie on the causal pathway between these factors and disability. The figures should be interpreted as indicating the approximate relative importance of the different factors.

There were strong univariate associations with age, income, length of education, and history of heart attack, stroke, angina, dyspnoea, diabetes, hypertension, and leg pain. A proportional hazards model was used to adjust for demographic features and comorbid chronic diseases. There was a linear relationship between the risk of immobility and the number of diagnoses recorded (a relative risk of 3 for those with four or more conditions compared with those with no conditions). Multivariate adjusted risks were also calculated for immobility after incident conditions (that occurred during the follow up period). These were 2·7 for stroke, 3·0 for hip fracture, 1·8 for cancer, and 2·0 for heart attack. For those with a history of hip fracture but who had recovered to full mobility at baseline no further increase in risk was observed, although numbers were small. Prevalent arthritis at baseline did not predict future immobility but 40% of the sample reported arthritis so the discriminating ability of this criterion may have been poor.

The same group examined behavioural and lifestyle risk factors for loss of mobility. Current smoking (relative risk (RR) 1·2–1·3), abstention from alcohol (RR 1·2), heavy alcohol consumption (RR 1·0–1·2), obesity (RR 1·2–1·4), and low physical activity (RR 1·7) were all associated with increased risk even among those reporting no chronic diagnoses or after adjusting for number of chronic conditions. Female ex-smokers were at less risk than current smokers, and male ex-smokers were at no increased risk compared with never smokers, emphasising the value of elderly people quitting smoking.[8]

Similar results were reported from another cohort, the Longitudinal Study on Ageing.[9] Ten per cent of 5151 community residents aged 70–74 lost the ability to walk 400 metres over two years of follow up. In multivariate analyses, being female, unmarried, not college educated, having diabetes, arthritis, stroke or visual impairment, and taking little regular exercise were all independently predictive of loss of function.

Other studies have documented the prevalence of various diagnoses in groups of disabled people defined without specific reference to locomotor disability but in whom it can safely be assumed that locomotor problems were very common. Campbell et al found heart failure (31%), osteoarthritis (26%), stroke and dementia (22% each), proximal femoral fracture, deafness, and psychiatric illness (14% each), macular degeneration and cataract (12% each), and lung disease, Parkinson's disease, and ischaemic heart disease (about 10% each) to be the most prevalent conditions amongst the most disabled 10% of their study population.[3] The OPCS survey reported the causes of disability (defined using a much lower threshold) as musculoskeletal (46%), ear (38%), eye (22%), cardiovascular (22%), neurological including stroke (13%), mental (including dementia) (13%), and respiratory (13%). For those in the severest disability categories (comprising 7% of all disabled subjects) a broadly similar pattern emerged but with somewhat greater prevalence of neurological disease (38%), eye problems (33%), and mental problems (22%).[2]

Among the most disabled people some diagnoses are much more important than is suggested by the results of studies of relatively fit community populations. Hip fracture[10] and stroke[11 12] are associated with particularly poor prognoses for locomotor disability.

Intervention

Given the numerous causes of and contributors to locomotor disability, a wide range of interventions may be used to prevent or relieve it.[13] Managing immobility plays an important part in acute illness, before pressure sores, muscle atrophy, joint contractures, pneumonia, and venous thrombosis supervene. Where the pathological process is irreversible it may be possible to reduce impairments (for example, reducing pain, improving muscle strength and cardiorespiratory fitness) or apply disease specific interventions (replacing hip or knee joints, removing cataracts, drugs for Parkinson's disease). Physiotherapy is often used to reduce residual locomotor disability. Supervised repeated practice of the target activity is the main strategy, together with the supply of aids and instruction in their use. Mobility handicap may be minimised by improvement in the physical environment (such as providing aids, ramps, rehousing).

Good team work is essential in rehabilitation. Assesssing and improving mobility, balance, transfers, stair climbing, walking outdoors, rising from the floor, and lifting are the natural province of the physiotherapist. However, in hospital nurses spend much more of the day with the patient than does the physiotherapist and at home relatives often play a similar role. Occupational therapists are generally responsible for seating and wheelchairs, and mobility is an important component of many of the activities they promote, such as dressing and cooking. A chiropodist and an optician may also contribute.

Formal evaluation of rehabilitation has proved difficult. This is in part due to the heterogeneity in the causes and characteristics of the affected group. Another problem has been difficulty in formulating adequate outcome measurements. Proportions of patients achieving specific tasks could, however, be measured (for example, "rise from a chair", "walk 400 metres", "climb 12 stairs"), and timed walking tests or treadmill exercise tolerance are sometimes used. Many interventions have been evaluated using aggregated disability scales, which are probably too insensitive for this purpose. Many therapy techniques have been difficult to test in randomised controlled trials because of difficulties in defining a control group (in whom complete neglect would be unethical) and the logistics of conducting the very large trials required to demonstrate moderate benefits in groups showing heterogeneous responses such as differing severities of stroke or arthritis, with differing degrees of comorbidity.

Trials have demonstrated better mobility as a result of a range of disease modifying or impairment relieving therapies. Exercise tolerance in heart failure is improved with angiotensin converting enzyme inhibitors compared with placebo.[14] Total hip arthroplasty improves six minute walking distance and other quality of life parameters.[15] Oral gold therapy in rheumatoid arthritis and selegiline in early Parkinson's disease improve mobility compared with placebo.[16 17]

Some good evidence on the effectiveness of rehabilitation services is available. Stroke units reduce both mortality and disability compared with general medical wards (see, for example, Indradavik et al[18] and Kalra et al[19]) suggesting that some combination of appropriate, enthusiastic, and careful medical, nursing, or therapy intervention is effective even in the absence of differences in quantity of input (defined in terms of therapy sessions, nursing numbers, or skill mix).[19] A randomised trial of physiotherapy assessment and advice long after a stroke showed small improvements in walking speed.[20] Some evidence has suggested that intensive outpatient therapy is more beneficial than less intensive therapy in a selected group of stroke patients.[21] Specialist orthogeriatric units are also effective in improving outcomes after hip fracture.[22] Randomised trials of treatment in osteoarthritis have been too few and too small to be conclusive.[23 24]

Another approach has been to evaluate generic interventions. Hart et al screened 545 subjects over 85 living at home; 118 (22%) were disabled and 79 were not receiving aids. A package of simple aids was provided to half these subjects, whose disability in the tasks targeted was less on reassessment than that of a control group.[25] A meta-analysis of results from a broad range of geriatric evaluation and rehabilitation trials demonstrated improved outcomes for those services with control over medical recommendations and long term follow up compared with "conventional" management.[26]

Health policy

Strategies for improving mobility reach across the whole spectrum of health services. Wide application of established and proven primary and secondary presentation for cardiovascular disease and osteoporosis could have a major impact on the prevalence of immobility. Exercise and avoidance of obesity may reduce the impact of osteoarthritis. Health promotion and disease prevention should not be neglected as they have the potential to have a far greater impact on locomotor disability than any intervention in established chronic disease.

With large and increasing numbers of patients presenting with locomotor disabilities, good rehabilitation services are essential. This requires easy, acceptable, and equitable access. Among the elements required are a responsive acute medical service, early involvement of expert geriatricians, multidisciplinary assessment and intervention, and community services for long term treatment and follow up. There should be a full medical assessment and trial of rehabilitation before institutionalisation. There is increasing evidence that these measures improve functional outcomes and reduce the need for institutional care.[26]

The aim of these services is to reduce handicap, and this will require close liaison with the social care and commercial sectors. Architectural and planning initiatives (access to public buildings, adapted pavements, road crossing facilities), and environmental alterations in the home are at least as important as medical therapies.

1 World Health Organization. *International Classification of Impairments, Disabilities and Handicaps.* Geneva: WHO, 1980.
2 Martin J, Meltzer H, Elliot D. *The prevalence of disability among adults.* OPCS Social Survey Division. London: HMSO, 1988.
3 Campbell AJ, Busby WJ, Robertson MC, Lum CL, Langlois JA, Morgan FC. Disease, impairment, disability and social handicap: a community based study of people aged 70 years and over. *Disabil Rehabil* 1994;**16**:72–9.
4 Guralnik JM, LaCroix AZ, Abbott RD, Berkman LF, Satterfield S, Evans DA, *et al.* Maintaining mobility in late life. 1. Demographic characteristics and chronic conditions. *Am J Epidemiol* 1993;**137**:845–57.
5 Heikkinen E, Waters WE, Brzezinski ZJ. *The elderly in eleven countries. A sociomedical survey.* Copenhagen: WHO Regional Office for Europe, 1983:56.
6 Andrews GR, Esterman AJ, Braunack-Mayer AJ, Rungie CM. *Aging in the western Pacific.* Manila, WHO Regional Office for the Western Pacific, 1986.
7 Clarke M, Hughes AO, Dodd KJ, *et al.* The elderly in residential care: patterns of disability. *Health Trends* 1979;**11**:17–20.
8 LaCroix AZ, Guralnik JM, Berkman LF, Wallace RB, Satterfield S. Maintaining mobility in late life. 2. Smoking, alcohol consumption, physical activity and body mass index. *Am J Epidemiol* 1993;**137**:858–69.
9 Mor V, Murphy J, Masterson-Allen S, *et al.* Risk of functional decline amongst well-elders. *J Clin Epidemiol* 1989;**42**:895–904.
10 Keene GS, Parker MJ, Pryor GA. Mortality and morbidity after hip fractures. *BMJ* 1993; **307**:1248–50.
11 Wade DT, Langton Hewer R. Functional abilities after stroke: measurement, natural history and prognosis. *J Neurol Neurosurg Psychiatry* 1987;**50**:177–82.
12 Collen FM, Wade DT. Residual mobility problems after stroke. *Int Disabil Stud* 1991;**13**: 12–5.
13 Ebrahim S. Rehabilitation. In: Brocklehurst JC, Tallis RC, Fillit HM, editors. *Textbook of geriatric medicine and gerontology,* 4th ed. Edinburgh: Churchill Livingstone, 1992: 1038–54.
14 CONSENSUS Trial Study Group. Effects of enalapril on mortality in severe congestive heart failure. *N Engl J Med* 1987;**316**:1429–35.
15 Laupacis A, Bourne R, Feeny D, Wong C, Tugwell P, Leslie K, *et al.* The effect of elective total hip replacement on health related quality of life. *J Bone Joint Surg [Am]* 1993;**75**: 1619–26.
16 Bombardier C, Ware J, Russell IJ, Larson M, Chalmer A, Read JL. Auranofin therapy and quality of life in patients with rheumatoid arthritis. *Am J Med* 1986;**81**:565–78.
17 Parkinson's Study Group. Effects of deprenyl on the progression of disability in early Parkinson's disease. *N Engl J Med* 1989;**321**:1364–71.

18 Indradavik B, Bakke F, Solberg R, Rokseth R, Haaheim LL, Holme I. Benefit of a stroke unit, a randomised controlled trial. *Stroke* 1991;**22**:1026–31.
19 Kalra L, Dale P, Crome P. Improving stroke rehabilitation: a controlled study. *Stroke* 1993;**24**:1462–7.
20 Wade DT, Collen FM, Robb GF, Warlow CP. Physiotherapy intervention late after stroke and mobility. *BMJ* 1992;**304**:609–13.
21 Smith DS, Goldenberg E, Ashburn A, *et al.* Remedial therapy after stroke: a randomised controlled trial. *BMJ* 1981;**282**:517–20.
22 Kenny DC, Reid J, Richardson IR, Kiamari AA, Kelt C. Effectiveness of geriatric rehabilitative care after fractures of the proximal femur in elderly women: a randomised clinical trial. *BMJ* 1988;**297**:1083–6.
23 Dieppe P, Cushnaghan J, Jasani MK, McRae F, Watt I. A two-year placebo controlled trial of non-steroidal anti-inflammatory therapy in osteoarthritis of the knee joint. *Br J Rheumatol* 1993;**32**:595–600.
24 Green J, McKenna F, Redfern EJ, Chamberlain MA. Home exercises are as effective as outpatient hydrotherapy for osteoarthritis of the hip. *Br J Rheumatol* 1993;**32**:812–5.
25 Hart D, Bowling A, Ellis M, Silman A. Locomotor disability in the very elderly: value of a programme for screening and provision of aids for daily living. *BMJ* 1990;**301**:216–20.
26 Stuck AE, Siu AL, Wieland GD, Adams J, Rubenstein LZ. Comprehensive geriatric assessment: a meta analysis of controlled trials. *Lancet* 1993;**342**:1032–6.

42 Confusion

LIN-YANG CHI, CAROL BRAYNE

While being regarded as one of the most commonly encountered mental problems in medical practice, particularly in the elderly, confusion itself entails puzzlement as a diagnostic term.

Confusion is a "disorientation resulting from memory impairment, hallucination, mistaken interpretation of events, and/or uncertainty about one's role or identity."[1] Impaired attention and concentration and inability to think, register, and recall are among its hallmarks. It can be divided into acute and chronic states according to the speed of onset. While most of the latter will be diagnosed as dementia, the former is regarded as equivalent to delirium. Between 50 and 75% of cases of dementia can be attributed to Alzheimer's disease, which is discussed in detail in chapter 29. Vascular dementia has emerged as the second most common cause. This chapter starts with acute confusional state (delirium) and then covers chronic confusional states other than Alzheimer's disease.

Acute confusional state (delirium)

Diagnostic criteria

Delirium is defined as a transient global disorder of cognition and attention accompanied by disturbed psychomotor behaviour and sleep–wake cycle.[2] Impaired conscious level is the central clinical feature, and the presentation is varied. The patient may be deluded or hallucinating, with either reduced or heightened activity and responsiveness. Disorientation in time is common, followed by impairment in place, and symptoms are likely to be worse in the late afternoon and at night.[3]

According to the fourth edition of the *Diagnostic and Statistical Manual of Mental Disorders* (DSM-IV),[4] delirium is a disturbance of consciousness and a change in cognition that cannot be accounted for by pre-existing dementia, developing over a short period of time (hours to days) and with evidence suggestive of a general physical condition. In the International Classification of Diseases (ICD-10),[5] in addition to the criteria mentioned above, disturbance of psychomotor activities and sleep patterns and deterioration in recent memory are listed as supportive of a diagnosis of acute confusion.

Delirium should be differentiated from dementia. Although they share some similar symptoms and can happen concurrently in the same person, the management and potentially reversible outcome of delirium distinguish it from dementia. The underlying physical causation of delirium in demented patients may be missed and should always be considered as a possibility when sudden deterioration has occurred. Clinically delirium tends to have a fluctuating course with quicker onset, shorter duration, and clouding of consciousness. In contrast, dementia is characterised by a deterioration of intellectual or cognitive function without disturbances of consciousness.

The particular importance of delirium lies in its potential treatment and reversibility. In some elderly people delirium may be the first or even the only clue to an underlying life threatening illness. In one series of patients with acute confusional states an organic cause was found in 85% of cases.[6] If an underlying physical condition cannot be identified, and the symptoms are exhibited as a consequence or with a history of other mental illnesses such as paranoia or psychosis, the diagnosis is unlikely to be delirium.

Magnitude of the problem

Although delirium is a major clinical problem, especially in geriatric medicine, few epidemiological studies have addressed this topic. Most studies of delirium have been based on sequential admissions to hospital. While patients of any age group can receive a diagnosis of delirium, the incidence is highest in the elderly. Studies reveal that about 30–50% of hospital inpatients aged 70 and over demonstrate evidence of delirium at some point of the admission.[7 8] Even higher ratios have been reported from a few studies. Gustafson and colleagues found 61% of elderly patients admitted for treatment of femoral neck fracture developed delirium during their stay in hospital.[9] Delirium has been consistently associated with high mortality, prolonged hospital stay (up to three or four times those non-demented), and admission to an institution (table 42.1).[10–12] The severity of the underlying physical illness as well as the delirium itself contribute to the poor prognosis.

Delirium is rarely detected in population studies of the elderly because the natural history of the condition is by definition relatively short with the resolution of recovery or death. Furthermore, such individuals tend to be protected by relatives or carers and participation in epidemiological studies may be refused.

Risk factors

Elderly people may be susceptible to delirium simply because of the age related accumulation of brain changes, which may be presented as dementia,[13] or the presence of systemic diseases, such as congestive heart failure[9] or pneumonia. Resistance to physical and psychological stresses is

Table 42.1   Combined outcomes of patients with delirium and control subjects

Outcome	Mean value (range)	
	Patients	Control subjects
Length of stay (days)	20·7 (12·1–30)	8·9 (7·2–14)
Rate of institutional care (%)		
at 1 month	46·5 (16–82)	18·3 (3·4–40·5)
at 6 months	43·2 (12–65)	8·3 (5–18)
Mortality rate (%)		
at 1 month	14·2 (3–25)	4·8 (1–12·5)
at 6 months	22·2 (14·3–27)	10·6 (0–13)

Adapted from Cole and Primeau[10] with permission of the publishers.

considered to be lowered with age. Thus dehydration, malnutrition, pre-existing multiple illnesses, and underload or overload of sensory stimuli can all trigger the development of delirium.[14] Intoxication by various substances, notably prescribed medicines, is another possibility.

In addition to the polypharmacy[15] often practised on the elderly, less efficient drug metabolism in the elderly can cause intoxication in doses regarded as normal for younger adults. Anticholinergic drugs, which can be found in many psychotropics, have been repeatedly shown to be the cause of delirium in elderly patients.[16 17] Withdrawal from addictive substances, such as alcohol or hypnotics, has also been found to be related to development of delirium. Poor eyesight and hearing can also lead to misuse of medicines. Although any single one of these, if severe enough, is capable of inducing delirium, multiple aetiology is more typical (see table 42.2[18] for review).

Treatment

There may well be a role for prevention in delirium and it should be emphasised, in view of the possible lethal consequences of the condition. Health education for the elderly, their families, and carers to understand and recognise possible risk factors, such as polypharmacy, could reduce the incidence of delirium.

The recognition and prompt treatment of delirium are, however, probably of most importance. Early diagnosis and treatment may be facilitated by programmes targeted at medical professionals[19] and nursing staff. Proper treatment includes identifying then correcting the aetiological factors, as well as symptomatic/supportive therapy.[2] A well lighted room with calendar and clock as well as adequate staffing are beneficial. As nocturnal exacerbation of symptoms is so typical, careful observation by night nursing staff can be very informative.

Table 42.2 Prospective studies of risk factors for delirium

Study	Population, age (years), sample size	Study type	Outcome	Independent predictors
Williams, 1985	Hip fracture patients, age ≥60, n=170	Prospective, daily ratings by nurses postop days 1–5	Postoperative confusion in 88 (51%), defined as the presence of any of four behaviours: disorientation inappropriate communication inappropriate behaviour illusions or hallucinations Incident confusion only	Age Preoperative poor performance on cognitive testing Low pre-injury activity level
Gustafson, 1988	Hip fracture patients, age ≥65, n=111	Prospective, daily observations	Delirium in 68 (61%) measured by the modified Organic Brain Syndrome Scale; "in accordance with DSM-III criteria". Did not separate prevalent and incident delirium	Age Dementia
Foreman, 1989	Medical patients, age ≥60, n=71	Prospective, daily observations	Acute confusion in 27 (38%), defined as the presence of any of 25 behaviours on the Clinical Assessment of Confusion checklist. Incident confusion only	Hypernatraemia Hypokalaemia Hyperglycaemia Hypotension Azotaemia High number of medications High confusion rating by nurses High number of orienting items in environment Low number of social interactions

Study	Patients	Method	Findings	Risk factors
Rockwood, 1989	Medical patients, age ≥65, n=80	Prospective, daily observations	Delirium in 20 (25%) measured by the Glasgow Coma Scale; defined by DSM-III criteria. Did not separate prevalent and incident delirium	Age Dementia Unstable condition on admission
Rogers, 1989	Elective hip or knee surgery patients, age ≥60, n=46	Prospective evaluations preop and postop (day 4)	Delirium in 13 (28%) by two psychiatrists based on DSM-III criteria. Incident delirium only	Use of scopolamine, propranolol, or flurazepam
Francis, 1990	Medical patients, age ≥70, n=229	Prospective evaluations every 48 hours	Delirium in 50 (22%), based on operationalised DSM-IIIR criteria. Did not separate prevalent and incident delirium	Abnormal sodium level Severe illness Chronic cognitive impairment Fever/hypothermia Psychoactive drug use Azotaemia
Schor, 1992	Medical and surgical patients, age ≥65, admitted from a long term care institution or the community of East Boston, MA, n=291	Prospective daily observations for 14 days	Delirium in 91 (31%) measured using the Delirium Symptom Interview; defined by DSM-III criteria. Incident delirium only	Age >80 years Chronic cognitive impairment Fracture on admission Neuroleptic or narcotic use Infection Male gender

DSM-III, *Diagnostic and Statistical Manual of Mental Disorders*, 3rd edition; DSM-IIIR, *Diagnostic and Statistical Manual of Mental Disorders*, 3rd edition revised; postop, postoperative; preop, preoperative. Reprinted from Inouye[18] with permission from *American Journal of Medicine*.

Health policy

There is no specific policy recommendation in relation to the confusional states. The most important action relates to adequate protection and recognition of underlying conditions. Policy makers should be aware that confusion is associated with increased health service costs.

Vascular dementia

Diagnostic criteria

Vascular disease of the brain is a major cause of chronic confusion second to Alzheimer's disease in many populations. Other terms have been used in the past, such as atherosclerotic dementia, psychosis with cerebral arteriosclerosis, and multi-infarct dementia. As with Alzheimer's disease, vascular dementia also suffers from diagnostic uncertainty. According to DSM-IV[4] and ICD-10[5] dementia is characterised by a cognitive decline together with memory and other higher cortical function impairments (such as aphasia, apraxia, and agnosia) interfering with usual activity. Three further features are needed for the diagnosis of vascular dementia: (a) stepwise deterioration with "patchy" distribution of deficits; (b) neurological symptoms/signs; and (c) significant cerebrovascular disease.[20] Obviously evidence of the relationship between cerebrovascular disease and dementia is crucial.[21] Methods of diagnosis, such as the widely used Hachinski ischaemic score,[22] remain uncertain in epidemiological settings.[23] Furthermore, Alzheimer's disease and vascular dementia can occur in the same patient with a mixed diagnosis.

Magnitude of the problem

Most community based studies have combined data on vascular dementia and mixed type dementia. Generally speaking the prevalence rates of "dementia with a vascular component" are between 1·2 and 4·2% for people aged 65 and over and between 2·4 and 5·6% for those 75 and over.[24] The prevalence of vascular dementia estimates have wide confidence intervals because of small numbers and rise with age, although less markedly than in Alzheimer's disease. More vascular dementia appears to be found in men (table 42.3) whereas more Alzheimer's disease is found in women; however, the pattern is not as clear for incidence as relatively little data are available. One of the few incidence studies that provides a rate of vascular dementia for those aged 75 and over reported it as 1%.[25] The proportion of dementia caused by vascular dementia varies considerably across studies, from 18% to nearly 50%; however, the ratio of vascular dementia to Alzheimer's disease decreases with age, reflecting the combined effects of different incidence and survival rates.

Table 42.3   Prevalence of vascular dementia (including mixed dementia) according to gender

Author (country)	Age (years)	Rate (%) Men	Women
Sulkava (Finland)	>65	2·6	2·7
Shibayama (Japan)	>65	3·3	2·4
Canadian study of health and ageing (Canada)	>65	1·9	1·2
O'Connor (England)	>75	2·3	1·9
Rocca (Italy)	>75	3·6	2·8
Fratiglioni (Sweden)	>75	2·3	3·0

Adapted from Herbert and Brayne[20] with permission of the publishers.

Methodological issues have major effects on the findings of epidemiological studies on dementia and this also affects studies of vascular dementia. All the following factors were found to have a significant influence on the overall prevalence: age structure, living area, types of investigator, sample source, and diagnostic criteria.[26] While community-based studies suffer from lack of thorough diagnostic procedures, clinic-based studies are liable to selection bias.

Risk factors

In addition to advanced age and familial factors, hypertension, male sex, smoking, cardiac diseases, and diabetes mellitus are reported risk factors for vascular dementia,[27] thus sharing risk factors with stroke. These factors partly determine the diagnosis of dementia subtypes—for example, "history of strokes" and "evidence of associated atherosclerosis"—and the exact relationship of these factors to the development of dementia is not yet known. The role of diet[28] and other factors[29] that reduce risk of cardiac diseases and stroke are not yet understood.

Treatment

It has been suggested that aspirin may be an effective treatment for cognitive impairment caused by vascular pathology, for which there is limited evidence.[30] As yet there are no large randomised control trials to confirm this. Furthermore, the widespread use of aspirin to prevent vascular events in the general population limits the opportunity of examining this possibility.

Health policy

All measures to prevent vascular events in younger age groups should yield dividends in older age groups, with a later reduction in cognitive

395

decline caused by vascular pathology. Longer survival in individuals with greater risk, however, may cause a paradoxical increase in vascular dementia.

Other types of dementia

Dementia can be caused by other events, such as alcoholism, head injury, thyroid disorders, and nutritional deficiencies (all of which can also cause acute confusional states). The importance of these varies enormously from country to country and may depend on economic and cultural factors. The size of the problem would be indicated by other measures, such as rates of major road trauma and deaths from alcohol related liver disease. These less common causes of dementia should also be considered in contemplating preventive strategies for specific populations.

1 Confusion. *Churchill's illustrated medical dictionary.* New York: Churchill Livingstone, 1989.
2 Lipowski ZJ. Delirium (acute confusional states). In: Copeland JRM, Abou-Saleh MT, Blazer DG, editors. *Principles and practice of geriatric psychiatry.* New York: Wiley, 1994: 257–60.
3 Hope RA, Longmore JM, Hodgetts TJ, Ramrakha PS. *Oxford handbook of clinical medicine,* 3rd ed. Oxford: Oxford University Press, 1993.
4 American Psychiatric Association. *Diagnostic and statistical manual of mental disorders,* 4th ed., Washington: APA, 1994.
5 World Health Organization. *International statistical classification of diseases and related health problems,* 10th revision. Geneva: WHO, 1992.
6 Rockwood K. Acute confusion in elderly medical patients. *J Am Geriatr Soc* 1989;**37**: 150–4.
7 Gillick MR, Serrell NA, Gillick LS. Adverse consequences of hospitalization in the elderly. *Soc Sci Med* 1982;**16**:1033–8.
8 Warshaw GA, Moore JT, Friedman SW, *et al.* Functional disability in the hospitalized elderly. *JAMA* 1982;**248**:847–50.
9 Gustafson Y, Berggren D, Brannstrom B, *et al.* Acute confusional states in elderly patients treated for femoral neck fracture. *J Am Geriatr Soc* 1988;**36**:525–30.
10 Cole MG, Primeau FJ. Prognosis of delirium in elderly hospital patients. *Can Med Assoc J* 1993;**149**:41–6.
11 Kolbeinsson H, Jonsson A. Delirium and dementia in acute medical admissions of elderly patients in Iceland. *Acta Psychiatr Scand* 1993;**87**:123–7.
12 Francis J, Martin D, Kapoor WN. A prospective study of delirium in hospitalized elderly. *JAMA* 1990;**263**:1097–101.
13 Inouye SK, Viscoli CM, Horwitz RI, Hurst LD, Tinetti ME. A predictive model for delirium for hospitalized elderly medical patients based on admission characteristics. *Ann Intern Med* 1993;**119**:474–81.
14 Lipowski ZJ. *Delirium: acute confusional states.* Oxford: Oxford University Press, 1990.
15 Stewart RB, Hale WE. Acute confusional states in older adults and the role of polypharmacy. *Annu Rev Health* 1992;**13**:415–30.
16 Blazer D, Federspiel C, Ray W, Schaffnar W. The risk of anticholinergic toxicity in the elderly: a study of prescribing practices in two populations. *J Gerontol* 1983;**38**:31–5.
17 Sumner AD, Simons RJ. Delirium in the hospitalized elderly. *Cleve Clin J Med* 1994;**61**: 258–62.
18 Inouye SK. The dilemma of delirium: clinical and research controversies regarding diagnosis and evaluation of delirium in hospitalized elderly medical patients. *Am J Med* 1994;**97**:278–88.
19 Rockwood K, Cosway S, Stolee P, Kydd D, Carver D, Jarrett P. Increasing the recognition of delirium in the elderly patient. *J Am Geriatr Soc* 1994;**42**:252–6.
20 Hebert R, Brayne C. Epidemiology of vascular dementia, a review. *Neuroepidemiology* 1995;**14**:240–57.

21 Roman GC, Tatemichi TK, Erkinjuntti T, *et al.* Vascular dementia: diagnostic criteria for research studies. Report of the NINDS-AIREN international workshop. *Neurology* 1993; **43**:250–60.

22 Hachinski VC. Differential diagnosis of Alzheimer's dementia: multi-infarct dementia. In: Reisberg B, editor. *Alzheimer's disease: the standard reference.* New York: Free Press, 1983: 188–92.

23 Dening TR, Berrios GE. The Hachinski ischaemic score: a reevaluation. *Int J Geriatr Psychiatry* 1992;7:585–9.

24 Jorm AF. *The epidemiology of Alzheimer's disease and related disorders.* London: Chapman and Hall, 1990, chapter 5.

25 Katzman R, Aronson M, Fuld P, *et al.* Development of dementing illnesses in an 80-year-old volunteer cohort. *Ann Neurol* 1989;**25**:317–24.

26 Jorm AF, Korten AE, Henderson AS. The prevalence of dementia: a qualitative integration of the literature. *Acta Psychiatr Scand* 1987;**76**:465–79.

27 Skoog I. Risk factors for vascular dementia: a review. *Dementia* 1994;5:137–44.

28 Omura T, Hisamatsu S, Takizawa Y, Minowa M, Yanagawa H, Shegematsu I. Geographic distribution of cerebrovascular disease mortality and food intakes in Japan. *Soc Sci Med* 1987;**24**:401–7.

29 Bucht G, Adofsson R, Winblad B. Dementia of the Alzheimer type and multi-infarct dementia: a clinical description and diagnostic problems. *J Am Geriatr Soc* 1984;**32**:491–8.

30 Meyer JS, Rogers RL, McClintic K, Mortel KF, Lofti J. Randomized clinical trial of daily aspirin therapy in multi-infarct dementia: a pilot study. *J Am Geriatr Soc* 1989;**37**:549–55.

43 Iatrogenesis

CAMERON G SWIFT

Definitions and diagnostic criteria

Iatrogenesis in its purely linguistic sense means the causation of disease by the process of diagnosis or treatment. The definition here will be limited to that of morbidity (adverse reactions) brought about by the therapeutic use of drugs, excluding all other forms of intervention. While this definition excludes trivial drug side effects, it is important to realise that some perceived generally to be trivial may assume greater clinical significance in older people, particularly those in poor general health.

Subdivision into two main categories of adverse reaction, type A and type B, is standard.[1] Type A reactions are attributable to accentuation of a drug's known pharmacological action(s), related to dose, predictable, therefore, and relatively common. Type B reactions are idiosyncratic, unrelated to dose, frequently unpredictable and of unknown mechanism, governed by host factors, such as genetics or allergy, less common, but often more serious.

The problem of establishing clear cause–effect relationships in the diagnosis of adverse drug reactions is well known. "Proof" requires a close qualitative and temporal association of the adverse event, distinct from underlying disease, and confirmed by its cessation on drug withdrawal and by its recurrence on rechallenge. This approach is seldom justifiable on an individual patient basis and patently inapplicable to epidemiology. The detection and quantification of iatrogenesis in patient populations (pharmacovigilance) therefore depends on a range of methods for demonstrating associations between drug utilisation and morbidity, which used appropriately are none the less of considerable power. The most useful have been reviewed by Rawlins[2] and include spontaneous reporting systems, case–control and case–cohort studies, case registers, and experimental and observational cohort studies (including record linkage schemes). As with all scientific enquiry, the validity of the method chosen depends on its precise applicability to the category of information sought and on its intrinsic reliability in the hands of the investigator. Hence critical interpretation of epidemiological data on iatrogenesis will depend on the capability of the method to detect and quantify reliably the adverse reactions under scrutiny and to distinguish them from non-drug related morbidity.

398

The widely held view that old age confers increased vulnerability to iatrogenesis hinges on a number of preconceptions: (a) the observation that ageing in man is in general characterised by reduction in the reserve capacity of those homeostatic mechanisms providing defence against environmental influences (of which foreign compounds are one example); (b) cumulative anecdotal evidence from clinical practice; (c) a limited and hitherto inadequate suppy of data from epidemiological studies. These sources have largely focused on type A reactions as the principal cause of concern, although age has occasionally (and intriguingly) emerged as a possible determinant of isolated type B reactions.

Magnitude of the problem

This is probably most usefully addressed in terms of either (a) the overall or drug specific prevalence of iatrogenesis in relevant older populations, or (b) the effect of increasing age on the risk of occurrence of various defined adverse reactions. With few exceptions most studies have pointed to a public health problem of significant proportions and to increasing age as a positive risk factor for iatrogenesis. Because of the diffuse nature of the problem and the limitations of the methods, however, no straightforward general approach to quantification is possible.

Studies of the prevalence in general of iatrogenesis have been few. A multicentre observational cohort study of 1998 patients consecutively admitted to departments of geriatric medicine in Britain identified adverse reactions in 248 (12·4%) and attributed hospitalisation solely or partly to drugs in 209 (10·5%) cases.[3] This study was based on observer recognition and attribution of adverse reactions by physicians specialising in the care of the elderly, there being no control population or other reference point for comparison. Thus, while observer competence is not in question, bias in attribution cannot be excluded.

A study of randomly sampled medical outpatients questioned by professional interviewers found self reporting of adverse symptoms in about 30% of the sample, with fewer overall (25·2%) reported by an older group (mean age 75·7) than a younger group (33·5%) (mean age 50·4), in spite of the fact that they were taking more medications on average (2·9 v 2·5) and more likely to be taking four or more medications (28·9 v 22·7%).[4] This finding contrasted with previous inpatient studies and was thought to reflect (a) no increase in susceptibility with age; (b) different susceptibility compared with the minority frailer inpatient population; (c) lack of self awareness of adverse drug reactions amongst the elderly because of concurrent non-drug symptoms; or (d) greater tendency for young outpatients to blame drugs for their complaints.

A general practice study of 817 patients given single drug treatment for the first time in a given year found (based on interview questionnaire) a 41% incidence of "certain" or "probable" adverse drug reactions, of which

90% had occurred by the fourth day of treatment.[5] Unfortunately the precise breakdown by age group is not reported in this study.

An early study of factors predisposing to adverse drug reactions in hospital inpatients showed a progressive increase in susceptibility with age from around 3% frequency in those aged 20–29 to about 22% in those aged 70–79.[6]

As a final example, spontaneous reporting ("yellow card") data submitted to the United Kingdom Committee on Safety of Medicines showed an increase from 24 to 35% in the proportion of reported adverse drug reactions attributable to the elderly over the period 1965–83.[7]

While much of this information concerns type A events, the occurrence of some of the more serious type B reactions has from time to time shown a defined focus towards the elderly (for example, benoxaprofen toxicity, mianserin related blood dyscrasias).

The overall clinical significance of this combined material in terms of real morbidity is difficult to interpret because of the variety of detection methods and evaluation criteria utilised in each study and the inherent biases. There is, however, some evidence that subjective recognition of adverse drug reactions is lower in older people, and that retrospective recall is a problem, particularly with central nervous system effects. The underreporting affecting spontaneous reporting systems is well recognised and these systems require only serious or unexpected events to be notified (except for new drugs). Hence an element of prospective surveillance involving one or more observers is probably more reliable in adverse drug reaction detection in this age group. Overall the available evidence probably underestimates rather than overestimates the problem.

Such information as is available suggests that the most common adverse drug reactions in descending order of frequency are those affecting the gastrointestinal, central nervous, and cardiovascular systems, with variable proportions of skin reactions.[3-5] This by no means gives a clear indication of the relative clinical importance of each category.

Similarly the hierarchy of "offending" drugs reported actually provides little information about the actual scale of morbidity, apart from attempts to identify the relative contribution of different classes to hospitalisation.[3] More precise information on the effect of age on susceptibility to adverse reactions has emerged from studies of specific drug classes.

Several studies have identified age as a clear positive risk factor for gastrointestinal bleeding due to non-steroidal anti-inflammatory drugs. These have included data derived from spontaneous reporting,[7] record linkage,[8] (fig 43.1) cohort studies,[9] and case–control studies.[10 11] In most of these, discriminant analysis has shown age to be highly important amongst a number of variables, although occasionally its contribution appears smaller.[11] The importance of this morbidity is exemplified by cost estimates. For the year 1987 the cost of non-steroidal anti-inflammatory drug treatment for arthritis was estimated at $844 million. Of this, 31% was spent on the treatment of iatrogenic disease—of which 42% was on

400

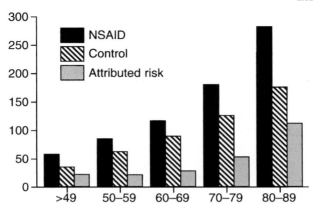

Fig 43.1   Gastrointestinal events per 1000 people in relation to age in non-steroidal anti-inflammatory drug (NSAID) takers and controls, showing the risk attributable to NSAID use. (Reproduced from Beardon et al.[8])

prophylactic medication (mainly misoprostol), 38% on hospital inpatient costs, and 20% on physician costs. It is also emphasised by the fact that when serious or life threatening reactions are separately identified the distribution curve moves sharply to the right along the axis of increasing age.[7]

The role of drugs acting on the central nervous system was particularly examined in the 1970s and 80s when levels of benzodiazepine prescription were higher than at present. Observational cohort studies of the Boston Collaborative Drug Surveillance Program (based on pharmacist identification substantiated by two independent clinician assessments) clearly demonstrated the positive relationship between increasing age and susceptibility to unwanted sedation from these compounds.[12 13] In addition to this approach, the wider implications for morbidity have been examined in terms of the association found between sedative/hypnotic use and the occurrence of falls in old age. In one study the use of long half life hypnotics was found to confer an 80% increase in the risk of hip fracture.[14]

With both the above drug classes and probably as a generality the time of greatest susceptibility has been found to be during the first few days of treatment. This is not to exclude the importance and seriousness of longer term adverse reactions (for example, tardive dyskinesia with neuroleptics, steroid osteoporosis in temporal arteritis or rheumatoid arthritis) but to stress the importance of an initial period of vigilance with some of the more common contributors to morbidity (for example, angiotensin converting enzyme inhibitors).

Determinants

The main determinants of iatrogenesis in the elderly may be usefully subdivided into factors extrinsic and intrinsic to the patient. The extrinsic factors are prescribing (scale and rationality) and compliance; the intrinsic factors are the effects of biological age associated processes on drug disposition (pharmacokinetics) and response (pharmacodynamics) and the effects of coexisting disease states.

Elderly people are the highest consumers of prescribed medication. Data from the Association of the British Pharmaceutical Industry showed that of the increase in annual prescription items in England and Wales of some 51 million over the years 1977–88 about 49 million (96%) were accounted for by prescriptions to people of pensionable age.[15] Cost related information for developed countries shows that in most cases 30–40% of prescriptions are for older people who constitute less than half these percentages of the population as a whole. These figures say nothing about the use of over the counter medication, although this is probably greatest in the 30–50 age group.[5]

The relationship, for example, between the total numbers of non-steroidal prescriptions and spontaneously reported episodes of upper gastrointestinal bleeding, both of which increase with age, has been shown to be remarkably close.[7] The likelihood of such a relationship would appear to be self evident. Other studies have highlighted the extent of prolonged and repeat prescribing for the elderly.

The rationality or quality of prescribing has proved much more difficult to measure but clearly if this is poor it would be logical to expect a higher level of adverse drug effects. An early community based study found an almost linear increase with age in the extent of prescribing of the three most commonly used classes of psychotropic compound (sedative/hypnotics, antidepressants, antipsychotics) in spite of sparse evidence for significant benefit to older people from any of the treatments concerned.[16] Similarly the place of non-steroidal anti-inflammatory drugs in the management of osteoarthritis, the most common and age associated indication for their use, remains highly controversial. Historically the research and drug development databases have contained sparse information with respect to ageing and older patients so the prescriber has been obliged to try and extrapolate from trials information in younger recipients—a poor rationale for the treatment of the elderly, particularly those who are frail.

The contribution of compliance problems has proved equally difficult to determine. Such evidence as there is indicates that elderly people as a group comply well with prescription advice, although age associated problems such as social isolation and longstanding illness cause them difficulty, poor professional communication and labelling are major stumbling blocks, impaired cognition when present indicates the need for third party involvement, and the multiple prescriptions and complex regimens with which they are assaulted inevitably promote higher error rates.[17]

The importance of intrinsic biological age associated changes in drug disposition and response is now well attested by a large literature and it is patently incorrect to attribute the burden of iatrogenesis solely or even predominantly to extrinsic factors. Epidemiologically, for example, the contributions of age *and* dose to the incidence of non-steroidal induced gastrointestinal bleeding have been repeatedly delineated[9-11] (figs 43.1 and 43.2). Equally the age associated susceptibility to unwanted sedation from benzodiazepines was one of the earliest phenomena clearly shown to be dose related,[12 13] as is the relationship to falls.[14] Far more examples have not been the subject of systematic epidemiological study but would undoubtedly include, for example, digoxin toxicity, diuretic related hypokalaemia, hyponatraemia and postural hypotension, first dose hypotension with angiotensin converting enzyme inhibitors, and the autonomic and CNS side effects of antidepressant and antipsychotic drugs.

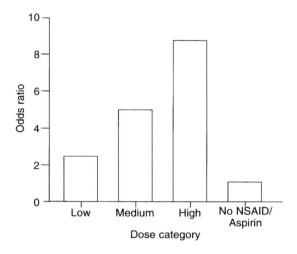

Fig 43.2   The effect of drug dose on the risk of ulcer complications with non-steroidal anti-inflammatory drugs (NSAIDs). (Reproduced from Langman et al.[11])

The mechanisms vary among and within drug classes and attempts to generalise have tended to be unhelpful, often allowing subtle but important age associated changes in pharmacokinetics and pharmacodynamics to be overlooked, with unfortunate consequences. Examples of some of the more important changes are shown in box 43.1. The reader is referred elsewhere for a more detailed consideration.[18]

Coexisting disease states increase in prevalence with the age of the population. The distinction between iatrogenesis and coexisting non-drug related morbidity may naturally prove difficult but a number of studies, particularly case–control studies and those with record linkage, have been able to demonstrate a clear effect of age on attributable risk for adverse drug reactions.[8 10] The contribution of disease states to alterations in drug handling and response is even more difficult to assess because of the increased heterogeneity, logistic difficulties in mounting the investigations, and a variety of other potential confounding factors. There is, however,

---

Box 43.1—Alterations in drug handling and response with increasing age

Physiological changes
Reduced glomerular filtration
Reduced tubular secretion
Reduced liver volume
Reduced liver blood flow
Reduced liver enzyme activity (frail elderly)
Increased relative proportion of body fat
Reduced albumin (frail elderly)
Reduced homeostatic reserve

Some consequences
Reduced clearance of renally eliminated drugs
Variable reduction in clearance of metabolised drugs
Greater reduction in hepatic clearance with frailty
Increased distribution volume of lipid soluble drugs
Reduced protein binding of extensively bound drugs
Greater susceptibility to (for example) postural instability or hypotension
Specific increase in sensitivity to some drugs (for example, warfarin)

---

evidence that subpopulations of "frail" institutionalised older people show additional and/or enhanced impairment of drug handling capacity and homeostatic reserve that heightens their vulnerability to iatrogenesis.[19]

Intervention

Achieving a reduction in drug related morbidity in the elderly will depend on a better understanding of the pharmacology of old age to inform drug development, the manufacture of better drugs more tailored to the needs of older people, and the achievement of more rational and circumspect prescribing. In spite of initiatives in all these areas there is as yet no hard evidence for any improvement, although it would be pleasant to speculate that, based on heightened awareness, this might be happening.

There remain many unanswered questions in pharmacology, particularly in the area of changes in pharmacodynamics and homeostatic mechanisms with age. In addition, drugs whose pharmacology is more complex (for example, those with chiral or enantiomeric properties, which account for about 30% of the pharmacopoeia) have been found to contribute unpredictably to reports of age related adverse reactions (on occasions resulting in withdrawal from the market) in recent years and are currently the subject of a programme of investigation in the author's department. Further work is required at this level. In addition, the development of new drugs with safer profiles holds promise. The developing track record of selective serotonin reuptake inhibitors for depression in the elderly awaits clarification, for example, and the possibility of selective inhibition of prostaglandin endoperoxidase synthase (cyclo-oxygenase) isoenzymes by novel non-steroidals is also of interest given the relative intrinsic deficiency of protective mucosal prostaglandins in the elderly.

It is not difficult to provide general guidelines for rational prescribing in the elderly and several have been proposed. These include such measures as particular care in diagnosis (particularly causes of symptoms), consideration of non-pharmacological alternatives (for example, sleep hygiene in insomnia, physical measures and counselling in osteoarthritis, advice slips in place of drugs), consideration of possible interactions (with drug or disease), time limited prescription of drug "courses", dose reduction where indicated (for example, warfarin), low initial dosage and titration where there is variability (for example, antidepressants and other metabolised drugs), early review for unwanted effects, and a clear plan or computer assisted strategy for discontinuation. A simple measure to assist with compliance is to require inspection and discussion of all drug supplies as an integral part of any consultation.

Health policy

The key health policy areas are in drug regulation, prescribing audit, and professional and public education.

The requirement by the regulatory bodies in developed countries for data in older subjects as a component of all relevant product licence applications has been a major step forward, triggered by the awareness of advanced age as an important determinant of a number of serious instances of drug safety regulation. This has provided an important stimulus to scientific enquiry not only into the characteristics of individual compounds but also into age related mechanisms in general. A potential risk of this requirement lies in its generalised prescriptive flavour, coupled with the time pressures facing companies in an already protracted premarketing development schedule so that key questions unique to individual drugs might receive less consideration. This tendency is possibly accentuated by the current drive to achieve harmonisation—for example, across the member states of the European Union, in the United States, and on the wider international front. The recently published International Conference on Harmonisation guidelines on required information in the elderly[20] cover the following ground:

- *Scope*—Significant use due to prevalence or age associated disorder (for example, Alzheimer's disease); new entities; new formulations or combinations; new uses or indications
- *Phase II/III clinical trials*—Meaningful numbers to permit comparison (for example, minimum 100 older subjects; higher percentage for Alzheimer's

disease); further studies if findings indicate need; separate older patient populations or part of all-age sample
- *Pharmacokinetic studies*—Formal studies (volunteers or patients: single/ multiple dose); pharmacokinetic screening as part of phase II/III trials; studies in renal and hepatic impairment
- *Interaction studies*

Careful tailoring of the requirements to individual compounds remains a clear necessity and will entail expertise together with an interactive approach involving companies, regulators, and clinical scientists in the field.

Organised therapeutic audit of prescribing in the elderly (and to some extent in general) is in its relative infancy. Self audit is available to prescribers through continuing medical education sources and it is important that this topic should receive adequate exposure within developing approved continuing medical education programmes, such as those for hospital doctors and general practitioners in the United Kingdom. A mechanism for peer audit exists within the work remit of formulary committees but its organisation is patchy. Economic audit has historically occurred in Britain, at least in general practice, through the mechanisms of the National Health Service Prescription Pricing Authority but is now a growing agenda of general management activity, both in hospital and community, and of the economics of fund holding general practices. It is questionable whether economic audit will contribute anything to the quality of prescribing for the elderly and there is a definite risk that patients might become deprived of the potential benefits of new and better drugs. The same holds true for the introduction of black and limited lists by governments and management authorities, although some appropriate general rationalisation has undoubtedly been achieved.

A major problem in therapeutic audit has been to agree on what data should be collected and how to interpret it. The author's research group is currently in receipt of a United Kingdom government grant to evaluate a number of possible screening markers that might provide a better clinical and scientific basis to assess prescribing quality in both hospital and primary care settings.

Finally, there is an ongoing need for public education in order to achieve a better informed expectation of the benefits and risks of modern drug therapy. Prescribers, particularly those in general practice (primary care), are in the forefront of demand from both patients and their carers. Some of the demand is built into cultural perceptions, is often fuelled by media material of dubious value, is difficult to withstand, and is an undoubted contributor to overmedication.

Conclusion

Iatrogenesis is a major issue of health care in late life. Much is preventable and there may already be some general improvement. It is important that adequate systems for adverse drug reaction detection are resourced and further developed and that there is a specific focus on old age to enable ongoing evaluation. It is also important that an accurate understanding of relative risk and benefit is promoted through research and education to ensure that older people are guaranteed the best possible outcomes from modern drug therapy.

1 Rawlins MD. Adverse reactions to drugs. *BMJ* 1981;**282**:974–6.
2 Rawlins MD. Pharmacovigilance: paradise lost, regained or postponed? *J R Coll Physicians* 1995;**29**:40–9.
3 Williamson J, Chopin JM. Adverse reactions to prescribed drugs in the elderly: a multicentre investigation. *Age Ageing* 1980;**9**:73–80.
4 Klein LE, German PS, Levine DM, Feroli R, Ardery J. Medication problems among outpatients. *Arch Intern Med* 1984;**144**:1185–8.
5 Martyrs CR. Adverse drug reactions in general practice. *BMJ* 1979;**2**:1194–7.
6 Hurwitz N. Predisposing factors in adverse reactions to drugs. *BMJ* 1969;**1**:536–9.
7 Castleden CM, Pickles H. Suspected adverse drug reactions in elderly patients reported to the Committee on Safety of Medicines. *Br J Clin Pharmacol* 1988;**26**:347–53.
8 Beardon PH, Brown SV, McDevitt DG. Gastrointestinal events in patients prescribed non-steroidal anti-inflammatory drugs: a controlled study using record linkage in Tayside. *Q J Med* 1989;**71**:497–505.
9 Fries JF, Williams CA, Bloch DA, Michel BA. Nonsteroidal anti-inflammatory drug-associated gastropathy: incidence and risk factor models. *Am J Med* 1991;**91**:213–21.
10 Griffin MR, Piper JM, Daugherty JR, Snowden M, Ray WA. Nonsteroidal anti-inflammatory drug use and increased risk for peptic ulcer disease in elderly persons. *Ann Intern Med* 1991;**114**:257–63.
11 Langman MJS, Weil J, Wainwright P, *et al.* Risks of bleeding peptic ulcer associated with individual non-steroidal anti-inflammatory drugs. *Lancet* 1994;**343**:1075–8.
12 Greenblatt DJ, Allen MD, Shader RI. Toxicity of high-dose flurazepam in the elderly. *Clin Pharacol Ther* 1977;**21**:355–61.
13 Greenblatt DJ, Allen MD. Toxicity of nitrazepam in the elderly: a report from the Boston Collaborative Drug Surveillance Program. *Br J Clin Pharmacol* 1978;**5**:407–13.
14 Ray W, Griffin M, Schaffner W, Baugh D, Melton L. Psychotropic drug use and the risk of hip fracture. *N Engl J Med* 1987;**316**:363–9.
15 Griffin JP, Chew R. *Trends in usage of prescription medicines by the elderly and very elderly between 1977 and 1988.* London: Association of the British Pharmaceutical Industry, 1990.
16 Skegg DCG, Doll R, Perry J. Use of medicines in general practice. *BMJ* 1977;**1**:1561–3.
17 Christopher LJ. Drug prescribing and compliance in the elderly. In: Swift CG, editor. *Clinical pharmacology in the elderly.* New York: Marcel Dekker, 1987:103–18.
18 Swift CG, editor. *Clinical pharmacology in the elderly.* New York: Marcel Dekker, 1987.
19 Woodhouse KW, James OFW. Hepatic drug metabolism and ageing. In: Denham MJ, George CF, editors. *Drugs in old age: new perspectives.* Edinburgh: Churchill Livingstone, 1990:22–35.
20 Food and Drug Administration, Department of Health and Human Services (USA). International Conference on Harmonisation; guideline on studies in support of special populations: geriatrics; availability. *Federal Register* 1994;**59**:33398–400.

44 Dying

ANN CARTWRIGHT

Dying comes under the heading of problems but it is not one that can be solved; death at some stage is the one certain and common event of life. Increasingly in advanced industrialised countries it is concentrated among the old. In 1992 in England and Wales death rates per 1000 were less than 1·0 for ages 1–34, rising to 266·0 for men aged 90 and over and 210·6 for women of that age.[1] So even for the oldest age group there was still a greater than 3:1 chance against death in a year. At younger ages death may be seen as a rarity, unfair, a tragedy, a problem, something society should strive to prevent; even at late ages when it might seem more natural it can still be somewhat unexpected and unwelcome and much effort and resources are devoted to trying to postpone it. One estimate is that in 1987 in England approximately 22% of occupied NHS bed days were taken up by people who would be dead within a year.[2]

For the most part death is a clearly defined and observable event; deaths are recorded, counted, and used as indicators of the health of groups, and societies. In addition, the process of dying and the way it happens can provide insights into the values and humanitarianism with which societies care for the old and the sick.

Rates

Uses

Death rates are one of the basic epidemiological tools. They are used in all the various fields of epidemiology described by Morris[3]: historical trends, the identification of community needs and problems, the search for causes, the assessment of individual chances, the identification of syndromes, putting clinical experiences into perspective, and the working of health services. They also enable comparisons to be made between countries and smaller areas.

They have been used in earlier chapters to illustrate gender differences, to demonstrate the relative importance of different diseases, and to assess risk factors and the usefulness of various interventions.

Age and gender

Among older people the gap between death rates for men and women narrows; between ages 55 and 79 rates for women in England and Wales in 1992 were between 57 and 59% of those for men but this proportion rose with increasing age after that: 64% for ages 80–84, 70% for 85–89, and 79% for those aged 90 or more.[1] Would equality be achieved around age 110? Another change in the pattern of deaths with increasing age is that death rates for single (never married) men were greater than for married men until age 84 but after that those for married men were somewhat higher than for single men. Marriage may be a protective factor for men up until that age but, if their wives survive, men may have to take on a caring role, which takes its toll in terms of their own survival.

Causes of death and age

Looking at broad causes of death among older compared with younger people, the proportion of those over 85 whose death is attributed to neoplasms is much lower, while proportionally more deaths are attributed to diseases of the respiratory system, to mental disorders, to diseases of the musculoskeletal system and connective tissue, and to signs, symptoms and ill defined conditions (fig 44.1). In addition, as Newens and colleagues have pointed out,[4] the underlying cause of death seriously understates the frequency of dementia but when the recording of other brain disease is taken into account the presence of potentially dementing brain disease is recorded much more frequently. They suggest that coding chronic conditions present at death, such as dementia, in addition to those causing or contributing to death would improve the value of death certificates for epidemiological purposes. Such a change would be particularly relevant for older people with multiple problems.

Goldacre[5] identified three patterns in the way different diseases were recorded on the death certificate among people dying within four weeks of admission to hospital: firstly, those usually recorded—for example, lung cancer, stroke, multiple sclerosis, myocardial infarction; secondly, those commonly recorded but often not as the underlying cause—diabetes, Parkinson's disease, hypertension, pneumonia; thirdly, those recorded in a minority of instances only—asthma, fractured neck of femur. One of the reasons he suggested for these variations was that conditions regarded as avoidable causes of death may have been under recorded on death certificates.

Geographical differences

There are a number of problems in allocating deaths to different areas. Should they be allocated to area of occurrence or to area of usual residence (the usual practice)? What should happen to residents from other countries and to people who have recently moved to long term institutions? Changes in practice can affect comparisons over time and there can be disputes over deaths from what are regarded as opprobrious causes. In making comparisons between geographical areas standardised mortality rates are

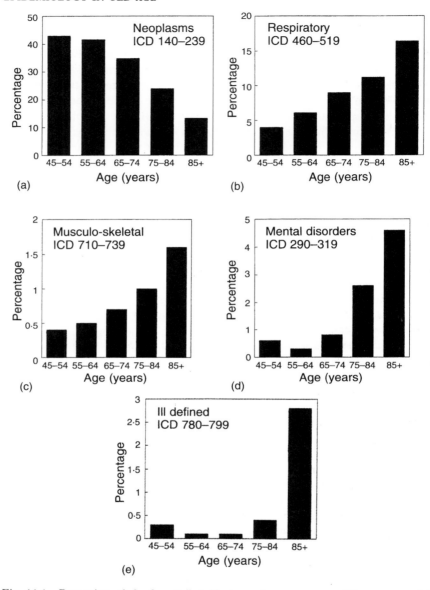

Fig 44.1 *Proportion of deaths attributable to various causes at different ages. (a) Neoplasms (ICD 140–239); (b) respiratory (ICD 460–519); (c) musculoskeletal (ICD 710–739; (d) mental disorders (ICD 290–319); (e) ill defined (ICD 780–799). Source: OPCS, Mortality Statistics, Cause 1992, HMSO, London, 1993.*

often used. These show death rates for a population with a standard age and sex distribution but they need to be interpreted with care. As Illsley and Le Grand[6] point out: "Since deaths at different ages have different causes, the aggregations of the experience of separate age groups into a

410

single figure means that the influence of different causes at different ages will be merged and their particular impact obscured." They go on to show how the use of standardised mortality rates has obscured differences in age specific death rates between regions and that simple conclusions about a north–south divide in Britain are not justified. In younger age groups it has disappeared, but it persists in older groups.

Studies of the quality of dying

What do we know about the process of dying and the disabilities, symptoms, and circumstances of people in the period before they die? How do our health and social services affect this process?

Studies of the quality of dying and of care in the last few weeks of life have concentrated almost exclusively on cancer deaths because these are the ones that can be identified. Only a quarter of deaths are, however, due to cancer and there are many aspects of these deaths that are atypical: those dying from cancer are relatively young; the deaths are more likely to occur in hospital; and nearly all those receiving care from hospices before they die have cancer or AIDS.

So while there is a substantial amount of research data about what happens in hospices (for review, see Seale[7]), and a number of studies of the experiences of patients with cancer, there is something of a dearth of information about deaths from other causes; therefore the experience of older people is underresearched.

Studies based on random samples of all deaths can, however, show the way in which a multitude of services function or fail to function as people are not identified because they were receiving care, although many obviously have great needs for care. The disadvantage of such studies is that they are retrospective and the views and experiences of the people who die cannot be obtained directly; information has to be collected from relatives and others close to the people who died. Various studies[8-10] have attempted to compare assessments made by patients shortly before death with those of relatives and carers made later and found little agreement. One of them[9] found that family members tended to be more critical of services and to report more symptoms.

Communication is one of the aspects of dying that has received much attention and open communication is one of the main tenets of the hospice movement. Although there has been a trend to more open communication in recent years,[2] there is still evidence that "next to pain, poor communication is the most important source of distress to the dying patient."[11] Many doctors say they are more likely to discuss a terminal prognosis with relatives than with the patient, and dying patients are still often left to surmise for themselves that they are dying.[2] The emotional isolation associated can only be guessed at.

411

Variations in the nature of the dying process

Data from two studies based on random samples of adult deaths in 1969 and 1987[2 12] showed few significant changes between the two points in time in the proportion for whom various symptoms were reported, but there was an increase among those with mental confusion, depression, and incontinence in the proportions who were reported to have had the symptom for a year or more, and mental confusion and incontinence were more common among the old. On both studies dying was often an unpleasant and painful process, although one in 10 of the deaths were unexpected, with no previous illness or warning (1969 definition), or sudden, with no illness or warning or time for care (1987 definition). These types of death were less frequent for older people.

The 1987 study also showed that people dying when they were old had greater needs, less support from relatives, and less medical and nursing care in relation to their needs than people dying at younger ages. Those aged 85 or more were less likely to die in a hospital or hospice or to have spent any of the last year of their lives in one than those dying at younger ages. In addition, the decline in home visiting by general practitioners over the years has hit the elderly and housebound particularly hard.

Dying at home has become less and less common over the years; people are slightly more likely to die in hospital and, although deaths in hospices have increased a great deal, proportionately they still accounted for only 4% of adult deaths in 1987.[2] The big increase is in people dying in residential and nursing homes. It is the old and very old who die in such places, partly because older people are more likely to live alone than they were in the past.

Euthanasia and living wills

Euthanasia and living wills can influence both the timing and the nature of death. Euthanasia, taking active steps to end a patient's life or allowing a patient to die through deliberate inaction, is illegal, and it is always difficult to measure the frequency of illegal activities but clearly it happens. A recent study of general practitioners and hospital consultants in one area of England[13] reported that 45% of the doctors said they had at some time been asked by a patient to hasten his or her death by active steps and another 14% had been asked to withdraw or withhold treatment. These proportions were higher for general practitioners than for hospital doctors. Of those who said they had been asked, 32% said they had at some time taken steps to bring about the death of a patient who had asked them to do so; this represents one in eight of those doctors who took part in the survey. The study gives no indication of the frequency with which such events happened.

In the Netherlands in the early 1990s modification of the law was under consideration and, although euthanasia was still a criminal act, prosecutions

412

were rare provided physicians abided by strict guidelines. A study carried out at this time estimated that euthanasia (terminating life at the patient's request) occurred in 1·8% of all deaths, assisted suicide (a physician intentionally prescribes or supplies lethal drugs but the patient administers them) in 0·3%, and in 0·8% drugs were administered with the explicit intention of shortening the patient's life without the strict criteria for euthanasia being fulfilled.[14] Other forms of medical decision about the end of life were more common: alleviation of pain and symptoms with opioids in such dosages that the patient's life might have been shortened were estimated to have occurred in 17·5% of deaths; and non-treatment decisions (the withholding or withdrawal of treatment in situations where treatment would probably have prolonged life) in another 17·5%. Altogether, therefore, some medical decision about the end of life was taken in 38·0% of deaths. This percentage varied little between age groups but euthanasia was less frequent among deaths of people aged 80 or more, while non-treatment decisions were more common. When cause of death was taken into account some type of medical decision about the end of life was taken in 59% of cancer deaths and in 43% of deaths from diseases of the nervous system, including stroke. Among the doctors, general practitioners were more likely than specialists to have practised euthanasia and nursing home physicians the least likely. On the other hand non-treatment decisions were taken twice as often by nursing home physicians as by general practitioners.

Living wills and advance directives are ways in which people seek to influence or initiate decisions made about the nature and timing of their death. The extent to which these are considered binding on doctors varies in different countries and is being contested in some. One randomised study,[15] in which the treatment group were given a package of preventive services, including counselling to complete advance directives, reported an excess mortality in the treatment group. Further analyses suggested that this could be explained in part by the lack of life sustaining treatment received by intervention participants, which may have arisen through advance directives limiting such treatment in the event of serious illness. Thus as the pressure for patient control increases and is accepted it seems likely that interventions related to the end of life will rise. This trend may be associated with an increasing expectation of life.

Policies

To some extent we are in a Catch 22 situation—the older people are when they die the more likely is their death to be preceded by a lengthy period of disability coupled with unpleasant symptoms. A study of changes in disability free life expectancy[16] concluded that Americans are not living longer healthy lives in the sense of being able to participate in the normal activities of everyday life. Additions to life expectancy between 1970 and 1980 were concentrated in disabled years. Once again it is the very old who

413

are disadvantaged: between 1970 and 1980 the proportion institutionalised increased among those 85 and over; among those under 80 it declined.

The emphasis on domiciliary care in Britain may reduce the proportion of older people who are in institutions but if the domiciliary services available to them do not improve then the quality of their life is likely to deteriorate.

The success of medical services at prolonging life seems almost inevitably to increase the extent as well as the length of disability before death. Just over a fifth of relatives and carers of a random sample who had died thought it would have been better if the person had died earlier; this proportion was higher for deaths of older people.[2]

Inevitably people will differ about the stage at which they view death as acceptable or even welcome for themselves and for those close to them, and it is argued that people are likely to change their views as circumstances alter. Some people regard the deliberate shortening of life as inappropriate in any circumstances and at the moment their views are generally upheld by the law. But is it reasonable to withhold choice from others? That is one facet of the current debate.

If the main goal is for a long, disability free life expectancy, services and research should be concentrating on the relief of chronic diseases and disability. For death with dignity, pain and symptom relief need to be combined with respect for the autonomy of the individual.

1 Office of Population Censuses and Surveys. *Mortality statistics 1992*. London: HMSO, 1994.
2 Seale C, Cartwright A. *The year before death*. Aldershot: Avebury, 1994.
3 Morris JN. *Uses of epidemiology*. London: Livingstone, 1957.
4 Newens AJ, Forster DP, Kay DWK. Death certification after a diagnosis of presenile dementia. *J Epidemiol Community Health* 1993;47:293–7.
5 Goldacre MJ. Cause-specific mortality: understanding uncertain tips of the disease iceberg. *J Epidemiol Community Health* 1993;47:491–6.
6 Illsley R, Le Grand J. Regional inequalities in mortality. *J Epidemiol Community Health* 1993;47:444–9.
7 Seale C. What happens in hospices: a review of research evidence. *Soc Sci Med* 1989;28: 551–9.
8 Ahmeddzai S, Morton A, Reid JT, Stevenson RD. Quality of death from lung cancer: patients' reports and relatives' retrospective opinions. In: Watson M, Greer S, Thomas C, editors. *Psycho-social oncology*. Oxford: Pergamon Press, 1988: 187–92.
9 Cartwright A, Seale C. *The natural history of a survey*. London: King's Fund, 1990.
10 Higginson I, Priest P, McCarthy M. Are bereaved family members a valid proxy for a patient's assessment of dying? *Soc Sci Med* 1994;38:553–7.
11 Rees D. Terminal care and bereavement. In: McAvoy B, Donaldson LJ, editors. *Health care for Asians*. Oxford: Oxford Medical Publications, 1990:304–9.
12 Cartwright A, Hockey L, Anderson JL. *Life before death*. London: Routledge and Kegan Paul, 1973.
13 Ward BJ, Tate PA. Attitudes among NHS doctors to requests for euthanasia. *BMJ* 1994; 308:1332–4.
14 van der Maas PJ, van Delden JJM, Pijnenborg L, Looman CWN. Euthanasia and other medical decisions concerning the end of life. *Lancet* 1991;338:669–74.
15 Patrick DL, Beresford SAA, Ehreth J, Diehr P, Picciano J, Durham M, *et al.* Interpreting excess mortality in a prevention trial for older adults. *Int J Epidemiol* 24(3):527–33.
16 Crimmins EM, Saito Y, Ingegneri D. Changes in life expectancy and disability-free life expectancy in the United States. In: Robine J-M, Blanchet M, Dowd JE, editors. *Health expectancy*. London: HMSO, 1992. (Studies in Medical Population Subjects, No 54.)

414

Epilogue

Epilogue: Intersection of epidemiology and ageing

ROBERT L KANE

Epidemiology has been responsible for much of the advance of knowledge in health related areas. Although most medical scientists hold the randomised clinical trial as the ultimate source of scientific knowledge, many areas are not easily tested in this manner. Instead, more deductive approaches are necessary. Both epidemiological and ageing science have grown enormously in the last several decades. New techniques have allowed more sophisticated levels of inference and helped to address some of the limitations of non-experimental inference.

An exciting development in epidemiology has been its expansion beyond its original uses for understanding the distribution and determinants of *disease* to encompass the distribution and determinants of *health*. In effect, rather than beginning with a search for risk factors for disease, the new epidemiology begins with the presence of disease and examines the potential effects of treatment. This new branch of epidemiology has been labelled "clinical epidemiology" by some and "health services research" by others. Its foundations can be credited to such pioneers as Cochrane[1] and Feinstein.[2 3] Clinical epidemiology has progressed to the stage where texts are written about it.[4 5]

The convergence of epidemiology and ageing has been quite fruitful. The intersection of these two fields has come a long way since the early meetings on this subject.[6 7] The importance of the field has been underscored by the development of specific methods for approaching the issues.[8 9]

More traditional epidemiological approaches have provided valuable insights into a number of areas; for example, epidemiological studies have shown a strong inverse relationship between years of schooling and the risk of developing dementia[10] and a positive relationship with general well-being.[11] Large scale epidemiological projects in defined catchment areas have been used to understand better the natural history of ageing.[12] Cohorts previously recruited for longitudinal studies of specific diseases, such as the Framingham study and the Alameda County study, have been converted to ageing studies as their samples age.[13 14]

National data sets have been established using epidemiological methods. For example, the national long term care survey collects information on

417

disabled older people to both trace their status over time and examine the relationship between disability and the use of services. Data from this study have been important in showing that becoming disabled in old age is not necessarily an irreversible event. Manton has demonstrated that even persons with substantial disability can improve their status. Among persons living in the community with impairments in five or six activities of daily living, he found that 42% had improved over a period of two years.[15] A parallel observation was made by Rogers, who expanded the concept of "active life expectancy", which essentially measured the time until a person became disabled,[16] to recognise the dynamic nature of functional incapacity whereby an older person could move in and out of states of dependency.[17]

Epidemiological methods can also make contributions on a new plane. The current interest in examining the effectiveness of medical care has spawned new applications for epidemiology. Randomised clinical trials alone will not be able to address a fraction of the clinical questions that need to be asked. Important among these is the effectiveness of care for older persons.[18] In the absence of good data older patients may be denied potentially useful care in the belief that such care would not be of great benefit to them. Because older persons use a disproportionately large share of health care, there is continuing pressure to find acceptable ways to limit their health care expenditures. Specific studies are needed to test the effectiveness, even the cost effectiveness, of offering various treatments to this age group. There is some reason to believe that age itself may not be the best basis on which to decide which patients are most likely to benefit from particular therapies. Rather, functional status or other clinical markers of risk may be more predictive of poor outcomes.

Historically, older persons have been systematically excluded from many clinical trials because they were judged to present too great a set of complications. Their comorbidities made it more difficult to separate the specific effects of the treatment under study. Their higher mortality rates meant a loss to follow up. Their multiple medications raised the possibility of drug interactions.

The rise of geriatrics in the last few decades has created new champions for older persons. The ironic state of affairs whereby those most likely to be using a therapy were specifically excluded from its testing is no longer tolerable. New studies that deliberately include older subjects will be needed to establish the risk:benefit ratio for new treatments and the areas where such care is effective. The skilful application of clinical epidemiological methods will be central to the success of these enterprises. Some will rely on traditional clinical trial methods but others will utilise epidemiological techniques, studying the results of actual care and relying on statistical methods to adjust for differences among those treated differently.

Epidemiology will also play an important role in improving the quality of care for older patients. The importance of clinical epidemiology increases in what may be termed "the age of effectiveness". Pressures to establish the effectiveness of various treatments have increased in the wake of growing

418

concerns about the rapidly rising costs of care. One attractive solution to controlling costs has been the idea of eliminating payment for those treatments that do not work. Unfortunately it is often difficult to establish just what type of care works for whom. It is rarely a question of whether a treatment is inherently good or bad. Those decisions have usually been made earlier. Rather, the distinction is about under what circumstances and in what types of patients is a certain approach to care successful. This question is especially hard to answer with older patients, who often present with complicated pictures because of multiple simultaneous problems. Thus clinical epidemiological techniques are particularly necessary with older patients.

Assessing outcomes requires some measure of change between the periods before and after treatment. Thus baseline status is important in directly measuring the effect; however, it is also important to determine the size of the effect because it may influence the amount of improvement or worsening possible. One can think of patient outcomes as being the result of four major forces: (a) baseline status, (b) patient factors, (c) environmental factors, and (d) treatment.

The patient factors include both clinical and demographic elements. Clinical factors important in establishing a prognosis or expected outcome include the traditional measures of diagnoses and comorbidities as well as measures of the severity of the individual problems. These may be reflected in laboratory values, history, or physical examination. Their clinical parameters may include the duration of the problem or the number of previous episodes experienced. Demographic factors may range from obvious measures, such as a person's age and gender, to more subtle items involving education and income or more amorphous areas like the extent of family and social support.

The environment of concern describes not only the physical environment but social and psychological aspects as well. Older persons are especially sensitive to their environments. Indeed one may describe one of the manifestations of senescence as the point where the person is less able to influence the environment and more likely to be influenced by it.

The goal of clinical epidemiology is to separate that component of outcomes attributable to treatment from the rest. This determination is essentially inferential. It requires statistical manipulation to identify what would be the expected outcome for patients with similar clinical, demographic, and environmental characteristics and contrasting the observed outcome with that expected. This procedure is quite comparable to what the epidemiologist does when he statistically adjusts rates to take into account differences in age, gender, and so on.

Because ageing is associated with increased variation, the process is even more complicated in examining the care of older persons, but the need for such approaches is all the more compelling. The same forces that encouraged closer examination of effectiveness are also fostering other approaches to reducing costs, among which is age based rationing.[19]

Geriatricians have an important role in advocating for older persons and hence must be at the forefront of efforts to resist the application of such simplistic but administratively attractive approaches. The best argument against such an approach to distributing scarce resources is to provide alternative ways to determine what really works for whom. Although there is growing evidence that technically intensive, and hence expensive, procedures developed for younger patients may be also effective on carefully selected older patients, arguments based on equity will be likely to favour younger groups unless compelling evidence of effectiveness is produced.

1 Cochrane A. *Effectiveness and efficiency; random reflections on health services*. London: Nuffield Provincial Hospitals Trust, 1972.
2 Feinstein AR. *Clinical biostatistics*. St Louis: Mosby, 1977.
3 Feinstein AR. *Clinimetrics*. New Haven: Yale University Press, 1987.
4 Fletcher RH, Wagner EH. *Clinical epidemiology*. Baltimore: Williams and Wilkins, 1988.
5 Weiss N. *Clinical epidemiology: the study of the outcome of illness*. New York: Oxford University Press, 1986.
6 Haynes SG, Feinleib M. *Proceedings of the Second Conference on the Epidemiology of Aging*. Bethesda, MD: National Institutes of Health, 1977.
7 Ostfeld AM, Gibson DC. *Epidemiology of aging*. Bethesda, MD: Department of Health, Education, and Welfare, 1975.
8 Brody JA, Maddox GL. *Epidemiology and aging: an international perspective*. New York: Springer, 1988.
9 Wallace R, Woolson R. *The epidemiologic study of the elderly*. New York: Oxford University Press, 1992.
10 Hill L, Klauber M, Salmon D, *et al.* Functional status, education, and the diagnosis of dementia in the Shanghai survey. *Neurology* 1993;**43**:138–45.
11 Guralnik JM, Land KC, Blazer D, *et al.* Educational status and active life expectancy among older blacks and whites. *N Engl J Med* 1993;**329**:110–6.
12 Coroni-Huntley J, Brock D, Ostfeld A, *et al. Established populations for epidemiologic studies of the elderly: resource data book*. Bethesda, MD: National Institute on Aging, 1986.
13 Jette AM, Branch LG. The Framingham disability study: II. Physical disability among the aging. *Am J Public Health* 1981;**71**:1211–6.
14 Kaplan G, Seeman T, Cohen R, *et al.* Mortality among the elderly in the Alameda County study: behavioral and demographic risk factors. *Am J Public Health* 1987;**77**:307–12.
15 Manton KG. A longitudinal study of functional change and mortality in the United States. *J Gerontol* 1988;**43**:S153–61.
16 Katz K, Branch LG, Branson MH, *et al.* Active life expectancy. *N Engl J Med* 1983;**309**: 1218–24.
17 Rogers A, Rogers RG, Branch LG. A multistage analysis of active life expectancy. *Public Health Rep* 1989;**104**:222–6.
18 Kane R, Pacala J. Geriatric clinical epidemiology. In: Vellas B, Albarde J, Garry P, editors. *Facts and research in gerontology 1994: epidemiology and aging*. New York: Springer, 1994: 5–11.
19 Callahan D. *Setting limits: medical goals in an aging society*. New York: Simon and Schuster, 1987.

Index